THE DEVERS MANUAL:

OPHTHALMOLOGY FOR THE HEALTH CARE PROFESSIONAL

DEVERS EYE INSTITUTE

Education, Research, Consultation

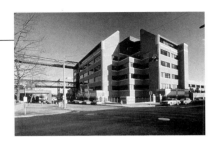

Devers Eye Institute is dedicated to developing new understanding about and treatments for potentially blinding eye diseases, while educating the professional and the public communities about ophthalmic disorders. Endowed in 1959 by Portland coffee merchant Arthur Henry Devers, the founding mission of the Devers Eye Institute was to provide eye care for people in need. Arthur Devers' personal struggle with the blinding disease retinitis pigmentosa made him acutely aware of the need for innovative ophthalmic research. With strong philanthropic support, Devers Eye Institute now provides a full range of diagnostic and treatment programs, and patient support services. The scope of the Devers Eye Institute's mission includes clinical care, community education, and ophthalmological research. The Institute boasts the region's most complete collection of research and patient education resources at the Merrill Reeh Ophthalmology Library. The Institute is the center of ophthalmologic services for Legacy Health System, one of the largest healthcare organizations in the Pacific Northwest. Patients come to Devers Eye Institute from throughout the region and from Pacific Rim nations for consultation by ophthalmologic subspecialists with fellowship training in glaucoma, retina, cornea, uveitis, oculoplastics, and neuro-ophthalmology. The Devers Eye Institute promotes and supports both basic and clinical research to further the understanding of ocular disease.

The Devers Manual is based upon a popular lecture series presented by the Devers Eye Institute's physicians and is designed for health care providers as a part of their ongoing professional education. The philosophy of *The Devers Manual* is to provide the primary care provider with an accessible and efficient summary of ophthalmic diseases, which are frequently seen in daily practice.

THE DEVERS MANUAL:

OPHTHALMOLOGY

FOR THE

HEALTH CARE

PROFESSIONAL

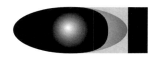

George A. Cioffi, MD

Director, Glaucoma Research
Devers Eye Institute
Legacy Portland Hospital
Portland, Oregon

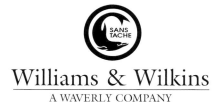

Williams & Wilkins

A WAVERLY COMPANY

BALTIMORE • PHILADELPHIA • LONDON • PARIS • BANGKOK
HONG KONG • MUNICH • SYDNEY • TOKYO • WROCLAW

Editor: Darlene Barela Cooke
Managing Editor: Frances M. Klass
Marketing Manager: Daniell T. Griffin
Production Coordinator: Danielle Hagan
Book Project Editor: Jennifer D. Weir
Illustrator: Timothy C. Hengst
Designer: Paul Fry
Illustration Planner: Lorraine Wrzosek
Cover Designer: Randy Rogers
Typesetter: BI-COMP, Inc.
Printer: Edwards Brothers, Inc.
Binder: Edwards Brothers, Inc.

351 West Camden Street
Baltimore, Maryland 21201-2436 USA

Rose Tree Corporate Center
1400 North Providence Road
Building II, Suite 5025
Media, Pennsylvania 19063-2043 USA

Accurate indications, adverse reactions and dosage schedules for drugs are provided in this book, but it is possible that they may change. The reader is urged to review the package information data of the manufacturers of the medications mentioned.

Printed in the United States of America

First Edition,

Library of Congress Cataloging-in-Publication Data

The Devers manual: ophthalmology for the health care professional /
  [edited by] George A. Cioffi. -- 1st ed.
      p. cm.
  Includes bibliographical references and index.
  ISBN 0-683-01690-3
  1. Eye--Diseases. 2. Eye--Diseases--Diganosis. 3. Diagnosis,
Differential. I. Cioffi, George A. II. Devers Eye Institute.
  [DNLM: 1. Eye Diseases--diagnosis. 2. Eye Diseases--therapy.
3. Diagnosis, Differential. WW 140 D491 1997]
RE46.D53   1997
617.7--dc21
DNLM/DLC
for Library of Congress   97-2483
                                                          CIP

The publishers have made every effort to trace the copyright holders for borrowed material. If they have inadvertently overlooked any, they will be pleased to make the necessary arrangements at the first opportunity.

To purchase additional copies of this book, call our customer service department at **(800) 638-0672** or fax orders to **(800) 447-8438.** For other book services, including chapter reprints and large quantity sales, ask for the Special Sales department.

Canadian customers should call **(800) 665-1148,** or fax **(800) 665-0103.** For all other calls originating outside of the United States, please call **(410) 528-4223** or fax us at **(410) 528-8550.**

Visit *Williams & Wilkins* on the *Internet:* http://www.wwilkins.com or contact our customer service department at **custserv@wwilkins.com.** Williams & Wilkins customer service representatives are available from 8:30 am to 6:00 pm, EST, Monday through Friday, for telephone access.

97 98 99 00
1 2 3 4 5 6 7 8 9 10

To the two individuals who made
The Devers Manual possible,

ARTHUR H. DEVERS
and
LINDA DRISLAN CIOFFI.

Through philanthropy,
Arthur Devers
provides eye care to thousands
of Oregonians in need.

Through patience, love, and support,
Linda
nurtured the atmosphere essential
to accomplish this project.

PREFACE

The Devers Manual: Ophthalmology for the Health Care Professional was conceived with three needs in mind: providing a differential diagnosis for common ocular disorders, establishing appropriate guidelines for the management of ocular disease, and strengthening communication between the primary care physician and the ophthalmologist. By meeting these needs, *The Devers Manual* hopes to enhance the care of individuals with eye disease.

The Devers Manual provides the nonophthalmic physician with the most common ocular diagnoses, their clinical manifestations, the appropriate treatment, and guidelines for their management. *The Devers Manual* is separated into four sections:

Section I: The Patient Calls: Common Ocular Complaints and Their Differential Diagnoses;
Section II: The Most Common Ocular Disorders and Their Management;
Section III: Specialized Ophthalmic Testing; and
Section IV: Appendix.

Section I, *The Patient Calls*, discusses the most common ocular complaints encountered in the primary care setting. This section reviews the most common etiologies of these complaints and lists the most important differential diagnoses. Section II, *The Most Common Ocular Disorders and Their Management*, addresses specific disease entities. This section is divided anatomically and reviews diseases which affect the ocular adnexa, the orbit, the ocular motility, the anterior segment of the eye, and the posterior segment of the eye. Each chapter in Section II includes:

(a) Introduction of the Pathophysiology
(b) Clinical Manifestations of the Disorders
(c) Differential Diagnosis
(d) Treatment
(e) Referral Guidelines and Tables
(f) Frequency of Visits
(g) Suggested Reading List.

The **Referral Guideline Tables** are meant to provide guidelines for the most efficacious and appropriate treatment of ocular disease by the healthcare professional. Each of these tables includes ICD-9 diagnostic codes. A list of the most common ocular diagnoses and their codes is also found in the Appendix.

Section III, *Specialized Ophthalmic Testing*, reviews the four most common specialized ophthalmic tests that ophthalmologists use in diagnosis and management of ocular disease. This section provides the primary care physician with a description of these tests and their indications.

Section IV, *Appendix*, provides a review of general orbital and ocular anatomy, as well as a "how to" section describing general examination techniques that are used by both the primary care physician and the ophthalmologist to evaluate the eye.

As editor, I wish to extend special thanks to each of the contributors. Their hard work cannot be overstated. I also wish to thank Suzanne Menks for extensive editorial review and manuscript preparation.

G.A.C.

ACKNOWLEDGMENTS

I would like to acknowledge the important contributions made by these individuals to the success of this book: Suzanne Menks, editorial assistant; Timothy C. Hengst, artist; and David Bacon and Milton Johnson, photographers.

CONTRIBUTORS

George A. Cioffi, MD
Director, Glaucoma Research
Devers Eye Institute
Legacy Portland Hospitals
Portland, Oregon

Roger A. Dailey, MD
Assistant Professor of Ophthalmology
Casey Eye Institute
Devers Eye Institute
Director, Oculoplastics
Portland Veterans Administration
  Medical Center
Portland, Oregon

Richard F. Dreyer, MD
Director, Vitreoretinal Service
Devers Eye Institute
Portland, Oregon

Colin Ma, MD
Vitreoretinal Service
Devers Eye Institute
Portland, Oregon

William T. Shults, MD
Chief of Neuro-Ophthalmology
Legacy Portland Hospitals
Portland, Oregon

Mark A. Terry, MD
Chief, Corneal Services
Devers Eye Institute
Legacy Portland Hospitals
Portland, Oregon

Andrea Cibis Tongue, MD
Pediatric Ophthalmologist
Legacy Portland Hospitals
Portland, Oregon

E. Michael Van Buskirk, MD
President & CEO, Devers Eye
  Associates
Chief of Ophthalmology
Devers Eye Institute
Legacy Portland Hospital
Portland, Oregon

Matthew W. Wilson, MD
Instructor of Ophthalmology
Casey Eye Institute
Portland, Oregon

CONTENTS ◖◗

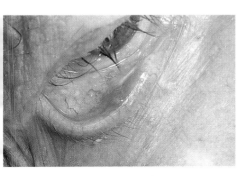

Figure 11.2   (See also page 37).

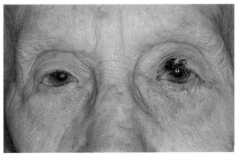

Figure 11.11   (See also page 48).

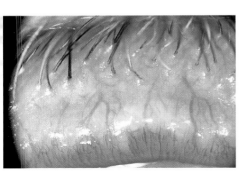

Figure 12.2   (See also page 53).

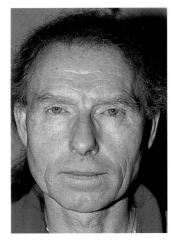

Figure 12.5   (See also page 55).

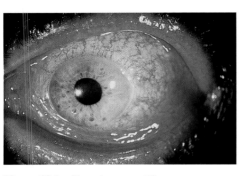

Figure 13.1   (See also page 62).

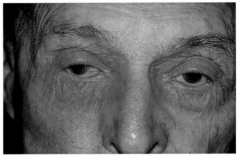

Figure 13.5   (See also page 70).

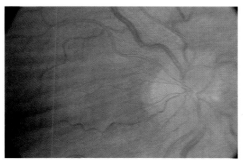

Figure 16.5 (See also page 98).

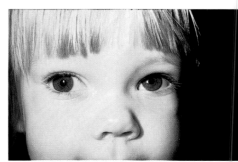

Figure 17.2 (See also page 112).

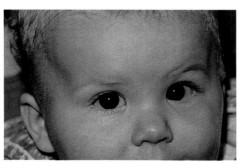

Figure 17.6A (See also page 117).

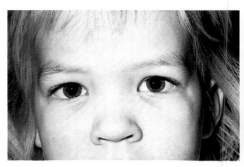

Figure 17.10A (See also page 126).

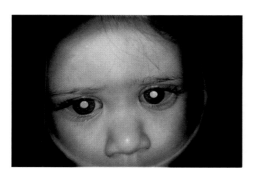

Figure 17.10B (See also page 126).

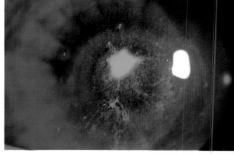

Figure 18.1 (See also page 132).

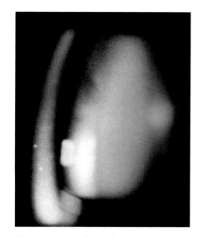

Figure 20.2   (See also page 148).

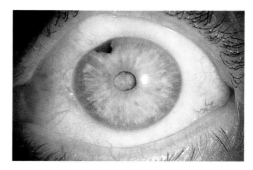

Figure 20.3   (See also page 148).

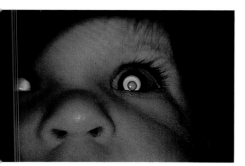

Figure 21.1   (See also page 157).

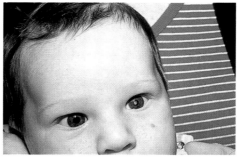

Figure 21.2   (See also page 157).

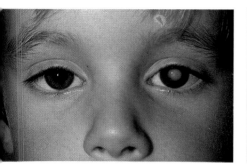

Figure 21.3   (See also page 157).

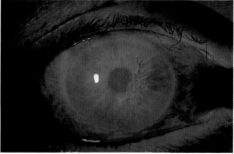

Figure 23.2   (See also page 182).

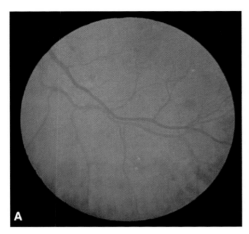

Figure 24.3A (See also page 193).

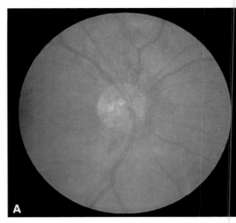

Figure 24.4A (See also page 194).

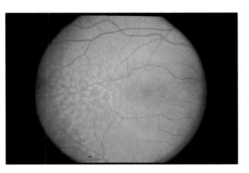

Figure 27.3 (See also page 221).

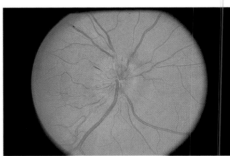

Figure 28.1 (See also page 230).

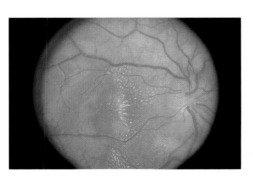

Figure 28.2 (See also page 231).

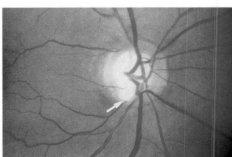

Figure 29.4 (See also page 257).

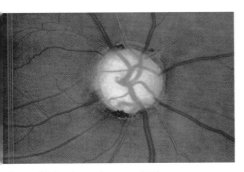

Figure 29.5 (See also page 257).

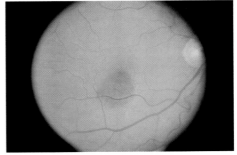

Figure 30.2 (See also page 275).

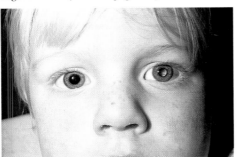

Figure 31.1 (See also page 280).

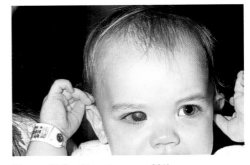

Figure 31.3 (See also page 281).

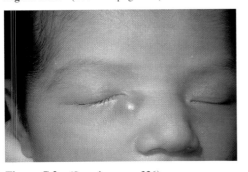

Figure C.2 (See also page 326).

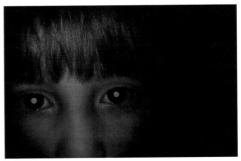

Figure C.6 (See also page 329).

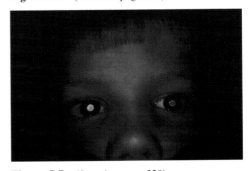

Figure C.7 (See also page 329).

THE PATIENT CALLS: COMMON OCULAR COMPLAINTS AND THEIR DIFFERENTIAL DIAGNOSIS

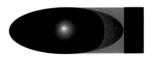

Chapter 1 ◖●◗
Blurry Vision

G. A. Cioffi

"Blurry vision" is a frequent complaint heard by both the primary care physician and the ophthalmologist. The etiology of blurred vision varies from simple to extremely complex and may be related only to the eye. However, it also may be related to a variety of systemic diseases. Several historical factors help determine both the etiology of the blurred vision and the severity of the problem. The onset of symptoms, whether gradual or rapid, helps determine a differential diagnosis. The duration of symptoms, whether transient or persistent, and whether the blurred vision is monocular or binocular, also may help in determining the etiology. Finally, the degree of blurred vision, ranging from mild to severe, will help the physician determine the seriousness of this common complaint. In general, the more rapid the onset of blurred vision and the more severe the loss of vision, the more urgent the need for a complete evaluation. Sudden, severe loss of vision, transient or permanent, is discussed in Chapter 2.

Simple techniques may be used to determine the degree of blurred vision. When newspaper print is held at a normal reading distance, a visual acuity of approximately 20/50 is required to read the print. It is often helpful to have patients determine their own extent of visual loss in each eye. It should always be remembered that spectacle correction, especially in older patients in whom bifocals are needed, should be worn during this test. Gradual, painless visual loss occurring over several weeks, months, or even years, is generally due to uncorrected refractive errors. In addition, this may be secondary to cataract formation. More ominous causes of long-term painless vision loss include open angle glaucoma and chronic retinal diseases, such as age-related macular degeneration and diabetic retinopathy. Finally, it should be remembered that a well-lubricated anterior ocular surface is needed for clear vision. Excessive tearing or deficient tearing may also cause blurred vision (see Excessive Tearing, Epiphora [Chapter 8]). Any significant vision loss (20/50 or worse) or vision loss associated with ocular pain should be evaluated promptly. Transient or intermittent blurred vision often is associated with systemic disease. Both hypoglycemia and hyperglycemia may cause visual fluctuations. These findings are usually binocular. Transient monocular visual changes should alert the physician to the possibility of regional blood flow alterations which may warrant a complete ocular, as well as systemic, workup.

Two simple techniques can be used during an office evaluation of a patient complaining of blurry vision. First, the pinhole technique allows the physician to determine if an uncorrected refractive error is a contributor to the blurry vision (see Appendix B). Patients with substantial improvement in their visual acuity when tested looking through a pinhole most likely have an uncorrected refractive error and require correc-

TABLE 1.1. Common Differential
Diagnosis—Blurry Vision
_____
Uncorrected refractive error*
Ocular surface disturbance (tearing or dry eyes)*
Cataract (crystalline lens opacification)*
Glaucoma
Diabetic retinopathy
Macular degeneration
_____
* Most common

tion. Second, a swinging flashlight test, used to check for a relative afferent pupillary defect (Marcus Gunn pupil), is useful in cases of monocular blurred vision (see Appendix B). Diseases of the neurosensory portions of the eye (the retina and optic nerve) will show a positive Marcus Gunn pupil in the affected eye. Any patient with a positive Marcus Gunn pupil warrants a complete ocular workup to establish the cause.

Chapter 2 ◖●❙
Sudden Vision Loss

C. Ma

"Clear vision" is a multifaceted perception which depends on the proper functioning of a complex organ and its relationship to the brain. Perhaps it is the richness of visual information which leads to the corollary that there are many ways in which patients describe altered vision. Symptoms are not usually sufficiently specific to reach a diagnosis, and serious diseases that require urgent treatment may, unfortunately, be accompanied by rather minor symptoms. Visual changes which are not accompanied by pain or irritation are usually referable to the posterior segment, where there is little somatosensory innervation. This portion of the eye is difficult for the primary care provider to examine; therefore, this chapter addresses symptoms that should alert the provider to evaluate, or refer the patient, as an emergency. In general, symptoms that develop rapidly (over hours or a couple of days), that are restricted to one eye, or part of the visual field in one eye are likely to be more serious than changes which have developed over several weeks, or that were only noticed when the patient incidentally covered the fellow eye (see also Chapter 4: "Ocular Pain and Redness").

Complete Loss of Vision

The sudden total loss of vision in one eye, to the extent of being unable to distinguish light and darkness, is most likely to be due to central retinal artery occlusion, causing ischemia of the entire retina. If the symptoms have lasted for less than 90 minutes, this is a true emergency as there may be some recovery of function if circulation can be restored. Branch retinal arterial occlusions cause equally severe loss of vision in one sector of the visual field, and should be evaluated and referred immediately. Patients with arterial occlusions often have a known history of carotid stenosis or peripheral vascular disease.

Transient blindness or amaurosis fugax may also result in sudden or complete sectional blindness. These symptoms may resolve spontaneously if the retinal embolus breaks up and moves downstream. Since there is almost always more material which may embolize to the eye or brain more permanently, these patients should still be evaluated urgently.

Infarction of the optic nerve, complete or sectoral, may cause similar symptoms, but is not reversible. Temporal arteritis is more likely to cause total infarction than ischemic optic neuropathy, and must be ruled out urgently to protect the other eye (see Chapter 28: "Optic Nerve Disorders").

5

TABLE 2.1. Common Differential
Diagnosis—Sudden Vision Loss

Central retinal artery occlusion*
Branch retinal artery occlusion
Ischemic optic neuropathy
Retinal vein occlusion*
Retinal detachment*
Macular degeneration*
Diabetic retinopathy

Most common

Faded Section of Vision

Sectional loss of vision is not a specific symptom because a wide variety of conditions may reduce the function of the retina or visual pathway. Typically, the affected area of the visual field is vaguely described as a gray shadow, or blurred area in which there may still be some perception of large objects or movement. Patients often find it difficult to describe which part of their vision is affected. The differential diagnosis includes retinal vein occlusion, retinal detachment, ischemic optic neuropathy and any maculopathy (Table 2.1). Individuals complaining of partial visual loss should be evaluated urgently if there is a history of sudden onset, or noticeable enlargement of the affected area, which may suggest a retinal detachment or vitreous hemorrhage. A helpful feature in the history would be a report of floaters or flashes prior to the loss of vision.

Distortion of Central Vision (Metamorphopsia)

If the patient reports that the outline of an object is interrupted by a gap or "kink," this is a fairly specific symptom for detachment, swelling or folding of the macula. The macula is the central zone of the retina, containing a high proportion of cone photoreceptors, which mediates the central 20° of the field of vision. This complaint should be evaluated urgently as it may be due to subretinal neovascularization, which is most often secondary to age-related macular degeneration in a patient older than 55, or similar diseases in younger patients.

Other, less urgent conditions, which may cause distortion of central vision, are central serous retinopathy, macular edema (e.g., due to background diabetic retinopathy, branch retinal vein occlusion, and postoperative cystoid macular edema), and epiretinal membranes.

Chapter 3 ◖●▮
Floaters and Flashes

C. Ma

"Floaters" are dark spots, strings, veils or "spiders" which seem to float in front of the patient. Floaters are caused by opacities in the vitreous cavity casting a shadow upon the retina. The essential element of the history is that floaters drift even when the patient does not move his eye, whereas a scotoma (blind spot) remains in exactly the same place relative to the center of the visual field. Normally, most people see some floaters, particularly in conditions of bright, even lighting (such as a clear sky, or against a blank piece of paper), but the presence of floaters are ominous if they have suddenly appeared. It is more significant if the floaters are small dots or specks, as these symptoms are likely to represent small droplets of blood in the vitreous cavity. Large floaters and ring-like shapes, especially those which the patient has had time to study and draw in elaborate detail, are more likely to be due to syneresis, the normal degenerative changes in the vitreous gel. With aging, the vitreous liquefies and the posterior vitreous pulls away from the anterior surface of the retina, known as a "posterior vitreous detachment." This normal process may result in both floaters and flashes and may be impossible to distinguish, symptomatically, from a retinal tear.

"Flashes" are bright visual phenomena which are not caused by external illumination. In the context of retinal disease, flashes occur when the retina is stimulated by vitreous traction, classically causing repeated "lightning streaks" which are seen in the patient's peripheral visual field. It is difficult for patients to determine in which eye the flashes occurred, and they may be very few in number.

Retinal Detachment

Floaters and flashes are the classic harbingers of peripheral retinal disease. Any patient who gives a good history of recent onset of these symptoms should be evaluated urgently (within the same day) with a dilated fundus examination. These symptoms may indicate a retinal tear, which may be treatable before it causes a frank retinal detachment. If, in addition, the patient notices peripheral loss of vision, suggesting that part of the retina may have detached, they should be seen quickly and evaluated, so that the detachment can be repaired before it involves the macula. Once the macula is detached, the chance for recovery of good central vision falls to 50%. Retinal detachment is more likely to occur in patients who are myopic (nearsighted), who have undergone eye surgery, or have suffered direct ocular trauma.

TABLE 3.1. **Common Differential Diagnosis—Floaters and Flashes**

Posterior vitreous detachment*
Retinal tear*
Retinal detachment*
Vitreous hemorrhage
Ocular trauma
Intraocular inflammatory diseases
Ocular migraine

* Most common

Vitreous Hemorrhage

In some patients, the number of floaters may increase rapidly and vision is obscured by a large amount of blood in the vitreous cavity. This can be accompanied by retinal detachment, and the patient, therefore, should be referred urgently to an ophthalmologist. If the fundus cannot be visualized, ultrasound examination is necessary. This situation is more common in diabetics with proliferative diabetic retinopathy.

Migraine

Patients with migraines may report flashes of light, associated with a blind visual spot. Migraines are associated with vision changes that are usually more central, bilateral, longer lasting, and often form a variety of geometric shapes, which gradually enlarge across the field of vision. There is usually a history of previous migraine episodes, and the symptoms are often followed by headache.

Chapter 4 ◖●❚
Ocular Pain and Redness

M. A. Terry

The inflammatory signs of pain and redness occur as the eye responds to internal or external adverse stimuli. The etiology is often quickly determined by the initial history and physical examination of the eye without the need for laboratory testing. The precise onset and duration of the symptoms, as well as a thorough examination of the eye (including level of vision), will help the physician to determine the severity of the disease.

The severity of the disease can be assessed using the following guideline:

1. *Visual Acuity:* Visual acuity is a critical component in the evaluation of the red or painful eye. If the vision of the eye is normal (or the same as the premorbid state) then the disease is unlikely to be serious enough to warrant immediate consultation. The worse and more rapid the deterioration of the vision, the greater the likelihood of serious ocular abnormality.
2. *Pain:* The level and the character of the pain can be a clue as to the severity of the disease. Pain described as "scratchy" or "itchy" usually indicates minor disease, while a "boring" or "aching" pain may herald severe disease. Deep-seated, boring pain is often a sign of intraocular inflammation. If the pain demonstrates significant progression or is associated with severe light sensitivity, then more thorough and urgent evaluation is warranted.
3. *Redness:* The distribution of the conjunctival redness can sometimes indicate the tissue level of disease. Generalized redness over the entire conjunctival surface with minimal pain can indicate superficial inflammation (e.g., simple conjunctivitis). Localized redness concentrated like a ring around the limbal area (the junction of cornea and sclera) is called "ciliary flush." This localized redness is often associated with photophobia (light sensitivity) and indicates intraocular, deep inflammation, and more serious disease.

Common causes of red eye which present to the primary care physician include conjunctivitis, corneal lesions, acute iritis, and acute glaucoma.

Conjunctivitis: Common conjunctivitis can be viral, bacterial, chlamydial, allergic or toxic. In simple conjunctivitis there is mild discomfort, generalized hyperemia, and watery or mucopurulent drainage. Importantly, the cornea is normal and the vision is never significantly impaired.

Corneal Lesions: The cornea is highly innervated and will respond to trivial or severe injury with pain and a "ciliary flush" redness at the limbus. Reflex tearing is common and photophobia (light sensitivity) can be severe. The level of vision decrease is determined by the location of the lesion. Central lesions overlying the pupil will decrease the vision and more aggressive therapy is warranted than for

TABLE 4.1. Common Differential
Diagnosis—Ocular Pain and Redness

Conjunctivitis*
Iritis/uveitis (intraocular inflammation)*
Ocular surface foreign body*
Corneal lesions (abrasion, ulcer)
Acute glaucoma

Most common

peripheral lesions. The most common corneal lesions that are encountered are corneal abrasions, corneal foreign bodies, and corneal ulcers.

Acute Iritis/Uveitis: The predominant symptom of uveitis is photophobia (light sensitivity). This is associated with aching pain, ciliary flush redness, mild to moderate decrease in vision and a clear cornea. Iritis can be secondary to trauma, external infection, and even idiopathic, but a major cause is autoimmune systemic diseases such as arthritis and sarcoidosis. Steroid treatment should be managed by an ophthalmologist to avoid the complications of glaucoma, cataract, and loss of vision.

Acute Glaucoma: When the drainage angle of the eye is occluded by peripheral iris, the intraocular pressure rises dramatically. This produces eye pain, as well as a frontal headache and ciliary flush redness. Nausea is commonly associated with acute glaucoma. The cornea may appear "steamy" (hazy with loss of normal sheen) and the pupil may be poorly reactive. Patients describe decreased vision with characteristic halos. With pressure over 50 mm Hg, permanent vision loss can occur rapidly (within hours) so immediate evaluation and therapeutic intervention are critical.

The ocular inflammation which produces pain or redness can be generated by the entire spectrum of ocular disease from the trivial to the acutely severe. Eliciting precise information from the patient regarding the type of pain and redness, the level of vision or visual loss, and the associated ocular and systemic symptoms is critical to determining the urgency of evaluation and treatment.

Chapter 5 ◐❚
Double Vision (Diplopia)

W. T. Shults

The perception of seeing two images is a difficult one for a patient to ignore, and it usually produces a prompt visit to the physician. It may be the result of a relatively minor ocular surface abnormality or something far more ominous such as a brain tumor. Obviously, it's important to recognize which patients merit further neurodiagnostic investigation and which can be dealt with by simple office procedures. Toward that end, it is helpful to divide diplopia patients into two groups: those with monocular diplopia and those with binocular diplopia.

MONOCULAR DIPLOPIA

Monocular diplopia exists when the patient's complaint persists when the patient views through one eye only. It is usually the result of the eye's inability to bend (refract) light appropriately, causing an imperfectly focused image to fall on the retina. Thus, tear film abnormalities, corneal scarring, lens opacities, or, more rarely, retinal diseases resulting in displacement of the rods and cones from their normal location can all produce monocular diplopia (Table 5.1). Such aberrant perceptions are more often described as ghost images rather than frank double vision.

A simple, yet elegant, method for determining whether the patient's monocular diplopia is refractive in origin is to have the patient view through a pinhole device. This tool will eliminate peripheral light rays which are most affected by the refractive problem and permit only the central rays through. As these rays are unaffected by refractive aberration, the image is sharply focused on the fovea and the ghost image created by the peripheral imperfectly refracted rays disappears, establishing the true origin of the patient's complaint. If this simple maneuver eliminates the patient's problem you can reassure the patient that the cure for the problem will likely be found in a new pair of glasses.

BINOCULAR DIPLOPIA

Binocular diplopia is eliminated by covering either eye and suggests that the origin of this symptom stems from the visual axes of the two eyes pointing in different directions. While the cause of such ocular misalignment is most often due to malfunction of one or more of the ocular motor nerves (III, IV, or VI) resulting from a host of etiologies, the problem may reside in other locations such as the ocular muscle itself (thyroid ophthalmopathy) or at the myoneural junction (myasthenia gravis) (Table 5.1). In sorting through the various causes of binocular diplopia, it is useful to keep

11

TABLE 5.1. Common Differential Diagnosis

Monocular diplopia
  Refractive Error*
  Cataract*
  Ocular surface disturbances*
  Corneal scars
  Macular disease
Binocular diplopia (ocular misalignment)
  Cranial nerve palsy*
  Strabismus*
  Ocular muscle restrictions (e.g., thyroid ophthalmopathy)
  Brainstem disorders
  Myoneural junction disorders (e.g., myasthenia gravis)
  Cerebral vascular accident
  Intracranial aneurysm

* Most common

in mind the anatomy of the ocular motor control pathways. Diplopia can result from diseases affecting the brainstem, ocular motor nerves, myoneural junction, or eye muscle.

Each of the ocular motor nerves originates in a cluster of cells called nuclei in the brainstem. The oculomotor nerve (III) and trochlear nerve (IV) originate from nuclei in the midbrain, while the abducens nerve (VI) derives from cells in the pons. The ocular motor pathways travel from these nuclei as fascicles within the brainstem to emerge from the stem as cranial nerves III, IV, and VI where they make their way to the cavernous sinus. Within the cavernous sinus, the ocular motor nerves are relatively close together and thus are susceptible to conjoint involvement from such disparate processes as aneurysms, inflammation, dural cavernous fistulas, and tumor. After passing through the superior orbital fissure at the back of the orbit, the nerves find their way to the appropriate ocular muscles (III to the superior rectus, medial rectus, inferior rectus, inferior oblique, and levator palpebrae superioris; IV to the superior oblique; VI to the lateral rectus). A knowledge of which nerves innervate which ocular muscles is necessary to ascribe patient complaints of diplopia to the proper muscle and ultimately to the correct etiology.

Binocular diplopia is usually abrupt in onset, although the patient may note visual blurring before frank doubling is appreciated. Characteristics such as the direction of image separation (vertical, horizontal, or torsional) and gaze direction producing the greatest degree of image separation, will often isolate the muscle or muscles involved and assist in defining the appropriate cranial nerve whose dysfunction is responsible for the patient's complaint.

Thus the "cross-eyed" elderly diabetic patient who complains of horizontal diplopia, greater at distance than at near and greater in left gaze than in right gaze, demonstrates the characteristics of limited abduction of the left eye likely resulting from a microvascular lesion of the left sixth cranial nerve. A middle-aged woman with prominent eyes and diplopia worse in upgaze than downgaze, most likely has a restrictive myopathy affecting the inferior rectus muscle, the result of lymphocytic infiltration in thyroid disease. Variable blepharoptosis and diplopia are the hallmarks of ocular myasthenia gravis, a disease which can occur at any age.

OVERVIEW

As these brief clinical vignettes imply, the cause of double vision in any given patient is often derived from the clinical setting in which the diplopia arises. By the same token, the extent to which neurodiagnostic testing is indicated often depends upon such things as the patient age and general state of health. The mere presence of diplopia is not an indication for neuroimaging studies. Thus, a child who develops an isolated sixth nerve palsy following a flu-like illness most probably has a postviral abducens nerve palsy and requires observation only. However, an 82-year-old with an isolated abducens palsy should, as a minimum, have a sedimentation rate (giant cell arteritis may present as an isolated abducens palsy) and assessment of glucose tolerance. Observation will be rewarded with spontaneous improvement over the course of several months in the majority of such patients.

The operative word is isolated. If the sixth nerve palsy is coupled with findings such as a Horner's syndrome or facial numbness, then the approach changes and neuroimaging of the cavernous sinus and skull base is warranted. A similar observation applies in the elderly patient with a pupil-sparing third nerve palsy since such a finding, even if accompanied by intense pain, usually is microvascular in origin and will resolve uneventfully over a period of several months. Pupillary involvement, however, changes the thrust of the evaluation as aneurysm (posterior communicating, internal carotid, or basilar tip) must be ruled out.

In a patient in whom myasthenia gravis is suspected, the gold standard is the edrophonium (Tensilon) test; however, this medication is not always readily available. Recently, a simple and highly effective alternative has been proposed, the "sleep test." After the examiner establishes which muscles are dysfunctional, the patient reclines with eyes closed for an uninterrupted period of some 20–30 minutes. It is not necessary that the patient fall asleep. The myasthenic patient, upon arousal, will usually exhibit short-lived, but nonetheless unequivocal, recovery of function in the affected muscles. This test is also helpful in clinical settings (such as patients with heart disease) where Tensilon testing may carry an increased risk. A positive sleep test in a patient with variable diplopia obviates an MRI scan at a considerable cost saving.

The extent to which one investigates a patient with binocular diplopia is often dependent upon the relative degree of comfort in ordering the various neuroimaging studies which may be required to properly assess such patients. While modern neuro-imaging techniques have greatly expanded our ability to diagnose, the misapplication of these tests can delay diagnosis and markedly increase the cost of medical care. The patient who has undergone an incorrectly targeted scan which was "negative" has been done a disservice because it is likely that the diagnosis has been delayed by the false sense of security engendered by the "normal" study. As implied in the above clinical scenarios, it is as important to know when neuroimaging is *not* warranted as it is to know which imaging techniques are optimal in assessing a particular patient. If the evaluating physician is uncertain, an appropriate consultation may be more cost effective than a single unwarranted scan. If the consultant determines a scan is indicated, it is more likely the scanning parameters chosen will optimize the data obtained and reduce or eliminate the need for repeat studies.

Patients with complaints of diplopia without obvious ocular misalignment require ophthalmic evaluation, since the assessment of subtle eye movement disorders usually requires specialized testing and measurement techniques.

◖◗ Chapter 6
Foreign Body Sensation

M. A. Terry

One of the most common complaints of the eye patient is, "I feel like something is in my eye." This "foreign body sensation" is often just that; a foreign object lodged on the surface of the globe or interior surface of the lid. Other etiologies are common, however, and must be considered in every patient with foreign body sensation.

The cornea, and to a lesser extent, the conjunctiva, is the most highly innervated surface tissue in the body. The corneal nerve endings lay within the superficial epithelial surface of the eye, and it is the impingement upon these nerves which causes the foreign body sensation. Minute particles or simply drying of the epithelial surface will cause foreign body sensation, and this can progress to frank pain if the epithelium is breached. The foreign body sensation persists long after the particle foreign body has washed out, until the epithelial surface has healed over the exposed nerves and the epithelial contour is smooth.

The etiology and importance of the foreign body sensation can usually be best assessed by a detailed history. Patients with chronic foreign body sensation over several weeks or months, usually represent chronic lid or tear film disease, which is best addressed on a routine basis. Patients with the acute onset of foreign body sensation represent a corneal or conjunctival lesion, which is best evaluated immediately.

The most common causes of foreign body sensation that the primary care physician will likely encounter include abnormalities of the lid, dry eye, and true foreign body. A common differential diagnosis of etiologies of foreign body sensation would include blepharitis, trichiasis, entropion, dry eye, and corneal or conjunctival foreign bodies.

ABNORMALITIES OF THE LID

Blepharitis is a common inflammation of the lid margin which often disrupts the tear film causing localized dry spots on the cornea and foreign body sensation. Bacterial blepharitis can create peripheral inflammation of the cornea resulting in epithelial breakdown and foreign body sensation.

Trichiasis is the misdirected lashes of the lid margin caused by a variety of lid inflammatory diseases. Mechanical irritation of the cornea by inward directed lashes causes foreign body sensation and is easily corrected by epilation of the offending lashes.

Entropion is a disorder of an inward-turned lid margin, resulting in the entire row of lashes touching the cornea or conjunctival surface. Therapy of the foreign body sensation requires corrective lid surgery appropriate for the disease causing the in-turned lid.

14

TABLE 6.1. Common Differential
Diagnosis—Foreign Body Sensation

Blepharitis*
Trichiasis*
Dry eye syndrome*
Ocular surface foreign body*
Entropion

Most common

DRY EYE

There are many causes of dry eye, and it is one of the most common ocular problems of the elderly. The most common cause of dry eye in the elderly is from the generalized decrease of tear production by the lacrimal gland associated with aging. This process can be accelerated in the systemic conditions of Sjögren's syndrome, rheumatoid arthritis, sarcoidosis, and Herpes zoster. The epithelial surface of the cornea is critically dependent upon the complex tear film, and any disruption of the normal wetting process will cause foreign body sensation. Besides the lack of production of tears, dry eye symptoms with foreign body sensation can result from normal evaporative breakup of the tear film. This can be caused by incomplete closure of the lids at night or irregularities of the surface of the eye. Conditions which affect the oil and mucin layers of the tear film will also destabilize the tear film and cause functional dry eye. These conditions vary from systemic diseases such as rosacea and Stevens-Johnson syndrome, to localized abnormalities of the lid such as blepharitis and scarring from chemical or thermal burns. Primary therapy of dry eye is with supplemental topical lubricants.

FOREIGN BODY

Foreign bodies of the eye usually present with a very distinct history. The patient usually knows exactly when and where the foreign body event occurred. The foreign body progresses to frank pain if the corneal epithelium is violated, and profuse tearing and photophobia are common. Most conjunctival foreign bodies washout spontaneously, but many corneal foreign bodies are embedded. The upper lid must be everted during the examination, as occasionally a foreign body becomes embedded in the upper tarsal plate, hidden from view. When a history of hammering "metal on metal" is elicited (such as hammering a nail), a high suspicion of deeper penetration of a high-velocity metallic particle must be held, and the possibility of an intraocular foreign body addressed.

Foreign bodies of the cornea can be removed with a wet cotton tipped applicator, a sterile spatula, or a needle using topical anesthetic drops, and loupe magnification. Great care should be taken to avoid damaging the underlying corneal tissue, especially in the central cornea. Metal foreign bodies should be removed completely to avoid rust ring scarring. After removal, the eye should be pressure patched over an antibiotic ointment. Prompt referral to an ophthalmologist should be done if there is difficulty with foreign body removal, a rust ring is present, if there is any evidence of infection or ulceration, or if an intraocular foreign body is suspected.

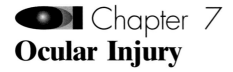 Chapter 7
Ocular Injury

M. A. Terry

Ocular trauma presents some of the most varied and challenging situations for the physician caring for eye problems. Each trauma setting is unique and the severity of the injury can range from trivial to sight-threatening. A calm and methodical approach to the ocular history and a complete physical examination will usually lead to an accurate assessment of damage and the appropriate course of therapy.

The most common ocular traumas presenting to the primary care physician are blunt trauma with ocular contusion, sharp object trauma with ocular laceration, and chemical burns. These categories of trauma are addressed in detail in Section II, but a common approach to all ocular trauma follows (Table 7.1).

HISTORY

The specific time and setting of the trauma should be recorded. Besides the obvious medical-legal implications of this information, the state of the eye at the time of examination will depend in large part on the amount of time since the injury, the relative cleanliness of the injury, and the force or potency of the injuring element. The presence and use of protective goggles at the time of injury should be recorded, especially for on-the-job injuries.

VISUAL ACUITY

The vision must be evaluated, even if it is no more than asking the patient "can you read your watch with your glasses on." Any loss of vision must be evaluated and explained. A drop of topical anesthetic should be used in a painful eye to properly assess the best level of vision. Relief of pain may allow the patient to concentrate on vision and may result in substantial visual improvement. The recorded vision at the initial examination documents the loss of vision from the preinjury state and provides a baseline vision against which to measure the success of therapy. In general, the severity of the loss of vision is indicative of the severity of the injury, but important exceptions exist.

LIDS

Blunt trauma often causes severe swelling and closure of the lids. If the patient reports an inability to open their swollen lids, a complete ocular examination is warranted.

16

TABLE 7.1. Important Aspects in the Evaluation of Ocular Trauma

Detailed history of injury
Documented visual acuity
Ocular motility testing
Thorough external periobital/lid examination
Pupillary response and symmetry assessment
Marcus Gunn pupil testing
Anterior segment evaluation
Dilated retinal examination

Upon examination, gentle manipulation of the lids must be done to allow vision testing and examination of the globe. Gentle palpation of the orbital rim for areas of irregularity or point tenderness should be performed. Abnormalities of the periorbital bony structures may necessitate further diagnostic evaluations, such as orbital x-rays or CT scans. Care should be taken to place minimal pressure on the globe; if this is not possible, then ophthalmology referral is recommended. In addition to assessing the ocular adnexa, ocular motility (the patients ability to look in all directions of gaze) should be evaluated. Eye movements should be full and conjugate, both eyes moving in symmetry. Restrictions of ocular movements may indicate bony or soft tissue injury in the orbit.

PUPIL

Symmetry of the size of the pupils may be an important indication of ocular health. The patient or an observer may report pupillary asymmetry. The pupils should be round and briskly reactive to light. A dilated or sluggish pupil may indicate damage to the iris sphincter muscle or intense ocular inflammation. A distorted pupil may represent a corneal laceration with peripheral iris plugging of the wound, direct iris laceration, or detachment of the iris from its base (iris dialysis). Testing for an afferent pupillary light defect (Marcus Gunn Pupil; see Appendix B) is also important.

ANTERIOR SEGMENT

Most patients are unable to see enough detail of the anterior segment of the eye to describe specific injury patterns over the phone. Therefore, any perceived discrepancy by the patient of the appearance of the injured globe to the uninjured eye should be evaluated immediately. Most injuries of the cornea and sclera can be directly viewed and assessed with loupes or the slitlamp microscope. Surface foreign bodies are frequently seen and are discussed in Section II. Small perforations from "metal on metal" hammering injuries must be meticulously looked for as they can be easily missed. Use of fluorescein dye to determine if aqueous is leaking from a corneal wound is a useful diagnostic technique.

RETINA

The general state of the retina following ocular trauma can be assessed by history, by asking the patient specific questions regarding the patient's central and peripheral vision. If the patient expresses absolutely no change in central or peripheral vision, then serious retinal injury is less likely. If the patient describes the acute onset of flashes, floaters, curtains, or veils in the peripheral vision, then immediate evaluation for possible retinal tears and detachment is warranted. When the patient is evaluated, an ophthalmoscope should be used to view the retina. The inability to view the optic nerve in the setting of reduced vision and a clear cornea may indicate the presence of blood in the vitreous cavity, a cataract of the lens, or blood in the anterior chamber (hyphema). Assessment of the retinal status may require referral to an ophthalmologist and specialized ultrasonographic testing.

TREATMENT

Patients reporting ocular trauma can be partially assessed over the telephone, but given the diversity and complexity of ocular injuries nearly all patients need to be examined. The patient should be instructed not to eat or drink anything on the way to the clinic so that any necessary emergency procedures will not be delayed and anesthesia risks can be avoided. The patient should be instructed to protect the eye from pressure or reinjury, and no drops should be instilled except by the physician. Once the physician has evaluated the injury, the acute therapy administered depends on the type and severity of the injury. Most surface abrasions and foreign bodies can be treated in the clinic and pressure patched. Chemical burns can be irrigated and referred. Perforating injuries of the globe should have a shield gently taped over the lids, avoiding pressure on the globe, and be referred immediately.

Critical to the management of any trauma case, however, is the meticulous documentation of the presenting history and physical at the initial examination by the treating physician.

Chapter 8 ◖●◗

Excessive Tearing (Epiphora)

G. A. Cioffi

Another frequent ocular complaint is excessive tearing, or "epiphora." Epiphora refers to tears rolling down the cheek and generally is caused by one of two mechanisms. Excessive tearing can be the result of sudden reflex tearing due to irritation of the ocular surface. It may also be the result of a blockage of the lacrimal drainage system.

Tears are produced both by the major lacrimal gland, located in the superior temporal quadrant of the orbit, and by accessory lacrimal glands, which are found along the internal surface of both the upper and lower eyelids. The accessory lacrimal glands are responsible for basic tear secretion, while the major lacrimal gland provides much of the aqueous portion of reflex tearing. Tears serve the useful purposes of maintaining a smooth optical surface on the anterior portion of the eye, as well as providing anti-infective agents and removing foreign particulate from the anterior surface of the eye. Tears are normally drained through two puncta at the medial aspect of each of the upper and lower eyelids. These puncta, or drainage holes, lead to a single canaliculus which drains into the lacrimal sac. The lacrimal sac is situated along the lateral nasal bridge and drains into the nasal cavity via the nasolacrimal duct. Blockage of the nasal excretory system at any point may result in excessive tearing.

REFLEX TEARING

Reflex tearing may be the result of a foreign body sensation created when any external irritant stimulates the conjunctival or corneal nerve endings. Both particulate matter and noxious vapors may cause such an irritation. Allergens such as pollens may, as well, stimulate an allergic inflammatory response resulting in tearing. Excessive tearing associated with allergy is usually accompanied by intense itching, especially at the medial canthal region of the eye. Epiphora associated with a foreign body sensation should alert the physician to the possibility of a corneal abrasion, ocular foreign bodies, lid abnormalities, and dry eye syndromes (see Chapter 6, "Foreign Body Sensation"). It seems a paradox that dry eye syndromes (inadequate basic tear secretion) may result in epiphora, but reflex tearing is often the result of foreign body sensations stimulated by inadequate ocular surface lubrication.

BLOCKAGE OF NASAL LACRIMAL DRAINAGE

Epiphora which results from a blockage of the nasal lacrimal excretory system may occur congenitally because of incomplete formation and opening of the drainage system. Although in many infants the lacrimal blockage will spontaneously open,

19

TABLE 8.1. Common Differential
Diagnosis—Epiphora

Reflex Tearing
    Allergic conjunctivitis*
    Ocular foreign body*
    Lid malposition*
    Noxious stimuli exposure
    Dry eye syndromes
    Corneal lesions
    Trichiasis
Blockage of Nasolacrimal Drainage
    Dacryocystitis*
    Infectious punctal occlusion*
    Traumatic punctal occlusion*
    Canaliculitis

* Most common

most will require irrigation and dilation of the lacrimal drainage system. In addition, infectious blockage of the system may occur in both children and adults. Tearing resulting from an infectious etiology most often is unilateral. This can be used as a generalized guide to separate tearing associated with irritation, which almost always is bilateral. Dacryocystitis is a common infection of the lacrimal sac which occurs most often in infants and postmenopausal women. The most common cause of dacryocystitis in children is *Haemophilus influenzae;* in adults, it is *Staphylococcus aureus.* Spontaneous resolution of dacryocystitis may occur. Conservative treatment with warm compresses may initially relieve symptoms, but recurrence is the rule. More often, relief of an obstruction of the nasolacrimal system and/or drainage of the infected nasolacrimal sac is required to eradicate dacryocystitis.

Blockage of the puncta may also occur from relatively minor trauma or infection. This often can be identified on clinical examination. Reopening of the puncta may be achieved with dilation in the office setting. Topical antibiotics and warm compresses may be effective in infectious punctal occlusion. Blockage of the canalicular system may also occur as a result of infection. A variety of topical (such as idoxuridine) and systemic (such as chemotherapy with fluorouracil) agents have also been cited as causes of canalicular obstruction. Canalicular obstruction is much less common than either punctal occlusion or dacryocystitis. Among the pathogens which cause canaliculitis and canalicular obstruction are *Actinomyces israelii, Candida albicans,* and *Aspergillus* species.

Chapter 9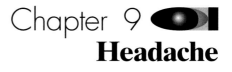
Headache

W. T. Shults

Headache is one of the most frequent maladies addressed in the physician's office. Over-the-counter headache preparation sales total over one billion dollars annually and almost 50 per 1000 patient visits to physicians are for this complaint. Often headache pain centers around or behind the eyes, prompting concern that ocular disease may be present. While that is sometimes the case, more often there is an extraocular cause.

OCULAR USE HEADACHE

While most headaches of any cause can be exacerbated by prolonged close work requiring accommodation, primary refractive or fusional disorders rarely produce headaches severe enough to cause the patient to seek medical attention. If the headache occurs primarily with intense and prolonged close work, then a refractive error or minimal vertical or horizontal phoria (tendency for the eye to deviate held in check by fusional mechanisms) may be present and is correctable by glasses. In general, such disorders are an overemphasized cause of headache.

HEADACHE ASSOCIATED WITH OCULAR AND ORBITAL DISORDERS

While local ocular and orbital diseases (such as conjunctivitis, corneal abrasion, iritis, optic neuritis, angle closure glaucoma, and inflammatory orbital pseudotumor) are all associated with ocular/orbital pain, the clinical signs and associated symptoms usually makes the relationship to the underlying disorder clear and should prompt referral for further management. Thus, a mucopurulent discharge coupled with conjunctival injection suggests conjunctivitis, while photophobia, circumlimbal injection and anterior chamber flare and cells (visible with a slitlamp) define iritis. Pain (particularly with eye movement) and acute monocular visual blurring implies optic neuritis, while nausea-inducing aching discomfort coupled with visual halos around lights accompanies acute angle closure glaucoma.

Up to one-half of patients with diabetic third nerve palsies will experience severe periorbital discomfort so intense as to be indistinguishable from that occurring with posterior communicating artery aneurysmal rupture. Photophobia may accompany the head pain associated with subarachnoid hemorrhage, migraine, or optic neuritis. Sudden onset of pain in the angle of the jaw radiating to the ipsilateral orbit and temple combined with an oculosympathetic paresis should raise concern regarding the possibil-

TABLE 9.1. Common Differential
Diagnosis—Headache Associated with Ocular
Disease

Ocular use headache*
Uncorrected/inadequately corrected refractive error*
Ocular irritation headache (e.g., corneal abrasion)*
Iritis/uveitis (intraocular inflammation)
Angle closure glaucoma
Optic neuritis
Inflammatory orbital pseudotumor
Diabetic cranial nerve III palsy
Migraine (common, classical, complicated)*
Cluster headaches
Trigeminal neuralgia
Temporal arteritis
Headache associated with increased intracranial pressure

---

* Most common

ity of spontaneous dissection of the carotid artery. Pain coupled with facial numbness in the distribution of one of the branches of the fifth cranial nerve, especially if occurring in a patient who has previously had a skin cancer removed from the face, suggests intraneural spread of cancer. Such patients may develop diplopia if the tumor tracks back along a sensory branch of the trigeminal nerve and enters the cavernous sinus (from which point it gains access to the ocular motor nerves). Orbital or ocular pain occurring in a setting devoid of examination abnormalities may have a functional origin and must always be kept in mind when the examination fails to define a cause for the patient's discomfort.

MIGRAINE

Migraine is a very common disorder which afflicts approximately 10% of people at sometime in their life. Although headache is a usual feature of migraine, its presence is not invariable and many patients experience other symptoms of migraine without experiencing any headache (so-called migraine equivalents). Migraine is traditionally divided into several types: common, classical, complicated.

Common Migraine

Unlike classical migraine, common migraine has no well-defined aura though it may be preceded by a vague prodrome including psychic phenomenon (such as depression) and fluid retention. The headache may start as unilateral, but may generalize to involve the whole head. It is not uncommonly throbbing, but may convert to a steady generalized aching discomfort. Nausea is a regular feature of common migraine, hence the term "sick headache." The pain lasts for a variable period of hours to days. Patients often gain relief by seeking a dark, quiet place.

Classical Migraine

A well-defined aura is what characterizes classical migraine. The aura is most often visual, but can be characterized by hemihypesthesia or aphasia. The visual changes can be highly variable, but most often the aura begins as a small grayish zone of impaired vision close to fixation. Over a 20–30 minute period, the zone of impairment grows and takes on a zig zag or "fortification" shape with vision recovering at the trailing edge as the leading edge expands. The fortification spectra may flicker, or shimmer, and appear brightly lit. The headache, which is often unilateral, begins as the aura fades and usually is more brief in duration than that associated with common migraine. That the aura is a cerebral rather than an ocular phenomenon is attested to by its persistence in patients who have no eyes. Migraine often begins in adolescence, decreases in frequency in the third and fourth decades, and may recur as isolated visual aura without headache in later years, when it may be difficult to distinguish it from a vertebrobasilar transient ischemic attack.

Complicated Migraine

The usual visual, and less common sensory and motor, auras of classical migraine are transient phenomena lasting 20–30 minutes before clearing. Occasionally, the visual, sensory and motor deficits persist, resulting in prolonged, or even permanent, defects of neurologic function. Thus, transient, and sometimes permanent, homonymous hemianopsia, hemiplegia, hemisensory loss, and alexia have all been ascribed to migraine. These deficits have now been documented with neuroimaging studies to arise from presumed focal cerebral infarctions. Complicated migraine should be part of the differential diagnosis in all young people suffering strokes.

The visual aura of migraine often favors one side. However, if it is monotonously unilateral, the possibility of an underlying structural abnormality, such as an arteriovenous malformation or tumor, must be considered and neuroimaging studies obtained. Ophthalmoplegic migraine is an uncommon variant of complicated migraine, generally having its onset in the first decade of life. In this type of migraine, the patient develops an oculomotor nerve palsy (usually involving the pupil) as the headache reaches its zenith. The paresis is transient at first, but with repeated episodes it may become permanent.

CLUSTER HEADACHE

Often considered a migraine variant, cluster headaches are characterized by recurrent episodes of severe unilateral head or face pain, typically occurring in "clusters": daily headaches occurring during a susceptible period of weeks to months, followed by quiescent periods when the patient is headache-free. The pain is quite severe, often leading the patient to contemplate suicide during the episode. Ipsilateral conjunctival injection and nasal congestion accompany the head pain, as well as ipsilateral oculosympathetic paresis, which may persist after the acute event has cleared. Cluster headache sufferers, who are predominantly males in the third to fifth decades of life, may be awakened from a sound sleep with intractable pain. Cluster headaches may occur in migraine sufferers and be admixed with common or classical migraine episodes.

TRIGEMINAL NEURALGIA

Typically described as lancinating, the pain of tic douloureux consists of recurrent brief stabs of intense pain in the second and third divisions of the trigeminal nerve followed by less intense lingering discomfort. Rarely, the first division of the trigeminal nerve is involved, but almost never in isolation. Unlike cluster headaches, which begin in the third and fourth decades, tic douloureux is generally a disorder of later life, having a peak incidence in the sixth and seventh decades. When it is seen in a younger person, consideration must be given to multiple sclerosis as a cause. In the older age range, the most commonly identified cause is cross-compression by a tortuous atherosclerotic vessel of the trigeminal sensory root at its point of entry into the brainstem.

TEMPORAL ARTERITIS

Headache is one of the most regular symptoms of temporal arteritis and is not solely isolated to the temples, but may be holocephalic in nature. Systemic symptomatology such as fever, weight loss, jaw claudication on chewing, and polymyalgia rheumatica will point the alert clinician toward the proper diagnosis in an elderly patient with a new onset headache and scalp tenderness.

HEADACHES WITH INCREASED INTRACRANIAL PRESSURE

Most patients presenting with a complaint of headache are worried about the possibility that they might harbor a brain tumor as the cause of their discomfort. The same might be said of the physician confronting such a patient for the first time. While headache is a common accompaniment of increased intracranial pressure, it is most often nonspecific and nonlocalizing. The headache is often moderate in severity and worsened by physical activity, coughing or straining and may be more prominent when the patient first awakens in the morning. If localizing neurologic findings or papilledema are present, neuroimaging studies should be performed to search for an intracranial mass.

THE MOST COMMON OCULAR DISORDERS AND THEIR MANAGEMENT

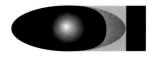

PART A
Disorders of the Ocular Adnexa

Chapter 10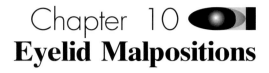
Eyelid Malpositions

M. W. Wilson and R. A. Dailey

INTRODUCTION

The eyelids are specialized structures designed to protect the eye and lubricate the cornea, while maintaining an aperture for vision. Malposition of the eyelids may interfere with these functions. A familiarity with the anatomy of the eyelid makes its malposition more easily understood. The eyelids measure approximately 30 mm in length horizontally. The palpebral fissure is the opening between the upper and lower eyelid, and it measures 10–12 mm in height. The eyelids are most simply thought of as opposing anterior and posterior lamella (Fig. 10.1). The anterior lamella is a myocutaneous layer composed of skin and the orbicularis oculi. There is keratinized epidermis overlying a modified dermis with associated skin appendages. The orbicularis oculi consists of pretarsal, preseptal, and orbital portions. Each contributes to proper eyelid closure. The pretarsal and preseptal portions help to form the medial and lateral canthal tendons which stabilize the eyelids. The orbital septum divides the anterior and posterior lamella. It arises from the periorbita (the periosteal lining of the orbit) and acts as a barrier against the spread of infection and the herniation of orbital fat. The posterior lamella includes the eyelid retractors, the tarsus, and the conjunctiva. The eyelid retractors are deep to the preaponeurotic fat. The upper eyelid retractors are the levator palpebrae superioris and Müller's muscle, also known as the superior tarsal muscle. The levator palpebrae superioris arises at the orbital apex from the lesser wing of the sphenoid. It overlies the superior rectus muscle. Anteriorly, the levator becomes an aponeurotic sheet that attaches to the medial and lateral orbital walls and to the anterior tarsal surface. Müller's muscle arises from the posterior surface of the levator aponeurosis and attaches to the superior tarsal border. The lower lid retractors are analogous to their upper lid counterparts. They, however, do not arise from the orbital apex, but rather originate from an anterior extension of the inferior rectus muscle known as the capsulopalpebral fascia.

The eyelid retractors are innervated by the third cranial nerve as well as sympathetics that travel with internal carotid artery and through the cavernous sinus. The levator palpebrae superioris is innervated by the superior division of the third cranial nerve. Müller's muscle and the inferior tarsal muscle receive sympathetic innervation. The

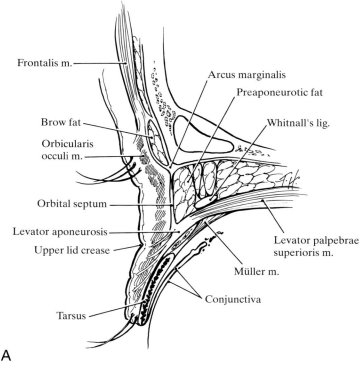

A

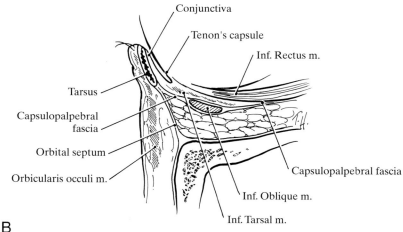

B

Figure 10.1. Upper (**A**) and lower (**B**) eyelid diagrams illustrating the anterior myocutaneous lamella, the orbital septum, and the posterior lamella consisting of the eyelid retractors, the tarsus, and the conjunctiva.

TABLE 10.1. Referral Guidelines

DIAGNOSIS (CODE)	TREATMENT	WHEN TO REFER
Ptosis (374.3)	Levator resection, mullerectomy, fascia lata sling	Visual disturbance, etiology unclear
Dermatochalasis (374.87)	Blepharoplasty	Visual disturbance, asthenopic symptoms
Entropion (374.0)	Horizontal shortening, mucous membrane graft, hard palate graft	Foreign body sensation, tearing, and red eye
Trichiasis (374.05)	Epilation, cryotherapy, electrolysis, radiofrequency	Foreign body sensation, tearing, and red eye
Ectropion (374.1)	Horizontal shortening, skin graft	Foreign body sensation, tearing, and red eye

tarsi are composed of dense connective tissue and give form to the eyelid. The tarsal plates border the eyelid margin. The superior tarsus measures 10 mm in height, while inferior tarsus measures 4 mm in height. Each of the tarsi contains meibomian glands that drain onto the eyelid margin. The conjunctiva is a mucosal surface tightly adherent to posterior tarsal surface. It joins with the skin on the lid margin and is reflected onto the ocular surface at both superior and inferior fornices. The accessory lacrimal glands of Krause and Wolfring are located within the conjunctival fornices.

CLINICAL MANIFESTATIONS

Eyelid malpositions may occur with a variety of signs and symptoms. Patients may complain of decrease visual acuity. This may be simply related to a droopy lid (ptosis) blocking the visual axis, or to a more serious problem such as corneal compromise secondary to eyelash abrasions or exposure. Patients with ptosis of the eyelids may also complain of eye strain or fatigue from the sustained effort of keeping the eyelids open. Tearing is a frequent complaint of patients with either ectropion or entropion (see later). The eye is frequently red and uncomfortable. Ectropions prevent the eyelids from adequately protecting the cornea. The cornea is subject to drying resulting in reflex tearing and the sensation of a foreign body being present. Entropions allow eyelashes to abrade the cornea disrupting its epithelial surface. The patient perceives this as a foreign body sensation and reflex tearing is stimulated. The compromised cornea is susceptible to subsequent epithelial erosion and infection. These symptoms are exacerbated in dry and windy conditions.

DIFFERENTIAL DIAGNOSIS

Malposition of the eyelid results from a deficiency or weakness of the layers described earlier. There are four basic malpositions of the eyelids: ptosis, dermatochalasis, entropion, and ectropion (Table 10.1).

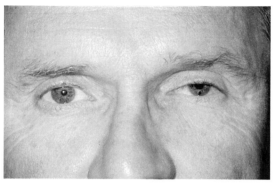

Figure 10.2.   Ptosis of the left upper eyelid. Note the absent corneal light reflex on the left as the upper eyelid cover the pupil and visual axis.

PTOSIS

Ptosis is a drooping of the upper eyelid margin caused by a failure of the upper eyelid retractors to raise the lid to its normal resting position at the superior limbus (Fig. 10.2). Patients with ptosis experience a restriction of their superior and temporal visual fields. In children, uncorrected ptosis may cause occlusion amblyopia with permanent visual loss. Ptosis may be aponeurotic, myogenic or neurogenic. Pseudoptosis may be caused by mechanical forces lowering the lid. Aponeurotic ptosis is caused by a thinning, stretching, or disinsertion of the levator aponeurosis from the tarsus of the upper eyelid. It is the most common cause of acquired ptosis. Involutional changes associated with aging are most commonly responsible, but trauma and surgery are also frequent causes. Aponeurotic ptosis is often seen in contact lens wearers who manipulate their eyelids frequently. A history of a progressive ptosis over months to years is commonly found. Aponeurotic ptosis does not vary during the day, and a superiorly displaced lid crease is seen on exam. Myogenic ptosis results from an abnormality of the levator palpebrae superioris. It is the most common cause of congenital ptosis. A prominent lid crease may be absent. The levator is poorly developed and may be infiltrated with fat. Muscular dystrophies and myotonic dystrophies both cause myogenic ptosis. Oculopharyngeal dystrophy is an autosomal dominant disease of variable penetrance first described in French Canadians. Myogenic ptosis may be the hallmark of the disease. Mitochondrial diseases such as chronic progressive external ophthalmoplegia, present with weakness of the levator initially, and later involve the other extraocular muscles. Systemic involvement may result in complete heart block, such as in Kearns-Sayre syndrome. Patients with myogenic ptosis tend to be younger than those with aponeurotic ptosis.

Neurogenic ptosis results from disruption of the normal neural stimulus to the upper eyelid retractors. The third cranial nerve innervates the levator palpebrae superioris and the sympathetic nerve innervates Müller's muscle. Supranuclear lesions of the third cranial nerve result in a contralateral ptosis. Nuclear lesions of the third nerve cause bilateral ptosis as there is only one midline subnucleus that controls both levators. Infranuclear lesions, those directly affecting the third cranial nerve, cause a complete ipsilateral ptosis in association with a palsy of the superior rectus, medial rectus, inferior rectus, and inferior oblique, and an efferent pupillary defect. Damage to the sympathetic innervation of Müller's muscle causes a ptosis of 2–3 mm, whereas disruption of the third cranial nerve may result in complete ptosis. Sympathetic ptosis may be associated with pupillary miosis and facial anhidrosis (Horner's syndrome). Lesions may occur in the first, second, or third order neurons. Pancoast tumors, neuroblastomas, and carotid artery dissection should be eliminated as possible etiologies in patients with sympathetic ptosis. Blockade of the neuromuscular junction occurs in myasthenia gravis, and ptosis may be the presenting sign. The ptosis is usually variable in nature, being worse at the end of the day. Patients may also complain of diplopia if other extraocular muscles are involved. Most patients respond to Tensilon testing. Of patients with myasthenia gravis having only ocular symptoms, 80% will develop systemic manifestations within 2 years. Eaton-Lambert syndrome is a paraneoplastic syndrome associated with oat cell carcinoma of the lung that mimics myasthenia gravis.

TREATMENT AND FREQUENCY OF VISITS

Examination should include measurement of the amount of ptosis and levator function. The position of the lid crease should be noted. If necessary, Tensilon testing should be performed to exclude myasthenia gravis. If Horner's syndrome is present, pupillary testing with 10% cocaine and 1% hydroxyamphetamine will localize the lesion (Fig. 10.3). If a third nerve palsy involves the pupil, an intracranial aneurysm should be excluded. Pupil-sparing third nerve palsies often result from microvascular disease. Formal visual fields showing less than 40° of superior visual field document significant ptosis. Photographs are often necessary for documentation. A second office visit may be needed to recheck for stability measurements before finalizing a surgical plan. Surgery to correct may be performed in the office with local anesthetic. An awake patient allows for a more precise correction. Many surgical techniques to correct ptosis have been described. The ptosis operation employed depends on the degree of ptosis, the etiology of the ptosis, and the surgeon. More complex surgeries with the harvesting of autologous fascia lata require an operating room and a general anesthetic.

DERMATOCHALASIS

Dermatochalasis is a redundancy of the skin of the upper and lower eyelids (Fig. 10.4). It may be associated with a weakening of the orbital septum and herniation of orbital fat into the eyelids. A concurrent ptosis due to the mechanical forces from extra skin or a weakened levator aponeurosis may occur. Associated lower eyelid laxity may cause either an entropion or ectropion. Although patients may complain that they look old or tired, their "baggy" upper eyelids can be more than a cosmetic problem. Dermatochalasis is a functional alteration in normal lid anatomy caused by aging, trauma, infection, inflammation, and neoplasms. Patients with dermatochalasis have superior visual field defects and the extra effort needed to keep the eyelids open causes asthenopic, headache symptoms. Changes in the position of the lower lid margin cause trichiasis, blepharoconjunctivitis, corneal exposure, and epiphora.

TREATMENT AND FREQUENCY OF VISITS

Examination should include evaluation for an aponeurotic ptosis. Malposition of the lower lid should be noted. One to two office visits are adequate to formulate a surgical

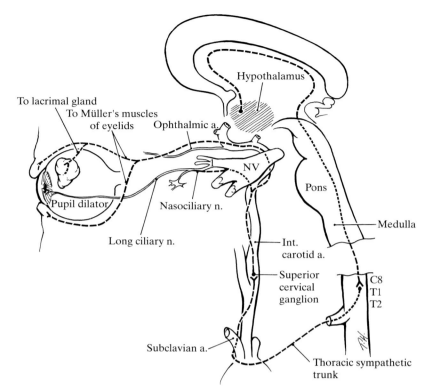

Figure 10.3.   Sympathetic pathway beginning in the hypothalamus, descending to the cervicothoracic spinal cord, ascending to the superior cervical ganglion, and finally traveling with the internal carotid artery to the eye.

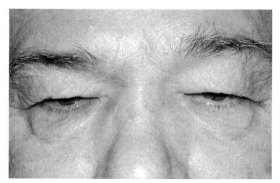

Figure 10.4.   Bilateral dermatochalasis. The upper eyelids block the visual axis secondary to the redundancy of the skin.

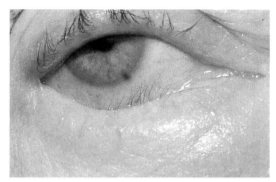

Figure 10.5. Entropion of the right lower eyelid. Note the trichiasis (misdirected eyelashes) abrading the corneal surface.

plan. Blepharoplasty (excision of redundant skin, muscle, and herniated orbital fat) may be performed in the office with local anesthesia. Patient anxiety may require the surgery be performed in the operating room with monitored anesthesia care and intravenous sedation. Newer techniques for blepharoplasty such as the carbon dioxide laser are often better performed with intravenous sedation. Surgeons must be judicious in their corrections to prevent postoperative complications such as corneal exposure and dry eye resulting from the overzealous removal of tissue. Hemostasis is essential and patients should be monitored postoperatively for bleeding, particularly for vision-threatening retrobulbar hemorrhages.

ENTROPION

Entropion is an inward rotation of the eyelid margin caused by a relative shortening of the posterior lamella in comparison to the anterior lamella (Fig. 10.5). The eyelashes abrade the cornea, and patients complain of a red eye and a foreign body sensation. Entropion more often involves the lower lid. Most entropion are involutional and are, therefore, more often seen in the elderly. A horizontal laxity of the lower lid and lower lid retractor disinsertion from the inferior tarsal border results in entropion. The preseptal orbicularis oculi overrides the pretarsal muscle. Cicatricial entropion is caused by a mechanical shortening of the posterior lamella, usually a result of scarring of the palpebral conjunctiva. It is found in patients with Steven-Johnson's syndrome, ocular cicatricial pemphigoid, alkali burns, and severe cases of adenoviral conjunctivitis. Spastic ectropion is caused by horizontal lid laxity and ocular irritation. The preseptal overrides the pretarsal orbicularis. The entropion is intermittent and best appreciated after forced eyelid closure. Congenital entropion is extremely rare. It is caused by dehiscence of the lower lid retractors.

TREATMENT AND FREQUENCY OF VISITS

A detailed examination evaluating lower lid laxity, position of the lower lid retractors, scarring of the conjunctiva, and corneal integrity is needed. Patients are at-risk to develop a secondary bacterial keratitis with devastating visual loss. As with other

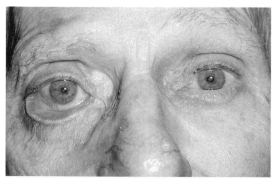

Figure 10.6.   Ectropion of the right lower eyelid secondary to Bell's palsy. The conjunctiva is inflamed and the inferior cornea is unprotected.

eyelid malpositions, preoperative photographic documentation is essential. Surgical management can usually be determined after initial consultation. Simple procedures such as horizontal lid shortenings can be performed in the office with local anesthetics. More complex operations involving mucous membrane grafts and hard palate grafts are best performed with monitored or general anesthesia. Postoperative follow-up is determined by the success of the surgery. Persistent malposition of the eyelashes must always be corrected. Trichiasis is a misdirection of the eyelashes so that they abrade the cornea (Fig. 10.5). Trichiasis is most commonly associated with entropion. If repair of the entropion does not fully correct the trichiasis, the eyelashes must be removed either by simple epilation or more elaborate means. Cryotherapy, electrolysis, and radio frequency epilation offer long-term relief from symptoms. Each procedure may be performed in the office with local anesthetic.

ECTROPION

Ectropion is an outward rotation of the eyelid margin caused by a relative shortening of the anterior lamella in comparison to the posterior lamella (Fig. 10.6). Patients present with a red eye complaining of epiphora (tearing) and a foreign body sensation in the eye. Ectropion may be involutional, paralytic, or cicatricial. Involutional ectropion is caused by horizontal lid laxity. Laxity of the medial and lateral canthal tendons of the eyelid also contribute. Paralytic ectropion results from a palsy of the seventh cranial nerve. Loss of orbicularis tone results in weakness of the anterior lamella of the lower lid and the eyelid margin rotates outward. Scarring of the anterior lamella (eyelid skin) causes vertical shortening, and may result in cicatricial ectropion as the lid is pulled externally. If the ectropion is severe enough to cause any symptoms (tearing and red eye), patients should be referred to an ophthalmologist. Eyes with ectropions are at risk of developing a secondary bacterial keratitis and corneal scarring due to exposure.

TREATMENT AND FREQUENCY OF VISITS

Examination should determine if there is horizontal laxity of the lower lid and laxity of the canthal tendons. The presence of scars should be recorded. Keratinization and edema of the externally rotated palpebral conjunctiva should be noted, as well as the position of the punctum of the lacrimal system. Corneal integrity should be assessed. Photographs are required to document findings. Surgical plans can usually be formulated after a single visit. Simple procedures such as horizontal tightening of the lower lid may be performed in the office with local anesthesia. Procedures involving full thickness skin grafts are best performed in operating room with either intravenous sedation or general anesthesia. Postoperative visits are dependent upon surgical success.

SUGGESTED READINGS

Anguilar GL, Nelson C. Eyelid and anterior orbital anatomy. In: Hornblass A, ed. Oculoplastic, orbital and reconstructive surgery. Baltimore: Williams & Wilkins, 1988:3–15.

Bartley GB. Functional indications for upper and lower eyelid blepharoplasty. Ophthalmology 1991;98:1461–1463.

Christenbury J. Aponeurotic ptosis. In: Bosniak S, ed. Principles and practice of ophthalmic plastic and reconstructive surgery. Philadelphia: WB Saunders, 1996:323–341.

Gilbard SM. Involutional and paralytic ectropion. In: Bosniak S, ed. Principles and practice of ophthalmic plastic and reconstructive surgery. Philadelphia: WB Saunders, 1996:422–437.

Long JA, Goldberg RA. Entropion. In: Bosniak S, ed. Principles and practice of ophthalmic plastic and reconstructive surgery. Philadelphia: WB Saunders, 1996:413–421.

Martin RT, Nunery WR, Tanenbaum M. Entropion, trichiasis and districhiasis. In: McCord CD, Tanenbaum M, Nunery WR, eds. Oculoplastic surgery. 3rd ed. New York: Raven Press, 1995:145–174.

Older JJ. Acquired ptosis. In: Hornblass A, ed. Oculoplastic, orbital and reconstructive surgery. Baltimore: Williams & Wilkins, 1988:341–353.

Rathbun JE. Entropion. In: Hornblass A, ed. Oculoplastic, orbital and reconstructive surgery. Baltimore: Williams & Wilkins, 1988:309–324.

Swartz NC, Murphy M, Cohen MS. Lower eyelid retraction and cicatricial ectropion. In: Bosniak S, ed. Principles and practice of ophthalmic plastic and reconstructive surgery. Philadelphia: WB Saunders, 1996:438–446.

Wesley RE. Ectropion repair. In: McCord CD, Tanenbaum M, Nunery WR, eds. Oculoplastic surgery. 3rd ed. New York: Raven Press, 1995:249–262.

◖◗ Chapter 11
Eyelid Lesions: Benign and Malignant

M. W. Wilson and R. A. Dailey

INTRODUCTION

The eyelids are host to a number of different lesions, both benign and malignant. Maculae, papules, plaques, and nodules may arise. These may be inflammatory, infectious, neoplastic, cystic, or degenerative in nature. Eyelid lesions are most simply categorized as benign or malignant. In examining patients, clinicians must be careful, as different lesions may have similar appearances. Malignant tumors may masquerade as benign and vice versa. As a rule, any suspicious lesion should be biopsied.

CLINICAL MANIFESTATIONS

Eyelid lesions may present with a variety of signs and symptoms. Infectious and inflammatory lesions will have associated erythema, edema, and pain. There may be diffuse swelling of the entire lid with focal tenderness and enlargement of a preauricular lymph node. Scaling and crusting may be present along the lid margin. Loss of eyelashes and conjunctival injection may also be noted. The patient typically complains of dry eyes with foreign body sensation or reflex tearing. Neoplasms may present as asymptomatic mass lesions. They are most often brought to the attention of the clinician because of cosmetic concerns. However, neoplasms may be erythematous and ulcerated. An associated ptosis, entropion, or ectropion may result from any eyelid lesion (see Chapter 10, "Eyelid Malpositions"). Loss of eyelashes and conjunctival injection may also be associated features with lid lesions. Degenerative and cystic lesions most frequently present as asymptomatic masses. Erythema and edema are rare. If the lid margin is involved, cysts may interfere with the visual axis. Additionally, both degenerative and cystic lesions may cause mechanical eyelid malpositions. The conjunctiva and cornea are usually spared by these processes.

DIFFERENTIAL DIAGNOSIS
BENIGN LESIONS (Table 11.1)
Inflammatory Eyelid Lesions

Blepharitis, the most common inflammation of the eyelids, is a diffuse inflammatory response of the eyelid margin which may be acute or chronic (see Chapter 12, "Blephari-

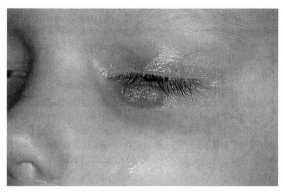

Figure 11.1. Child with external hordeolum. Note the large area of erythema and edema.

tis"). The cause may be allergic or infectious. Staphylococcal blepharitis results from an overgrowth of bacteria along the lid margin and an allergic reaction to the released exotoxin. Seborrheic blepharitis has a chronic course and is usually associated with scalp dandruff. External hordeolums, or "styes," are acute infections of either the apocrine sweat glands or sebaceous glands of the anterior lamella of the eyelid, Moll's glands, and Zeis' glands, respectively. Erythema and edema surround a raised nodule along the lid margin (Fig. 11.1) Focal tenderness is a common feature. Internal hordeolums are acute or chronic infections of the meibomian glands (the sebaceous glands of the tarsal plate) caused by staphylococcus. A tender, inflamed nodule is seen on the anterior lid surface. Diffuse edema of the eyelid may be present. A chalazion is a chronic lipogranuloma of the meibomian glands presenting as painless thickening of the tarsal plate (Fig. 11.2). Multiple chalazion may occur within a short period of time.

Pyogenic granulomas are eyelid lesions which are neither infectious or granulomatous. Instead, they are exuberant granulation tissue. The clinical appearance is a red, fleshy, highly vascular growth occurring on the palpebral (inside the eyelid) conjunctiva. They may be seen after trauma and surgery or in association with chalazion that

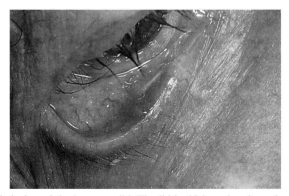

Figure 11.2. Chalazion of the lower eyelid. The lid is thickened and a palpable nodule can be identified by everting the lid. (See also color section.)

◼▮ TABLE 11.1. Referral Guidelines—Benign Lesions

DIAGNOSIS (CODE)	TREATMENT	WHEN TO REFER
Blepharitis (373.00)	Lid scrubs, topical antibiotic ointment at bedtime	Failure to respond to therapy
External hordeolum (373.11)	Warm compresses, topical antibiotics	Failure to respond to treatment
Internal hordeolum (373.12)	Warm compresses, topical antibiotics, incision & drainage	Failure to respond to conservative therapy, incision & drainage
Chalazion (373.2)	Warm compresses, steroid injections, incision & curettage, TCN 500 mg QD	Failure to respond to therapy, multiple or recurrent lesions
Pyogenic granuloma (686.1)	Topical steroids, excision	Initial management
Molluscum contagiosum (078.0)	Excision, cryotherapy, incision & drainage	Initial management
Verruca vulgaris (078.0)	Observe, excision	Excision
Herpes simplex (054)/ herpes zoster (053)	Oral acyclovir, topical antivirals, analgesics, possible steroids	Initial management
Preseptal cellulitis (373.13)	Oral or I.V. antibiotics	To exclude orbital cellulitis
Fungi (117.9)	Oral or I.V. antibiotics	Biopsy
Sarcoidosis (135)	Oral or topical steroids, excision, systemic evaluation	Biopsy or excision
Amyloidosis (277.3)	Observe, excision, systemic evaluation	Excision
Milia (374.05)	Observe, excision	Excision
Subdoriferous cyst (374.84)	Observe, excision	Excision
Sebaceous cyst (374.84)	Observe, excision	Excision
Epidermal inclusion cyst (706.2)	Observe, excision	Excision
Epidermoid/dermoid cyst (706.2)	Observe, excision	Excision
Seborrheic keratosis (702.19)	Observe, excision	Excision
Keratoacanthoma (238.2)	Excision	Excision, rule out squamous cell carcinoma
Actinic Keratosis (702.0)	Excision	Excision, rule out squamous cell carcinoma
Inverted follicular keratosis (264.8)	Excision	Excision, rule out squamous cell carcinoma
Cutaneous horn (702.8)	Excision	Excision, rule out squamous cell carcinoma
Xanthelasma (272.2)	Observe, excision, rule out diabetes and hyperlipidemia	Excision
Capillary hemangioma (M9131/0)	Observe, oral or local steroids, interferon, excision	Rule out amblyopia, steroids, interferon, excision

◼◼ TABLE 11.1. (continued)

DIAGNOSIS (CODE)	TREATMENT	WHEN TO REFER
Cavernous hemangioma (M9121/0)	Observe, excision	To assess visual acuity, confirm diagnosis, excision
Nevus flammeus (757.32)	Observe, argon or tuneable dye laser	Rule out or follow for glaucoma, laser therapy
Sebaceous adenoma	Observe, excision	Excision
Trichoepithelioma	Observe, excision	Excision
Trichofolliculoma	Observe, excision	Excision
Tricholemmoma	Observe, excision	Excision
Pilomatrixoma	Observe, excision	Excision
Freckle (709.09)	Observe	
Nevus (224)	Observe, excision	Excision
Nevus of Ota (216.1)	Observe	Exam every 1–2 years to rule out uveal melanoma & glaucoma

have spontaneously drained. Local excision or topical steroids are possible treatment alternatives. Viruses may also cause benign eyelid lesions. Molluscum contagiosum is an umbilicated growth usually on the external eyelid caused by a pox virus. Single or multiple lesions may occur on the eyelids and elsewhere on the body. Viral particles shed by these lesions cause a follicular conjunctivitis and keratitis. Verruca vulgaris of the eyelid is caused the human papilloma virus (Fig. 11.3). Amelanotic growths with papillomatous surfaces are characteristic. Lesions may be solitary or multiple.

Herpes simplex and herpes zoster both cause a vesicular blepharoconjunctivitis with or without an associated keratitis (see Chapter 23, "Ocular Herpetic Infections"). Herpes simplex typically has mild-to-moderate pain with a paucity of vesicular lesion scattered along the eyelid margin or in the lateral canthus. Herpes zoster causes an eruption of vesicles usually affecting the dermatome of the first division of the fifth cranial nerve. Involvement of the tip of the nose indicates an increased likelihood of

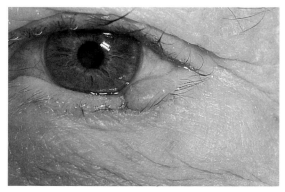

Figure 11.3. Verruca vulgaris of the eyelid is caused by the human papilloma virus. Note the raised amelanotic lesion.

ocular involvement. Pain is usually marked to severe. Scarring of the lids with resultant lagophthalmos, cicatricial ectropion, and trichiasis may occur.

Bacterial infections of the eyelid may cause a preseptal cellulitis characterized by diffuse erythema and edema. An antecedent history of skin trauma is usually present. Erysipelas and impetigo may also trigger a preseptal cellulitis. In infants and children, the possibility of *Haemophilus influenzae* as a causative organism must be considered, as it can spread quickly to the orbit and the central nervous system.

Fungi rarely result in infections of the eyelids. Candida, coccidioidomycosis, blastomycosis, and sporotrichosis have all been reported to infect the eyelid. Sarcoidosis is another inflammatory condition that may affect eyelids, as well as virtually all the internal structures of the eye. Erythematous umbilicated papules and nodules may be present on the lids. These lesions are usually asymptomatic and respond to both systemic and topical steroids. Sarcoid granulomas may also be found on the palpebral conjunctiva. Biopsy of these lesions may assist in confirming a diagnosis of sarcoid. However, random biopsies of the conjunctival are of limited value in diagnosing sarcoidosis.

TREATMENT

Eyelid scrubs with baby shampoo remove scales and crust, decrease bacterial flora, and improve the quality of the tear film in cases of blepharitis (see Chapter 12, "Blepharitis"). Antibiotic drops and ointment help control symptoms. Warm compresses applied for 15–20 minutes four times daily will encourage drainage of a hordeolum. Bacitracin or erythromycin ophthalmic ointment may be prescribed on a temporary basis to decrease bacterial flora and prevent recurrences. As with external hordeolums, warm compresses with topical antibiotics are standard therapy for internal hordeolum. Warm compresses, local steroid injections, and incision and curettage are recommended treatments for chalazion. Surgical therapy is necessary when conservative treatment fails to resolve the chalazion. Recurrent chalazion should be sent to pathology to exclude possible malignancies such as sebaceous cell carcinoma. Oral tetracycline 500 mg per day may prevent new chalazion from forming by decreasing the viscosity of meibomian secretions. Incision and drainage are occasionally indicated. Patients with blepharitis, hordeolum or chalazion should be instructed in lid hygiene to minimize recurrences.

Local excision usually results in complete resolution of pyogenic granulomas and verruca vulgaris. Local excision, incision and curettage, and cryotherapy are most common treatment modalities for viral eyelid lesions. The application of caustics such as liquefied phenol, silver nitrate, and trichloroacetic acid has also been described.

Treatment of both herpetic conditions includes oral acyclovir and analgesics (see Chapter 23, "Ocular Herpetic Infections"). Topical antiviral ointments may be needed in herpes simplex infections. Close observation by an ophthalmologist is needed to monitor adverse sequelae including corneal scarring, uveitis, and possible glaucoma.

In cases of preseptal cellulitis in children, aggressive broad spectrum, intravenous antibiotic therapy is needed. In adults, oral antibiotics with Gram-positive efficacy should suffice.

Degenerative Eyelid Lesions

The skin of the eyelids is the most common and most characteristic site for the involvement of primary systemic amyloidosis. Lesions are typically bilaterally, symmetric single or multiple confluent papules exhibiting a yellowish or waxy appearance. Ptosis or complete external ophthalmoplegia secondary to amyloid infiltrates may accompany skin lesions. Additionally, purpura may be seen on the eyelid as well as elsewhere on the body due to fragility of blood vessels from amyloid deposits. A confirmatory biopsy may be needed to establish the diagnosis. An underlining hematologic malignancy should be excluded. Secondary localized amyloidosis is found in association of a number of lesions including basal cell carcinoma, Bowen's disease, and seborrheic keratoses.

Cystic Eyelid Lesions

Milia are keratin-filled cysts most commonly seen in newborns. They are also found postoperatively along surgical incisions or after carbon dioxide superpulsed laser resurfacing. Sudoriferous cysts, or cysts of Moll, are fluid-filled, translucent, blister-like elevations of the epidermis resulting from a blockage of the gland of Moll. These cysts are found along the eyelid margin. Sebaceous cysts are white to yellow bumps occurring beneath the normal skin of the eyelid. Obstruction of Zeis' glands, the meibomian glands, or the sebaceous glands associated with eyelash follicles may precipitate formation of these lesions. Epidermal inclusion cysts occur on the skin surface of the eyelid. These cysts arise from either the infundibulum of the eyelash follicles or from the implantation of epidermis into the dermis from trauma. Multiple inclusion cysts may be a hallmark of Gardner's syndrome.

Epidermoid and dermoid cysts are choristomatous lesions. Choristomas occur along lines of embryonic fissure closure. Surface ectoderm and its associated dermal appendages are trapped within the deeper mesenchymal tissue. An epidermal-lined cyst with or without dermal appendages results. The cyst is filled with keratin. The frontozygomatic suture is the most typical location for these choristomas. Lesions are usually fixated to bone. In childhood, epidermoid and dermoid cysts present as painless masses. In adults, the cysts frequently rupture and are painful, inflamed tumors.

TREATMENT

For most simple cystic lesions, excision is curative. However, complete excision of the entire lesions is needed for resolution of cysts associated with glandular obstruction and eyelash follicles abnormalities. Without complete excision, recurrences are common. Both epidermoid and dermoid cystic lesions should be excised intact, as release of the keratin debris will incite a granulomatous inflammatory reaction.

Neoplastic Eyelid Lesions

Benign neoplasms arise from both the skin and adnexal structures of the eyelid. These neoplasia may be either pigmented or nonpigmented, and many are associated with inflammatory lesions. Some eyelid neoplasias contain aberrant vascular elements. Differentiation of various neoplastic lesions is important because many are associated with other diseases, both ocular and systemic, and some are predecessors of malignant lesions.

Seborrheic keratosis is a waxy lesion of variable pigmentation with a verrucous surface affecting patients most commonly after the sixth decade. These lesions are

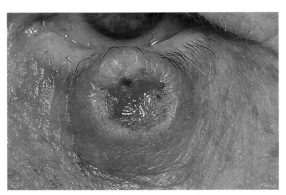

Figure 11.4. Keratoacanthoma is a rapidly growing umbilicated tumor with a keratin- filled center.

said to have a "stuck on" appearance. These growths are hyperkeratotic, acanthotic lesions with no malignant potential. Keratoacanthoma is a rapidly growing umbilicated tumor with a keratin-filled center (Fig. 11.4). It resembles squamous cell carcinoma, but pursues a different clinical course, which may include spontaneous resolution. History is paramount in establishing the correct diagnosis.

Actinic keratosis or solar keratosis occur on sun-exposed surfaces, such as the eyelids, as flat, scaly erythematous plaques. These lesions are dysplastic and may give rise to invasive squamous cell carcinoma. Inverted follicular keratosis is a hyperkera- totic neoplasm with a predilection for the face. It is usually solitary with a varied clinical appearance. It may be nodular, papillary, and verrucous. Inverted follicular keratoses are thought to be induced by a virus. Cutaneous horn is a descriptive term and not a diagnosis (Fig. 11.5). It refers a hyperkeratotic growth overlying a number of different epidermal neoplasms, both benign and malignant, including seborrheic keratosis, verruca vulgaris, squamous cell carcinoma, and basal cell carcinoma. The base of the lesion must be biopsied to establish the correct diagnosis.

Xanthelasmas are dermal tumors of the eyelid. Solitary or multiple elevated yellow plaques occur most commonly in the medial canthal area. These tumors are composed of an aggregation of lipid-laden histiocytes. There is an increased incidence of diabetes and hyperlipidemia (types II and III) in patients with xanthelasma of the eyelids.

Capillary hemangioma, or strawberry nevus, is the most common benign vascular tumor of the eyelid (Fig. 11.6). Capillary hemangiomas are composed of small endothe- lial lined vascular spaces. Tumors are reddish-purple growths with small surface invagi- nations and have a soft consistency. Tumors appear in infancy and may initially increase in size before regressing later in childhood. If the hemangioma compresses the eye or occludes the visual axis, the child is at risk of developing amblyopia. Cavernous hemangiomas are rarely found in the eyelids. These tumors occur more frequently as intraconal orbital tumors in adults, where they may produce axial proptosis and refrac- tive changes in the eye. They are composed of large dilated vascular spaces.

Nevus flammeus, or port-wine stain, is the vascular anomaly found in association with Sturge-Weber syndrome that may involve the eyelids (Fig. 11.7). The lesion is present at birth. Unlike a capillary hemangioma, a nevus flammeus does not blanch with pressure. It neither increases in size nor spontaneously involutes. Patients with

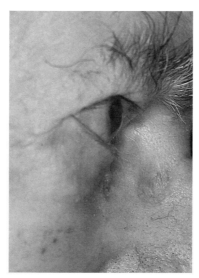

Figure 11.5. Cutaneous horn. This hyperkeratotic growth extends from the eyelid and may overlie a variety of different epidermal neoplasms, both benign and malignant.

involvement of the eyelids are at-risk to develop glaucoma and should be evaluated and followed by an ophthalmologist.

Sebaceous adenomas are raised yellow papules occurring on the eyelids and nose of elderly patients. Tumors arise in the sebaceous glands of the caruncle, Zeis' glands, and the meibomian glands. There is an association between multiple sebaceous adenomas and visceral malignancies known as Muir-Torre syndrome.

Four benign tumors arise from the hair follicles of the eyelid. These lesions are usually asymptomatic nodules that are best treated by simple excision. Trichoepithelio-

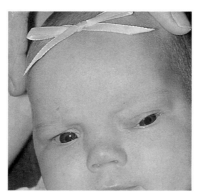

Figure 11.6. Capillary hemangioma, or strawberry nevus, in an infant (left medial upper eyelid). Tumors are reddish-purple growths and may initially increase in size before regressing later in childhood. Tumors may enlarge and cause occlusion amblyopia.

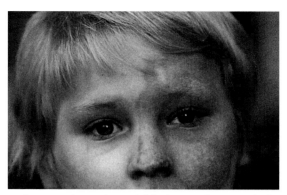

Figure 11.7.   Nevus flammeus (port-wine stain) is the vascular anomaly found in association with Sturge-Weber syndrome. Note the distribution of the hemangioma along the left trigeminal nerve in this child, with associated glaucoma in the ipsilateral eye.

mas are elevated skin-colored nodules occurring along the eyelid margin. Multiple trichoepitheliomas are inherited in an autosomal dominant manner with incomplete penetrance. Trichofolliculomas are small elevated nodules with a central umbilication filled with keratin. The presence of a protruding white hairs helps to establish the correct clinical diagnosis. Trichilemmomas arise from the sheath of the hair follicle. These lesions may be solitary or multiple and are usually asymptomatic. Pilomatrixomas, or calcifying epitheliomas of Malherbe, are solid, freely movable subcutaneous nodules in the eyelid or brow of children or young adults. The tumors are reddish-purple in color with subepithelial patches of yellow. Pilomatrixomas grow at a moderate rate and rarely recur after excision.

Benign pigmented lesions of the eyelids arise from both epidermal and dermal melanocytes. Freckles (ephelis) are reddish-brown maculas scattered over sun-exposed surfaces. Sunlight darkens these patches. Nevocellular nevi vary in their clinical appearance. Nevi occur frequently on the surface of the eyelid and eyelid margin. Histologically, nevi can be separated into three groups. Junctional nevi arise from melanocytes of the deep epidermis. These lesions are flat, pigmented maculae. Compound nevi have both epidermal and dermal components. These nevi appear as slightly elevated pigmented growths that have a papillomatous surface. Both junctional and compound nevi have malignant potential. Intradermal nevi are the most common and benign of the nevocellular nevi. These tumors are elevated amelanotic growths that may be nodular, pedunculated, or papillomatous in appearance. Hairs may protrude from the surface of the lesions.

Nevus of Ota, or oculodermal melanocytosis, is a pigmented lesion of the eyelid arising from deep dermal melanocytes. There is an associated increased pigmentation of the sclera and uveal tract, which produces a bluish hue over the white of the eye. In African-Americans, there is an increased incidence of glaucoma. In Caucasians, there is an increased frequency of both uveal and orbital malignant melanoma.

TREATMENT

Seborrheic keratosis may be either observed or excised. However, inflamed seborrheic keratosis often presents a diagnostic dilemma both clinically and pathologically. Al-

TABLE 11.2. Referral Guidelines—Malignant Lesions

DIAGNOSIS	TREATMENT	WHEN TO REFER
Basal cell carcinoma (M8090/3)	Mohs' excision + reconstruction, radiotherapy	Initial management for diagnostic biopsy
Sebaceous cell carcinoma (M8410/3)	Mohs' excision + reconstruction, exenteration	Initial management, diagnostic biopsy
Squamous cell carcinoma M8073/3	Mohs' excision + reconstruction	Initial management, diagnostic biopsy
Malignant melanoma (M8090)	Mohs' excision + reconstruction	Initial management, diagnostic biopsy
Lymphoma (202.8)	Biopsy, cryotherapy, radiotherapy, systemic evaluation	Biopsy, referral to radiation oncologist as needed
Rhabdomyosarcoma (M8900/3)	Biopsy, chemotherapy, and radiotherapy	Immediate biopsy
Metastases (M8000/3)	Biopsy, locate primary if unknown	Biopsy

though keratoacanthoma is classically thought to be a benign lesion with no malignant potential, debate has arisen in recent years as to whether it may give rise to squamous cell carcinoma. Excisional biopsy is recommended and is curative. Treatment of actinic keratosis includes excision of the lesion and cryotherapy to the base of the lesion because of the malignant potential. Patients should be followed closely for future sun-induced neoplasms. Xanthelasma lesions may be simply excised for cosmetic reasons. Sebaceous adenomas may be observed or excised, but must be differentiated from sebaceous cell malignancies.

Capillary hemangiomas may be observed if they pose no threat to vision. If vision is threatened, oral steroids or local steroid injections may be used to involute the tumor. Interferon injections have also been used successfully in shrinking the size of the lesions. Local excision maybe needed, but is often difficult. A preoperative arteriogram with embolization of an arterial feeder may be therapeutic or facilitate surgery. Cavernous hemangiomas are excised if vision is threatened. Argon or pulsed tunable dye laser therapy provides good aesthetic results in patients with nevus flammeus, by decreasing the red coloration of these lesions.

MALIGNANT LESIONS

Malignant tumors of the eyelid may be primary or metastatic (Table 11.2). Primary tumors arise from the skin and its appendages. Metastatic lesions to the eyelid are rare and most commonly are carcinomas. Breast, lung, stomach, colon, thyroid, parotid, and pharynx are reported primaries. Metastatic malignant melanoma to the eyelids has also been reported. Malignant eyelid tumors are very rare in children. Rhabdomyosarcoma occurs most frequently as a orbital mass in childhood. It may present as a lid or conjunctival mass. The tumor may rapidly enlarge and immediate diagnosis is critical. There are three histologic variants: embryonal, pleomorphic and alveolar. Combination therapy with chemotherapy and radiotherapy achieves 80% survival at 5 years.

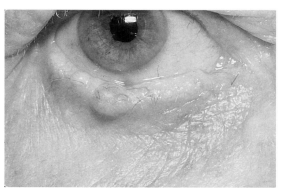

Figure 11.8. Basal cell carcinoma is the most common tumor of the eyelid. Note the nodular, "pearl-like" appearance.

The most common malignant eyelid lesions in adults are basal cell carcinoma, squamous cell carcinoma, sebaceous cell carcinoma, malignant melanoma, and lymphomas.

Basal Cell Carcinoma

Basal cell carcinoma is the most common tumor of the eyelid (Fig. 11.8). It accounts for 90% of all eyelid malignancies. These lesions tumors occur more commonly on the lower eyelid and in the medial canthus. The upper lid and lateral canthus are less frequently involved. Cumulative sun exposure seems to be a predisposing risk factor. Basal cell carcinomas occur most frequently in the sixth, seventh, and eighth decade of life.

Basal cell carcinomas may have a variety of clinical appearances. There are four distinctive patterns of growth that closely correlate with histologic findings. Nodular tumors are firm and indurated with fine telangiectatic vessels overlying. These neoplasms are usually painless and asymptomatic. Ulcerative tumors have a central crater with raised pearly margins. An inflammatory reaction is usually present. These tumors represent the classic rodent ulcer. The morphea (sclerosing) pattern appears clinically as a pale indurated plaque. It may be associated with eyelash loss along the lid margin or cause an ectropion or entropion. The morphea basal cell carcinoma is an aggressive tumor that deeply infiltrates the dermis and subcutis. The multicentric pattern has irregular nodular surface with telangiectatic vessels and there is diffuse multicentric involvement of the epidermis extending into the dermis. Nodular basal cell carcinoma may be safely excised with wide surgical margins. However, the ulcerative, morphea, and multicentric forms may extend beyond the margin of clinical involvement. Basal cell carcinomas rarely metastasize, and tumor deaths are unusual. Death most often results from neglected tumors that invade the orbit and the brain.

Sebaceous Cell Carcinoma

Sebaceous cell carcinoma is a rare tumor with a predilection for the ocular adnexa (Fig. 11.9). It arises from the meibomian glands, Zeis' glands, and the sebaceous glands

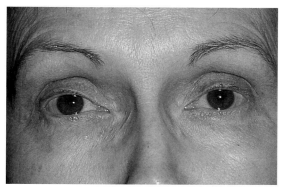

Figure 11.9. Sebaceous cell carcinoma is a rare tumor with a predilection for the ocular adnexa, most commonly the upper eyelid.

of the caruncle. The tumor may be multifocal in origin. Sebaceous cell carcinoma accounts for 1–3% of all eyelid malignancies. It more commonly involves the upper eyelid. Patients in the sixth to seventh decade are most frequently affected. Sebaceous cell carcinoma has a varied clinical appearance. It may be a small, firm nodule of the tarsus resembling a chalazion or a diffuse thickening of the tarsus. Patients may also present with an unilateral blepharoconjunctivitis that does not respond to antibiotics. There may be associated eyelash loss. Sebaceous cell carcinomas are aggressive malignancies with a tendency for widespread metastases. Pagetoid spread along the lid margin makes clinical determination of tumor extent difficult. Features associated with a poor prognosis include tumor location in the upper lid, greater than 10 mm in maximal diameter, origin from the meibomian glands, duration of symptoms greater than 6 months, infiltrative growth pattern, and moderate-to-poor sebaceous differentiation. Additional features typically associated with a poor prognosis are multicentric origin, pagetoid spread, and invasion of vascular structures, lymphatic channels, or the orbit.

Squamous Cell Carcinoma

Squamous cell carcinoma accounts for less than 5% of eyelid malignancies (Fig. 11.10). It more commonly involves the upper than the lower eyelid and may arise from preexisting lesions such as actinic keratosis. Tumors may also develop following radiotherapy and in patients with xeroderma pigmentosum. Clinically, squamous cell carcinoma appears as a raised indurated papule. Ulceration may also be present. These lesions have metastatic potential.

Malignant Melanoma

Malignant melanoma comprises 1% of all eyelid malignancies (Fig. 11.11). The clinical features, histologic findings, biologic behavior, and prognosis of eyelid malignant melanoma parallel those of other cutaneous melanoma. There are four types of primary cutaneous melanoma. Lentigo maligna melanoma arises from lentigo maligna, a flat,

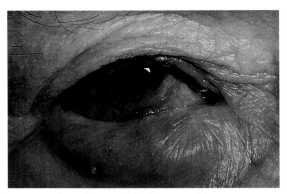

Figure 11.10.   Squamous cell carcinoma of the lower eyelid.

variably pigmented lesion with irregular borders found on sun-exposed areas of elderly patients. Involvement of the lower lid and canthal regions is common. Peripheral extension of the lesion may occur over years with waxing and waning of its borders. The vertical growth phase signals malignant transformation. The lesion develops an irregular nodular surface. Superficial spreading melanoma occurs in younger patients and primarily affects unexposed areas of the skin. It appears as a spreading pigmented lesion of varied color with irregular outlines and faintly palpable borders. Nodular melanoma is a small blue-black or amelanotic nodule. It occurs most often in the 40–50-year-old age group, and affects men twice as often as women. It occurs on both exposed and unexposed skin surfaces. Nodular melanoma has a rapid rate of growth with extensive invasion of deeper tissues. Acral lentiginous melanoma occurs on the palms, soles, distal phalanges, and mucous membranes. It appears as a macula of varying pigmentation ranging from tannish-brown to black. All four growth patterns may arise from preexisting nevi. Changes in color, size, surface, and surrounding skin herald malignant transformation. Malignant melanoma may also arise on the palpebral conjunctival surface of the eyelid. This tumor usually occurs in the presence of primary acquired melanosis with atypia.

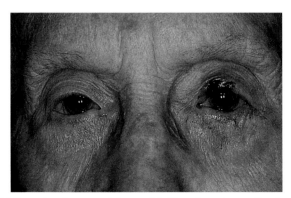

Figure 11.11.   Malignant melanoma of the eyelid. (See also color section.)

Lymphoma

Lymphomas may involve the eyelid. Conjunctival lymphomas appear in the fornices of the upper and lower eyelids as salmon-colored patches. These are most typically low-grade B cell tumors with no associated systemic disease. Cutaneous lymphomas again are mostly low-grade B cell lymphomas. There is approximately 40% chance that the patient will develop disease elsewhere. These lesions respond well to radiotherapy. All patients should be referred to an oncologist for a systemic evaluation. T cell lymphomas may affect the eyelids. These lesions present as raised erythematous plaques as part of mycosis fungoides.

TREATMENT

Basal cell carcinoma is treated by local excision of the entire lesion. However, clear surgical margins may be difficult to achieve as the tumor may extend beyond the clinically evident margins. These tumors are best excised under frozen section control. Mohs' micrographic surgery provides the highest cure rate. This technique is performed by a surgeon trained in utilizing frozen section monitoring to minimize tissue loss. Reconstructive procedures are usually performed by the ophthalmologist shortly after the tumor is excised. Recurrent tumors should be excised using the Mohs' micrographic resection as well. Radiotherapy is an alternative modality when Mohs' resection cannot be performed.

The optimal treatment of sebaceous cell carcinoma is complete surgical excision with wide surgical margins. Whether this is best accomplished by local excision using the Mohs' technique or by orbital exenteration is subject to debate and dependent on the extent of tumor involvement. Squamous cell carcinomas should be promptly excised because of their metastatic potential. Mohs' surgery is usually curative.

Malignant melanoma is best managed by wide local excision. Clark and Breslow classifications provide prognostic information. Tumors invading into the subcutaneous tissue or to a depth of 1.5 mm have a 50% survival over 5 years. Nodular tumors have the worst prognosis of the four growth patterns. This relates to its rapid vertical growth phase. These tumors have less than a 50% 5-year survival. Local excision of malignant melanomas of the conjunctiva with cryotherapy of the surgical base may be curative, but patients have a predisposition towards forming new malignant melanomas.

SUGGESTED READINGS

Biro L, Price E. Benign eyelid lesions of the eyelid. In: Hornblass A, ed. Oculoplastic, orbital and reconstructive surgery. Baltimore: Williams & Wilkins, 1988:212–221.

Conlon MR, Leatherbarrow B, Nerad JA. Benign eyelid tumors. In: Bosniak S, ed. Principles and practice of ophthalmic plastic and reconstructive surgery. Philadelphia: WB Saunders, 1996:323–341.

Doxanas MT. Malignant epithelial eyelid tumors. In: Bosniak S, ed. Principles and practice of ophthalmic plastic and reconstructive surgery. Philadelphia: WB Saunders, 1996:342–351.

Folberg R, Bernardino VB, Bernardino EA. Pigmented eyelid lesions. In: Hornblass A, ed. Oculoplastic, orbital, and reconstructive surgery. Baltimore: Williams & Wilkins, 1988:259–270.

Font RL. Eyelids and lacrimal drainage system. In: Spencer WH, ed. Ophthalmic pathology: an atlas and textbook. 4th ed. Philadelphia: WB Saunders, 1996:2218–2437.

Older JJ. Eyelid tumors: clinical diagnosis and surgical treatment. New York: Raven Press, 1987.

Reifler DM, Hornblass A. Squamous cell carcinoma of the eyelid. In: Hornblass A, ed. Oculoplastic, orbital, and reconstructive surgery. Baltimore: Williams & Wilkins, 1988:222–231.

Reifler DM, Hornblass A. Sebaceous gland tumors of the eyelid. In: Hornblass A, ed. Oculoplastic, orbital, and reconstructive surgery. Baltimore: Williams & Wilkins, 1988:232–238.

Tanenbaum M, Grove AS, McCord CD. Eyelid tumors: diagnosis and management. In: McCord CD, Tanenbaum, Nunery WR, eds. Oculoplastic surgery. 3rd ed. New York: Raven Press, 1995:145–174.

Chapter 12 ●◖❙
Blepharitis

M. A. Terry

INTRODUCTION

Blepharitis is a spectrum of diseases which produce either an acute or a chronic inflammation of the eyelids. Blepharitis accounts for over 50% of all cases of ocular complaints presenting to the primary care physician. An understanding of the pathophysiology of this group of disorders is crucial to its successful and cost-effective management.

The eyelids are complex structures with an anatomy composed of diverse elements including (from anterior to posterior) skin, lashes, the pilosebaceous base of the lash, the firm cartilage-like structure of the tarsal plate, 15–20 meibomian glands in each tarsal plate, and the conjunctival mucous membrane covering the posterior surface of the lid. The eyelids protect the eye in three ways: as a mechanical barrier; by spreading the tear film evenly to keep the surface of the eye wet; and by providing the critical lipid component of the tear film to prevent evaporation and drying. Depending upon the severity and chronicity of the inflammation associated with blepharitis, one or more of these functions can become compromised, placing the eye in jeopardy.

Over the years, several classification systems have evolved for blepharitis. The most clinically useful was described by Wilhelmus. In this system, blepharitis is classified based upon an anatomic separation of the lid margin into an anterior lamellae and a posterior lamellae. The anterior lamellae contains skin, muscle, eyelash follicles and associated glands of Zeis. The posterior lamellae contains the tarsal plate, meibomian glands, and eyelid conjunctiva. The location of the primary inflammation determines whether the patient has an "anterior blepharitis" or a "posterior blepharitis." This classification is clinically useful in that the etiology and appropriate therapy for anterior and posterior blepharitis is different, despite the similarities of presenting symptoms.

CLINICAL MANIFESTATIONS

Blepharitis may be asymptomatic and present as a chronic, low-grade inflammation of the lid margins seen only on careful magnified inspection. As the inflammation worsens and affects the tear film, the patient may complain of mild ocular irritation, foreign body sensation, burning, redness, and crusting of the lids in the morning. Occasionally, itching and photophobia are reported. In severe blepharitis, the tear film may be totally disrupted and the ocular surface may become vascularized from chronic inflammation. This may lead to irritation of the central cornea, and the patient may report decreased vision in addition to these other complaints.

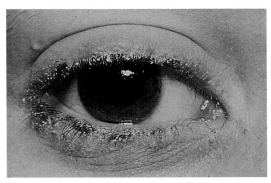

Figure 12.1.   Anterior blepharitis from *S. aureus*. Note crusting of lid, ulceration of lid margin, and lash loss.

ANTERIOR BLEPHARITIS

Anterior blepharitis is essentially a chronic infectious process punctuated by acute exacerbations. Initially thought to be nearly entirely due to staphylococci, more recent studies have identified additional organisms of *S. epidermidis, P. acnes*, and corynebacterium as being present significantly more often and in higher concentrations in blepharitis patients than in controls. Staphylococcal blepharitis is more common in women (80% of patients are female), and this is most likely related to the vector of eye makeup. The classic sign of a staphylococcal blepharitis is the presence of a hard, fibrinous, crusty scale on the anterior lid margin that surrounds the individual eyelashes and is described as a "collarette." In addition, the lid margin becomes red from inflamed surface vessels. As a staphylococcal infection becomes more severe and chronic, the lash follicles become affected, resulting in white lashes (poliosis), misdirected lashes (trichiasis), loss of lashes (madarosis), and even ulceration and notching of lid margin tissue (tylosis) (Fig. 12.1). A lid abscess can form as the staphylococcal organism gains access to and forms a purulent occlusion of the glands of Zeis (external hordeolum) or the meibomian glands (internal hordeolum).

The inflammation of the anterior staphylococcal blepharitis can go on to affect the posterior lid margin, conjunctiva, and cornea. The most common conjunctival finding is mild-to-moderate hyperemia. The conjunctival inflammation is felt to be a reaction to the liberation of staphylococcal toxins, leukocidins, and enterotoxin, and does not exhibit a purulent discharge. There are three characteristic corneal complications associated with staphylococcal blepharitis: punctate epithelial keratitis, marginal corneal infiltrates, and phlyctenular keratitis. Punctate epithelial keratitis appears on slitlamp biomicroscopy as pinpoint, flat, epithelial lesions which stain with fluorescein and are distributed evenly across the inferior third of the cornea. These result from a toxic reaction to the staphylococcal exotoxin and produce burning, photophobia, and tearing. Resolution occurs with control of the blepharitis. Marginal corneal infiltrates are seen on biomicroscopy as white infiltrates in the anterior corneal stroma of the limbal cornea, separated from the sclera by a clear zone. The overlying corneal epithelium is intact and these white infiltrates represent a hypersensitivity reaction to the staphylococcal antigens whereby an antigen-antibody reaction leads to complement activation and neutrophil infiltration. The third corneal complication of staphylococcal

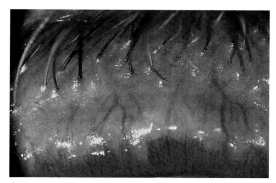

Figure 12.2.   Posterior blepharitis–obstructive meibomian gland dysfunction. Note the inspissated and pouting orifices of meibomian glands with extensive vessel engorgement on the posterior surface of the upper eyelid. (See also color section.)

blepharitis, phlyctenular keratitis, is also a hypersensitivity reaction, particularly to the cell wall antigen of the staphylococcal organism. This condition results in the formation of elevated, inflamed nodules which ulcerate and spread over the peripheral cornea and adjacent conjunctiva. Once healed, the lesions leave characteristic wedge-shaped vascularized scars. Although marginal infiltrates and corneal phlyctenules rarely threaten long-term loss of vision, their presence should alert the primary care physician to the presence of a severe underlying blepharitis.

POSTERIOR BLEPHARITIS

The posterior lamellae contains the tarsal plate and the critical oil-producing meibomian glands. Inflammation of this region involves meibomian gland dysfunction rather than a frank infectious process. The two basic forms of meibomian gland dysfunction (MGD) are the hypersecretory form and the obstructive form. In the hypersecretory form (also called "meibomian seborrhea"), the glands produce an excess of oils with very little inflammation present, but bloated glands are seen on lid eversion and a frothy foam is often present in the tear film. These patients primarily complain of burning and irritation of the eyes without redness. In the obstructive form of meibomian gland dysfunction, there is a stagnation and solidification of the oils which results in inspissated plugs of meibomian gland orifices (Fig. 12.2). As the oil backs up in the gland, it can leak through the walls of the engorged gland and cause a noninfectious, granulomatous response in the surrounding tarsal plate tissue. The resultant lid mass is a chalazion ("stye") which initially is red and tender before it resolves or becomes a fibrous lump in the lid (Fig. 12.3). The patients with obstructive meibomian gland dysfunction will complain of burning, mattering, grittiness, and tearing. On examination the posterior lid margin will reveal the red pouting orifices of the meibomian glands. Unlike the hypersecretory form, it is quite difficult to express the oils from the glands in obstructive meibomian gland dysfunction and pressing the lid margin has been described as "pushing out toothpaste from a tube." As the severity and chronicity of the condition worsens, the posterior lid margin becomes thickened, ulcerated and chronically hyperemic.

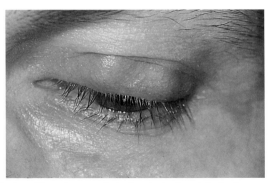

Figure 12.3.   Chalazion. Note the two chalazion (raised nodules) of upper lid in this patient with posterior blepharitis of obstructive meibomian gland dysfunction.

The effect of meibomian gland dysfunction on the tear film is the most critical concern in this disease. A smooth and consistent surface oil layer is essential for a normal functioning tear film (see Chapter 14, "Dry Eye Syndrome"). In meibomian gland dysfunction, especially the obstructive form, there is a qualitative alteration of meibomian gland secretions with a decrease of the normal lipids and an increase in free fatty acids and esterified cholesterols. This results in a very sparse tear oil layer and rapid evaporation of the tear film. The "tear breakup time," measured by slitlamp biomicroscopy, is severely reduced, and this results in chronic drying of regions of the cornea. The free fatty acids can be directly toxic to the epithelium and in combination with the unstable tear film the corneal epithelial surface can break down, vascularize and even ulcerate (Fig. 12.4). The etiology of meibomian gland dysfunction is still obscure, but it is known that meibomian gland dysfunction has a strong association with seborrheic dermatitis patients, as well as those suffering from even mild forms

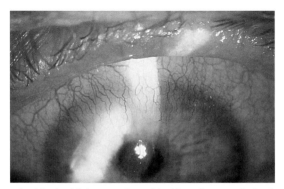

Figure 12.4.   Posterior blepharitis/rosacea keratitis. Note the vascularization of the peripheral cornea from ocular rosacea meibomian gland dysfunction.

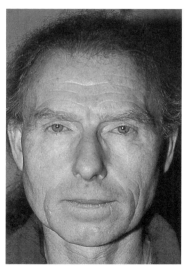

Figure 12.5.   Patient with acne rosacea. Note the characteristic telangiectatic vessels of nose and cheeks. (See also color section.)

of acne rosacea (Fig. 12.5). Finally, patients with infective anterior blepharitis will often have an exacerbation of meibomian gland dysfunction due to the action of microbial lipases, which split toxic free fatty acids from the triglyceride found in normal meibomian excreta. The inflammation produced allows stagnation of meibomian secretions and cellular debris, which then are utilized as a rich nutrient for further bacterial proliferation. The overlap in inflammatory synergism of anterior blepharitis and posterior blepharitis can now easily be appreciated.

DIFFERENTIAL DIAGNOSIS

Dry eye presents with many of the same complaints of blepharitis, such as burning and grittiness (Table 12.1). Indeed, because of the dysfunctional tear film, patients with blepharitis may have an associated dry eye from the evaporative effects rather than insufficient aqueous component. The clinician may be able to differentiate a primary dry eye patient from a primary blepharitis patient by careful examination of the patient with fluorescein staining and a slitlamp biomicroscopy. The corneal fluorescein staining in the dry eye patient will usually be located in the horizontal, interpalpebral region of the cornea, while the blepharitis patient will usually show fluorescein staining over the inferior third of the cornea all the way down to the limbus. Mucus filaments are also more characteristically seen with dry eyes than with blepharitis. Finally, it should be remembered that primary dry eye and blepharitis frequently occur simultaneously and the patient may require treatment for both conditions concurrently or sequentially.

Herpes simplex conjunctivitis can mimic simple anterior blepharitis. Herpes conjunctivitis is a primary infection in children and is usually markedly asymmetric. The onset of symptoms is acute rather than chronic. The lid margin may be red and the

◖◗ TABLE 12.1. Referral Guidelines—Blepharitis

DISEASE (CODE)	SIGNS & SYMPTOMS	TREATMENT	WHEN TO REFER
Anterior blepharitis (373.00)	Chronic irritation, redness, grittiness, burning and crusting of lids; occasional itching and photophobia; collarettes seen with slitlamp	Hot compresses and aggressive lid hygiene; initially, eliminate or minimize eye makeup; erythromycin ointment after lid scrubs	Inadequate response after 6 weeks of therapy; skin vesicles of herpes simplex; any visual loss or presence of corneal vessels or opacities
Posterior blepharitis (372.20)	Chronic burning and redness; chalazion formation; look for rosacea signs in skin of nose and cheeks; meibomian glands orifices plugged	Aggressive hot compresses; lid hygiene; oral tetracycline 200 mg q.i.d. or doxycycline 100 mg/day	Inadequate response after 6 weeks of therapy; persistent or recurrent chalazion ("styes"); any vision loss or presence of corneal vessels or opacities

patient's complaints similar to blepharitis, but the small, clear vesicles of herpes simplex often help make the differential diagnosis. These patients should be put on topical antivirals and, of course, steroids for this "blepharitis" are strictly contraindicated.

Molluscum contagiosum is an asymptomatic, nodular, umbilicated lesion with a central ulceration that sits on the lid like a wart. It is caused by a pox virus and may mimic a unilateral blepharitis. It creates a chronic follicular conjunctivitis. Excision of the lesion resolves the inflammation.

Allergic blepharitis can occur with external contact caused by drugs, cosmetics, chemicals, animal dander, and plants. The skin is often erythematous, edematous, and scaly, and the patient will primarily complain of itching and pain. The preservatives in eye drops and ointments (even those used to treat anterior blepharitis) are frequently causative agents.

Parasitic blepharitis is a rare, but often overlooked, form of lid inflammation. A thin, transparent mite known as *Demodex folliculorum* is present as an infestation of the sebaceous follicles of most adults and of 100% of individuals over 70 years of age. When present in abnormally abundant numbers, the mite causes dead epithelial cells to wrap like a tubular "sleeve" around the base of each lash, and the inflammatory reaction may cause itching and irritation. Another parasitic blepharitis, phthiriasis palpebrarum, is caused by pubic lice (*Phthirius pubis*), that may infest the eyelashes as well, because the spacing of the lashes is similar to the spacing of pubic hair follicles, allowing the adult louse to adhere firmly to adjacent cilia. A severe itching blepharoconjunctivitis results secondary to toxic feces of the louse released into the tear film. The louse eggs (nits) cemented onto the lashes present a striking appearance under the slitlamp biomicroscope, while the adult is relatively transparent and difficult to see (Fig. 12.6). Treatment is with mechanical removal of the nits and suffocation of the adults with topical physostigmine ointment. All the patient's family members and sexual contacts should be examined and treated as well.

Sebaceous gland carcinoma is a rare adnexal tumor that can mimic blepharitis. It presents as a persistent or recurrent unilateral lid inflammation and often there is a history of recurrent chalazion (see Chapter 11, "Eyelid Lesions: Benign and Malig-

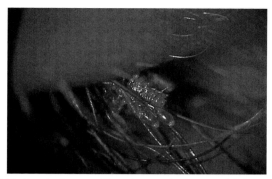

Figure 12.6. Phthiriasis palpebrarum. Note the translucent eggs (nits) attached to the midlash and the adult louse attached just above the base of the lashes.

nant"). The malignancy can be solitary, nodular, or multicentric, and a delay in diagnosis of greater than 6 months can reduce the 5-year survival rate by 50%. All recurrent chalazion should be biopsied and sent for histopathologic evaluation and curative surgical excision performed as indicated.

TREATMENT

The treatment of blepharitis involves an initial treatment of the acute condition for 2–8 weeks followed by maintenance treatment of this chronic disease indefinitely. Treatment begins with education of the patient. Once the diagnosis has been made, the patient must be thoroughly counseled and informed that blepharitis is a disease which can be controlled but not cured, and the aim of therapy is to relieve symptoms and prevent lid and corneal complications.

ANTERIOR BLEPHARITIS TREATMENT

The most important part of anterior blepharitis treatment is the conscientious use of warm compresses and lid hygiene. Without good lid cleaning, medication is ineffective in this disease. Warm compresses act to heat the solidified oils above their melting point and loosen the crust and cellular debris from the lid margin. Lid scrubs utilizing baby shampoo allow soaps to lyse bacterial cell membranes, reducing bacterial counts and also removing the blepharitic debris that serves as a bacterial nutrient. Patients are instructed to do the lid hygiene routine twice a day for severe cases of blepharitis until the condition improves, and then once a day to once every other day for maintenance therapy.

Before the lid hygiene routine, all eye makeup must be removed and no eye makeup should be used at all during the acute treatment of blepharitis. The patient takes a clean face cloth and wets it with hot water from the tap or basin, wrings out the cloth, and then applies the hot, moist compress to the closed lids for 5–10 minutes, rewarming the compress as it cools. After compresses, the patient should digitally massage the meibomian glands with small circular motions near the lid margins, pressing the lid against the globe. This massage allows the flow of normal meibomian gland oils now that the hot packs have melted the plugs from the gland orifices. The lids are thoroughly cleaned of all this oil and debris by using lid scrubs of the lid margins and lashes. A nonirritating shampoo (e.g., Johnson and Johnson's "No More Tears" baby shampoo) is diluted 50% with warm water, and the tip of a washcloth, a cotton ball, or a cotton-tipped applicator is used to gently scrub the lashes and lid margins of all four lids. The lids are then thoroughly rinsed with warm water.

Topical antibiotics are also used in the treatment of acute exacerbations of anterior blepharitis. The predominant organisms are *S. aureus, S. epidermidis, P. acnes, Moraxella* species, and corynebacterium species. The drugs of choice are ophthalmic preparations of erythromycin ointment or bacitracin ointment. This ointment is applied after the lid hygiene by placing a small amount on a washed finger tip and gently wiping it along the lash line of each lid. Antibiotic ointment is applied with the same frequency as the lid scrubs for 2 weeks and discontinued until the next exacerbation. Cultures are usually not performed unless the patient's condition does not improve on initial treatment and other etiologies of blepharitis have been dismissed.

The complications and associated conditions of anterior blepharitis may also require additional treatment. Internal and external hordeolums will usually resolve over several days with more prolonged (20 minutes) and more frequent (four times a day) applications of hot compresses. A course of systemic antibiotics such as erythromycin 250 mg four times a day, or tetracycline 250 mg four times a day, is also frequently indicated for these lid abscesses. Occasionally, surgical drainage is indicated and a referral to an ophthalmologist is warranted. Dry eye in a setting of blepharitis may benefit from nonpreserved ocular lubricants concurrent with the blepharitis treatment. Finally, although steroids have no place in the treatment of uncomplicated blepharitis, they may be briefly utilized by the ophthalmologist to prevent corneal scarring and vascularization when nodular phlectenules and corneal marginal infiltrates are severe. The significant steroid related complications of glaucoma, cataracts, and opportunistic infections should always be kept in mind when these agents are utilized.

POSTERIOR BLEPHARITIS TREATMENT

The cardinal defect in posterior blepharitis is the dysfunction of the meibomian glands secretory process. The obstructive forms of meibomian gland dysfunction is much more common than the hypersecretory or seborrheic form. Therefore, posterior blepharitis therapy is primarily directed toward relieving the lipid obstructions of the orifices, allowing a free flow of normal meibomian gland secretion, and reducing the inflammation of the glands. The same lid hygiene instructions for anterior blepharitis are given for the posterior blepharitis patient, and the emphasis is placed on more frequent and prolonged hot compress applications. The lid scrubs are less emphasized, but are still necessary to remove the lipolytic bacteria that feast on the stagnant oils and release the free fatty acids and other toxic byproducts. A mainstay of posterior blepharitis treatment is systemic tetracycline. Tetracycline has been shown to reduce the production of lipase in both sensitive and resistant strains of *S. epidermidis* and *S. aureus*. It has also been shown to inhibit the keratinization which contributes to meibomian gland orifice obstruction. The treatment regimen of tetracycline is 250–500 mg four times a day for several weeks, then tapering the dosage for 3 months. Once controlled, the maintenance dose is 250 mg per day and this is continued for years in many cases. Alternatively, doxycycline in one tablet of 100 mg each day is sometimes better tolerated and more convenient for some patients. In patients where a tetracycline antibiotic is contraindicated (e.g., children under the age of 14 and pregnant women), erythromycin 250 mg four times a day may be substituted with a similar tapering off schedule.

The complicated and associated conditions of posterior blepharitis should also be addressed. The chalazion, or "stye" should initially be treated aggressively with hot compresses as long and as frequently as the patient possibly can, but at least four times a day for 20 minutes each application. Tetracycline 250 mg four times a day or doxycycline 100 mg twice a day should be prescribed. Topical antibiotics are generally ineffective as this is a sterile granuloma. If the inciting meibomian gland can be induced to open up and drain with hot packs, then the chalazion will resolve without fibrosis within 7–10 days. If compress treatment is delayed or inadequate, then a posterior lid surgical incision may be necessary and ophthalmic referral is warranted.

REFERRAL GUIDELINES

Most patients with blepharitis can be educated and treated by their primary care physician and do not require a referral to an ophthalmologist (see Table 12.1). However, if the patient has not had an adequate response and relief of symptoms within 6 weeks of lid hygiene therapy and systemic antibiotic therapy, then referral to an ophthalmologist for further evaluation and therapy is reasonable. Certainly, if the diagnosis is in question or if the patient has recurrent and persistent chalazion (i.e., sebaceous gland carcinoma is ruled out) then routine referral for a comprehensive evaluation by an ophthalmologist with possible culture and biopsy is warranted. Finally, if the patient complains of mild vision loss or if corneal changes are found on examination, then the patient should be referred within 7 days for evaluation.

FREQUENCY OF VISITS

The patient with routine blepharitis without other complicating conditions should be seen initially for a full evaluation of the lids, tear film, and cornea. After extensive education of the patient regarding lid hygiene, hot compresses, and so on, the patient is reevaluated in 6–8 weeks. If the condition is controlled, the patient is reevaluated once a year, but more frequently if complications or exacerbations are encountered.

SUGGESTED READINGS

Coston T. *Demodex folliculorum* blepharitis. Trans Am Ophthalmol Soc 1967;65:361–92.

Cullen S, Crounse R. Cutaneous pharmacology of the tetracyclines. J Invest Dermatol 1965;45:263–268.

Dougherty J, McCulley J, Silvany R, et al. The roles of tetracycline in chronic blepharitis. Inhibition of lipase production in staphylococci. Invest Ophthalmol Vis Sci 1991;32:2970–2975.

Edward RS. Ophthalmic emergencies in a district general hospital casualty department. Br J Ophthalmol 1987;71:938–942.

Groden L, Murphy B, Rodnite J, et al. Lid flora in blepharitis. Cornea 1991;10:50–53.

McCulley J, Dougherty J, Peneau D. Classification of chronic blepharitis. Ophthalmology 1982;89:1173–1180.

Norn M. *Demodex folliculorum:* incidence and possible pathogenic role in the human eyelid. Acta Ophthalmol Scand Suppl 1979;108:1–85.

Pablo G, Homman A, Bradley S, et al. Characteristics of the extracellular lipases from corynebacterium acnes and staph epidermidis. J Invest Dermatol 1974;63:231–238.

Rao N, McLeod I, Zimmerman L. Sebaceous carcinoma of the eyelids and caruncle: correlation of clinicopathologic features with prognosis. In: Jakobiec F, ed. Ocular and adnexal tumors. Birmingham, AL: Aesculapius Publishing, 1978:461.

Smith R, Flowers C. Chronic blepharitis: a review. Contact Lens Assoc Ophthal (CLAO) 1995;21:200–207.

Thygeson P. Etiology and treatment of blepharitis. A study in military personnel. Arch Ophthalmol 1946;36:445–457.

Wilhelmus KR. Inflammatory disorders of the eyelid margins and eyelashes. Ophthalmol Clin North Am 1992;5:187–194.

Chapter 13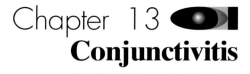
Conjunctivitis

M. A. Terry

INTRODUCTION

Conjunctivitis refers to a diverse group of inflammatory problems that affects the conjunctiva. Although most forms of conjunctivitis are self-limited, some may cause serious ocular complications through chronic inflammation and scarring. Conjunctivitis can be classified as infectious or noninfectious, and acute or chronic. Common causes of conjunctivitis encountered by the primary care physician include the infectious forms of viral, bacterial, and chlamydial, and the noninfectious forms of allergic and toxic conjunctivitis. Special consideration should also be given to neonatal conjunctivitis and its prophylaxis. Through the correct diagnosis and classification of conjunctivitis, the primary care physician can yield cost-effective therapy yet refer those cases requiring specialist treatment before long-term disability occurs.

DIFFERENTIAL DIAGNOSIS

Infectious Conjunctivitis (Table 13.1)

Viral Conjunctivitis

One of the most common forms of acute conjunctivitis is viral conjunctivitis. This has commonly been referred to as "pink eye" and is recognized by the schools and day care centers as extremely contagious. Viral conjunctivitis is generally caused by an adenovirus. Adenovirus types 8 and 19 cause the highly contagious epidemic keratoconjunctivitis (EKC) and types 3, 4, and 7 cause the less common pharyngeal conjunctival fever (PCF).

CLINICAL MANIFESTATIONS

The typical history with adenoviral conjunctivitis is that the patient or a family member has recently suffered a "cold" or "flu." The complaints are of eye redness, matting of the lids in the morning and watery discharge affecting one eye initially, then the fellow eye several days later, but to a lesser extent. There is no loss of vision and no significant pain. There may be some lid edema, irritation, and even subconjunctival hemorrhage (Fig. 13.1). An enlarged preauricular node is often present in viral, but not bacterial, conjunctivitis.

◘▮ TABLE 13.1. Referral Guidelines: Infectious Conjunctivitis

DISEASE (CODE)	SIGNS & SYMPTOMS	TREATMENT	WHEN TO REFER
Viral conjunctivitis (077.99)	Acute, bilateral; watery discharge; vision normal; minimal pain; preauricular node; highly contagious	Prevent spread of disease; cold compresses; gentamicin ointment at hour of sleep; resolves in 10–14 days	No referral for routine case; refer in 24 hours if severe pain or any decrease in vision
Bacterial conjunctivitis (372.11)	Subacute, bilateral; purulent discharge; minimal pain; vision normal	Gentamicin solution every 2 hours; resolves in 10–14 days; gram stain if gonococcus suspected	No referral if routine; refer immediately if patient has history of corneal transplant or glaucoma surgery
Chlamydial conjunctivitis (077.98)	Subacute onset; chronic redness for months; watery discharge	Doxycycline 100 mg twice daily; erythromycin ointment at hour of sleep for 21 days; resolves in 3–4 weeks; treatment of sexual partners	Referral for diagnostic testing or if no response to medication

TREATMENT

Viral conjunctivitis is self-limited and resolves completely in 10–14 days. Therapy, therefore, is directed toward limiting the spread of the disease and preventing bacterial secondary infection. The patient is informed of the extreme contagious nature of adenovirus (contagious for 14 days after the onset of symptoms) and is instructed to not share wash towels or makeup and to practice frequent handwashing. Healthcare workers should avoid patient contact during the contagious period. For comfort the patient can use cold compresses. A broad spectrum antibiotic such as gentamicin can be applied at night to prevent secondary bacterial infection.

Although viral conjunctivitis resolves without sequelae in most patients, complications resulting in vision loss can occur. Inflammation of the cornea (keratitis) during the initial stage of viral conjunctivitis may become so intense that epithelial sloughing and surface scarring may occur. Intraocular inflammation (uveitis) may occur, but is

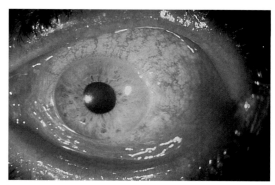

Figure 13.1.   Viral conjunctivitis. (See also color section.)

usually mild; yet, adhesions of the iris and elevations of intraocular pressure (glaucoma) can occur in selected patients. The most common cause of visual loss after adenovirus conjunctivitis is from the complication of late subepithelial corneal opacities. These opacities result from the chronic infiltration of white blood cells within the superficial cornea and occur several weeks after the acute infection. This is an autoimmune response to viral antigens in the cornea. Cautious use of topical steroids is necessary if vision is significantly reduced.

REFERRAL GUIDELINES

Routine viral conjunctivitis is most commonly addressed by the primary care physician. However, if the patient's symptoms do not improve after 1 week, consultation with an ophthalmologist should be considered. Despite a normal duration of 10–14 days, most cases of viral conjunctivitis improve over the first week. Finally, if the patient suffers from severe pain, photophobia, or any significant reduction in vision, ophthalmic consultation should be sought within 24 hours.

The frequency of follow-up for a viral conjunctivitis patient depends upon the severity of the inflammation and the stage of the disease. Uncomplicated cases should be seen 3 days after the diagnosis and again at 1 and 2 weeks. The patient should be advised to return for an examination should late photophobia (light sensitivity) or diminishment of vision occur, as these are symptoms associated with intraocular inflammation and corneal involvement. Patients referred to an ophthalmologist for complications of viral conjunctivitis may need to be seen weekly or biweekly for several months until stabilized.

Bacterial Conjunctivitis

Bacterial conjunctivitis can occur as a primary infection of the eyes or as a secondary infection in the compromised host, often following a viral illness. In the adult, bacterial conjunctivitis is usually subacute in onset and infects bilaterally, although often asymmetrically.

CLINICAL MANIFESTATIONS

Bacterial conjunctivitis presents with complaints of ocular irritation and redness, and the patient may note that the lids are matted shut in the morning. In contrast to the watery discharge associated with viral conjunctivitis, there is a mucopurulent discharge. The vision is usually normal. There is no palpable preauricular node as is found in viral conjunctivitis. The most common organisms found in bacterial conjunctivitis are staphylococcus, streptococcus, and hemophilus.

TREATMENT

Primary treatment of routine bacterial conjunctivitis is with a broad spectrum topical antibiotic solution such as gentamicin, applied every 2 hours for the first several days then tapered to four times daily for 7–10 days. Routine cultures are usually not necessary but should be utilized if there is poor response to the initial therapy. Most

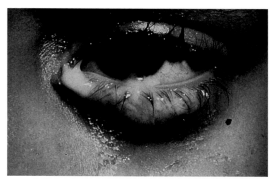

Figure 13.2.   Gonococcal conjunctivitis.

routine bacterial conjunctivitis cases will respond to appropriate antibiotics quickly with resolution of purulent drainage in 24–48 hours and complete resolution of symptoms in 10–14 days. Although conjunctivitis scarring can occur in severe cases, most patients heal without sequelae.

Referral Guidelines

The primary care physician should consider referral of a patient with bacterial conjunctivitis to an ophthalmologist if the patient does not improve in 2 or 3 days of therapy. Referral should be immediate if there is significant pain or visual loss. Patients with copious amounts of purulent discharge should have a Gram stain and culture performed for gonococcus, as this organism can rapidly progress to corneal ulceration and perforation, and requires intensive topical and parenteral antibiotics for adequate treatment (Fig. 13.2).

Finally, any patient that has had ocular surgery for corneal transplant, or filtration surgery for glaucoma at any time in the past, should be referred immediately at the onset of any conjunctivitis. Following these surgeries, the normal anatomy of the eye has been permanently altered. The eye is at a much greater risk of bacterial invasion (endophthalmitis) with severe loss of vision which may occur within hours of the onset of symptoms. Any "red eye" in this setting should be considered a medical emergency.

Patients with routine bacterial conjunctivitis (i.e., those with no previous history of corneal or glaucoma surgery) should be seen 2 days after the initial visit to assess the response to therapy. No further visits are necessary unless the patient experiences the onset of pain or visual loss after therapy has been initiated. Patients referred for complications of bacterial conjunctivitis (e.g., corneal ulceration or endophthalmitis) may require hospitalization and daily evaluation until the infection is stabilized and eradicated.

Chlamydial Conjunctivitis

Chlamydia is an obligate intracellular organism with a propensity for symptoms involving the mucus membranes, yet it is a systemic disease. The neonatal form is acquired

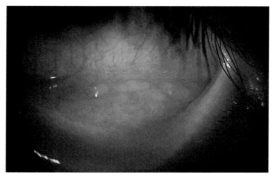

Figure 13.3. Follicles on a tarsal plate.

during passage through the vaginal tract. The adult form is a sexually transmitted disease.

CLINICAL MANIFESTATIONS

Adult chlamydial conjunctivitis is a disease that often is misdiagnosed and undertreated. The patients symptoms can mimic those of viral and allergic conjunctivitis though with a subacute onset. There is a watery discharge, irritation, chronic redness, and occasional photophobia. The vision is normal, and there is no significant pain. Unlike viral conjunctivitis, the symptoms can persist for weeks to months without appropriate treatment. Slitlamp examination reveals a chronic follicular conjunctivitis, often with mild cicatricial changes. Follicles are a lymphocytic inflammatory response, seen as gelatinous bumps on the palpebral conjunctiva (conjunctiva lining the inside of the lid) (Fig. 13.3). The diagnosis is confirmed with an immunodiagnostic test of a scraping from the conjunctival surface.

TREATMENT

Treatment must be systemic and topical. The drugs of choice are doxycycline 100 mg orally twice a day for 21 days with erythromycin ointment applied to the eyes at bedtime. Alternatively, tetracycline 500 mg orally four times a day, or erythromycin 500 mg orally four times a day, for 21 days may be substituted. The patient should be counseled regarding the transmission of this pathogen and that treatment of sexual partners is essential to minimize recurrence and spread of the disease.

REFERRAL GUIDELINES

As in other cases of chronic conjunctivitis, the primary care physician may prefer that the patient be managed by the ophthalmologist, and ophthalmic referral is best made on a routine basis when the diagnosis of chlamydia is suspected. The equipment and facilities for conjunctival cultures needed to make the diagnosis usually are only available to an ophthalmologist.

Adult chlamydial conjunctivitis will respond slowly to treatment over several weeks, therefore the uncomplicated patient need not be reevaluated for 3–4 weeks after initiation of therapy unless complications of medical therapy (allergy, side effects) occur. Referred patients may require examination biweekly for several visits until the disease and complications are resolved. Neonatal chlamydial conjunctivitis involves many special considerations and is best treated by an ophthalmologist. These infants may require daily examinations until stabilized.

Neonatal Conjunctivitis

Ophthalmic neonatorum is usually defined as a conjunctivitis occurring within 1 month of birth. This form of conjunctivitis is much different than adult conjunctivitis, in that the organisms are usually contracted from the vaginal passage and untreated can often cause blindness, especially if the organism is *Neisseria gonorrhoeae.* In 1881, Karl S. Credé introduced the therapy of 2% silver nitrate solution. This single prophylactic application to the eyes of newborns reduced the incidence of blinding neonatal conjunctivitis from 10% to 0.3%. Since that time, the United States and other countries have mandated prophylactic treatment of neonatal conjunctivitis. The more virulent pathogens of neonatal conjunctivitis include *Neisseria gonorrhoeae, Chlamydia trichomatous,* and herpes simplex type II. To provide better coverage for chlamydia, tetracycline or erythromycin ointment have been substituted for the more irritating silver nitrate prophylaxis. Recently, a single application of 2% povidone-iodine solution has been shown to be more effective and less toxic than any previous method of sterilizing the newborn conjunctiva.

Clinical Manifestations

Despite prophylaxis, neonatal conjunctivitis still occurs. The time of onset after birth of the conjunctivitis may give a clue to the etiology of eye inflammation in the newborn. In the first 24 hours, the infant may have mild redness and scanty discharge from a sensitivity reaction to the prophylactic antibiotic applied (chemical conjunctivitis). However, a profuse, mucopurulent discharge in the first few days of life is very suggestive of the highly virulent gonorrhoeae organism. Any newborn with red eyes and purulent drainage should be evaluated by an ophthalmologist. If Gram stain and cultures demonstrate gonococcus, then immediate therapy with ceftriaxone 25–50 mg/kg/d I.V. for 7 days is recommended to prevent acute perforation and blindness, as well as prevention of systemic infection.

Unlike gonorrhoeae, the inclusion conjunctivitis of chlamydia will have a delayed inflammation producing redness and watery discharge 5–7 days after birth. Chlamydial conjunctivitis is readily diagnosed in the infant with chlamydial cultures and immunodiagnostic stains. Treatment of neonatal chlamydia should consist of erythromycin syrup orally 50 mg/kg/d in four divided doses for 2 weeks.

The conjunctivitis in the newborn resulting from maternal genital herpes simplex can become systemic and fatal. The onset of redness, tearing, and a corneal epithelial defect usually does not occur for 7–10 days after birth. The geographic lesions of herpes simplex keratitis may be misdiagnosed as "abrasions," with disastrous ocular consequences. Any nonhealing "abrasion" in the newborn should be evaluated by an

◼︎ TABLE 13.2. Referral Guidelines: Noninfectious Conjunctivitis

DISEASE (CODE)	SIGNS & SYMPTOMS	TREATMENT	WHEN TO REFER
Allergic conjunctivitis (372.14)	Acute, bilateral; itching; watery discharge (beware of vernal in children)	Cold compresses; naphazoline HCL gtt; pheniramine maleate; ketorolac tromethamine; Iodoxamide tromethamine	No referral for routine "hay fever" patients; refer in 48 hours any child with "abrasion" and allergic conjunctivitis (vernal)
Toxic conjunctivitis (130.1)	Lid edema and redness; watery discharge; chronic topical medication use (iatrogenic)	Discontinue topical medications; cold packs; preservative-free lubricants	Refer if not better in 48 hours, if cornea is affected, or if vision declines

ophthalmologist. Systemic treatment with acyclovir and topical trifluridine (Viroptic) is effective in preventing systemic and ocular morbidity.

TREATMENT

The best "treatment" of neonatal conjunctivitis is its prevention with prophylactic antibiotic ointment (erythromycin or tetracycline) or 2% povidone-iodine solution. If, despite prophylaxis, ophthalmia neonatorum occurs, then immediate treatment for the specific etiology should be instituted as outlined earlier. With treatment, the vast majority of patients will be cured without sequelae. Any delay in therapy risks corneal scarring, perforation, and lifelong blindness.

REFERRAL GUIDELINES

Infectious conjunctivitis in the newborn represents a serious threat to the life and vision of the patient. Any newborn with purulent discharge or a nonhealing epithelial defect should be referred immediately. While treatment of adult conjunctivitis is entirely within the purview of the primary care physician, the role of the primary care physician in neonatal conjunctivitis is the prophylaxis and prompt referral of these complex and devastating conditions.

Every newborn should be evaluated within 24 hours of birth for evidence of gonorrhea conjunctivitis, then again at 7–10 days for chlamydia or herpes simplex conjunctivitis. Newborns with purulent conjunctivitis should be examined daily until the eye is clear. Herpes simplex cases should be seen at 24 and 72 hours after the initiation of therapy, and then weekly for several weeks. Chlamydia conjunctivitis cases should be evaluated 48 hours after initiation of therapy and then weekly for several visits.

NONINFECTIOUS CONJUNCTIVITIS (Table 13.2)

Allergic Conjunctivitis

One of the most common forms of conjunctivitis is allergic conjunctivitis. As a mucous membrane with constant contact with the external environment, the conjunctiva is

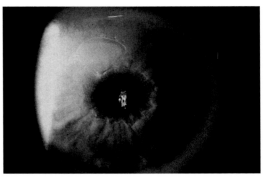

Figure 13.4.   Corneal shield ulcer of vernal keratoconjunctivitis.

often the first tissue to signal the body's allergic reaction to external antigens with a histamine release. This triggers the inflammatory cascade which results in the symptoms of the condition. The mildest and most widespread form of allergic conjunctivitis is found in the common seasonal "hay fever" patient. Although not vision-threatening and ultimately self-limited in duration, hay fever allergic conjunctivitis can be annoying and occasionally debilitating. Allergic conjunctivitis can also be chronic and unrelated to the seasonal pollens. Common antigens which can produce allergic conjunctivitis include house dust, mold spores, animal dander, feathers, and perfumes. The most severe form of allergic conjunctivitis is vernal conjunctivitis, which occurs primarily in children.

CLINICAL MANIFESTATIONS

The cardinal symptoms of allergic conjunctivitis are itching, redness, and watery eyes. Allergic conjunctivitis, whether seasonal or related to a specific antigen, does not cause significant pain or vision loss. However, vernal keratoconjunctivitis is one form of allergic conjunctivitis, usually in children, that can cause vision loss through persistent corneal epithelial breakdown, ulceration, scarring, and even perforation of the globe (Fig. 13.4) All forms of allergic conjunctivitis can be confirmed as an allergy reaction by a conjunctival scraping which will demonstrate the presence of eosinophils in the Giemsa stain testing.

TREATMENT AND PROGNOSIS

Seasonal allergic conjunctivitis is a self-limited disease and therapy is directed to relief of symptoms. While systemic antihistamines are effective, simple cold compresses and topical vasoconstrictors can also reduce swelling and relieve symptoms. For moderately severe acute allergic conjunctivitis, topical medications that combine a vasoconstrictor with an antihistamine are often useful (e.g., naphazoline HCL with pheniramine maleate). However, these medications should not be prescribed indiscriminately as their effectiveness decreases if used more than four times a day. Allergic conjunctivitis due to a specific antigen requires a detailed history to identify the inciting agent responsible for the acute onset of the patient's symptoms. Elimination or reduction of exposure to the offending antigen is often curative. Treatment with topical cromolyn sodium to inhibit the release of histamine from mast cells is of great benefit in reducing the severity of chronic forms of allergic conjunctivitis. Finally, the most recent additions of topical antiprostaglandins, such as ketorolac tromethamine 0.5% and lodoxamide tromethamine 0.1%, have extended the arsenal of treatment for more severe forms of allergic conjunctivitis.

Vernal keratoconjunctivitis, the most severe and intractable form of allergic conjunctivitis, often does not respond to conservative medical therapy. Topical corticosteroids may be required in the treatment of vernal disease. However, the use of steroids should be monitored by an ophthalmologist, because of the potential for adverse side effects, including glaucoma and cataracts.

REFERRAL GUIDELINES

Routine "hay fever" patients should respond well to treatment and generally do not require specialty consultation. Antigen-specific allergic conjunctivitis cases that are resistant to the usual therapy may require referral to an allergist for skin testing to identify the offending agent. Vernal keratoconjunctivitis is the one allergic condition that can cause visual loss in children. Therefore, any child or teenager with chronic allergic conjunctivitis with an epithelial defect of the cornea should be referred within 48 hours to an ophthalmologist for evaluation and therapy.

The chronic conditions of allergic conjunctivitis usually require minimal visits to the primary care physician and only one or two consultative examinations by the ophthalmologist for cases resistant to therapy. Cases of vernal, however, need to be followed closely, with visits every 3–7 days for several weeks until the corneal surface is healed and the inflammatory condition is stabilized. Once stabilized on a medication regimen, vernal patients are seen about once a month during the active season.

Toxic Conjunctivitis

Toxic conjunctivitis results from sensitivity to substances found in the tear film. Chemical toxic conjunctivitis has a distinct history of onset, and the patient can often correlate the onset of symptoms with the time of exposure to the offending drug or chemical. Many causes of toxic conjunctivitis are iatrogenic. Two common antibiotics used for bacterial conjunctivitis, sulfacetamide and neomycin, each have a 10–20% incidence of toxic and allergic conjunctivitis. Topical atropine drops, used for cycloplegia and pain relief in patients with iritis or uveitis, often cause toxic conjunctivitis. Idoxuridine (Viroptic) drops are effective in treating herpes simplex, but when used for longer than 3 weeks may result in a toxic keratoconjunctivitis that mimics the original disease. The preservatives found in many ophthalmic preparations are often the cause of toxic conjunctivitis. The preservative thimerosal is notorious for causing toxic and allergic conjunctivitis, especially in contact lens patients. However, even the relatively benign preservative of benzalkonium chloride found in many artificial tear preparations may be toxic to the conjunctiva when the drops are applied more often than four times a day.

CLINICAL MANIFESTATIONS

The patient with toxic conjunctivitis will usually present with lid erythema and edema, vascular injection and chemosis of the conjunctiva, and a watery discharge (Fig. 13.5).

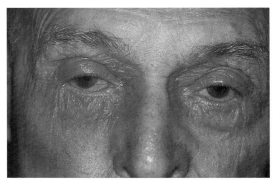

Figure 13.5.   Toxic blepharoconjunctivitis from neomycin. (See also color section.)

Except in cases of severe chemical trauma with acid or alkali, the cornea will show little involvement other than trace punctate fluorescein staining. The patient will have minimal pain or loss of vision, but may complain of photophobia and burning, or foreign body sensation.

TREATMENT

The treatment of toxic conjunctivitis is the same as the treatment of allergic conjunctivitis, removal of the offending agent. In any conjunctivitis which shows initial improvement on appropriate therapy, but which worsens on prolonged therapy, the diagnosis of iatrogenic toxic conjunctivitis should be considered, and the initial topical therapy discontinued, or at least reevaluated. Cold packs and the application of preservative-free lubricants often give symptomatic relief until the inflammation resolves. Severe cases of toxic conjunctivitis should be referred to an ophthalmologist for appropriate evaluation and possible steroid therapy.

REFERRAL GUIDELINES

Patients with toxic conjunctivitis should improve in 24–48 hours and no referral is necessary. If the cornea is involved, inflammation worsens or vision declines, then the diagnosis should be questioned and the patient referred for ophthalmologic evaluation.

Routine toxic conjunctivitis should be reevaluated 48 hours and 1 week after initiation of therapy. Mild chemical burns may require daily evaluation until stabilized.

SUMMARY

The diverse group of inflammatory conditions that we term "conjunctivitis" has been described and categorized in this section. In general, the forms of conjunctivitis which are benign and self-limited produce a mild injection of the conjunctiva, a watery discharge, have minimal pain, and the vision is normal. These benign forms of conjunctivitis include viral, adult chlamydial, allergic, and mild toxic conjunctivitis. More virulent forms of conjunctivitis may result in a mucopurulent discharge, corneal involvement, some pain, and, oftentimes, a reduction in vision. These virulent forms of conjunctivitis include gonococcal bacterial conjunctivitis, neonatal conjunctivitis, vernal keratoconjunctivitis, and toxic chemical burns. Overlap between these categories is common, and with the absence or delay of appropriate therapy, "benign" forms of conjunctivitis may cause permanent loss of vision.

SUGGESTED READINGS

deToledo A, Chandler J. Conjunctivitis of the newborn. Infect Dis Clin North Am 1992;6:807–813.

Ehlers W, Donshik P. Allergic ocular disorders: a spectrum of diseases. J Contact Lens Assoc Ophthal 1992;18:117–124.

Friedlander M. A review of the causes and treatment of bacterial and allergic conjunctivitis. Clin Ther 1995;17:800–810.

Friedlander M. Management of ocular allergy. Ann Allergy Asthma Immunol 1995;75:212–222.

Liesengang T. Disorders of the cornea, conjunctiva, and lens. In: Bartley G, Liesengang T, eds. Essentials of ophthalmology. Philadelphia: J.B. Lippincott, 1992;81–86.

Steinert RF. Current therapy for bacterial keratitis and bacterial conjunctivitis. Am J Ophthalmol 1991;112:105–145.

Syed NA, Hyndiuk R. Infectious conjunctivitis. Infect Dis Clin North Am 1992;6:789–805.

Terry A, Bruner W, Cobo M, et al. Conjunctivitis: referral practice pattern–San Francisco, CA. Am Acad Ophthalmol 1991;1–12.

Vaughan D. Bacterial conjunctivitis. In: Vaughan D, Asbury T, Tabbara K, eds. General ophthalmology. San Mateo, CA: Appleton & Lange, 1989:78–79.

Wegman D, Guinee V, Millian S. Epidemic keratoconjunctivitis. Am J Public Health 1970;60:1250–1257.

◑◗ Chapter 14
Dry Eye Syndrome (Keratoconjunctivitis Sicca)

G. A. Cioffi

INTRODUCTION

Dry eye syndrome is usually a bilateral, chronic condition in which there are multiple ocular surface changes resulting from insufficient tear production or instability of the tear film. This can lead to desiccation of the conjunctiva and cornea. Keratoconjunctivitis sicca is often a lifelong disease and is more common and more severe in the elderly population. This condition may be punctuated by periods of exacerbation, which may be associated with weather or seasonal changes, as well as heat, wind, smokey environments, air conditioning, low humidity, or intense eye use. Although the prognosis for most patients is excellent, severe cases, if left untreated, may lead to blinding complications.

The tears have multiple functions, which include lubrication of the anterior ocular surface, anti-infectious properties, removal of foreign particulate and creation of a smooth optical interface. Tears are composed of three basic components which are layered on the external surface of the eye: the oil layer, the aqueous layer, and the mucin layer. The outermost layer is oily and is produced by the meibomian glands at the edge of the upper and lower eyelids. The middle layer is watery and is the principal component of the tears. Most of the aqueous or middle layer is produced by the accessory lacrimal glands located on the inner surface of the eyelids. The large lacrimal gland, located under the superior lateral portion of the upper eye lid, produces the bulk of reflex tearing (Fig. 14.1). Immunoglobulin A, lysozymes, and other anti-infective agents are found in this middle layer. This layer also serves to cleanse the eye as well as wash away foreign matter. The outer, oily layer serves as a smooth optical interface and decreases the evaporative loss of the middle, watery layer. The innermost layer is comprised principally of mucin. This layer is produced by goblet cells located within the conjunctiva. The mucin allows the tear film to distribute evenly over the cornea. Without mucin, the tear film readily breaks apart over the hydrophobic corneal epithelium, resulting in irritation and blurring. A disturbance of any of these three layers may result in dry eye symptoms. The most common cause of keratoconjunctivitis sicca is absence or deficiency of the middle, watery layer.

CLINICAL MANIFESTATIONS

As with most chronic diseases, a detailed history will help to establish the etiology in many individuals presenting with dry eyes. The key symptoms associated with

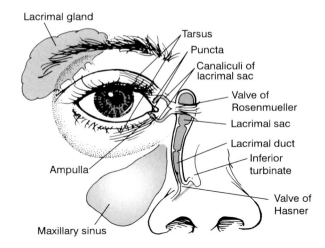

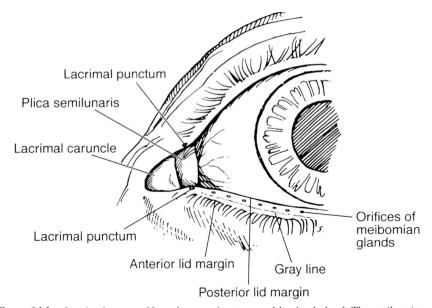

Figure 14.1. Lacrimal system. Note the superior temporal lacrimal gland. The meibomian glands are in the upper and lower eyelids and their orifices empty at the lash line. The accessory lacrimal glands are in the superior lid fornix and the goblet cells are located in the conjunctiva. (Reprinted by permission from Sires BS, Lemke BN, Kincaid MC. Orbital and ocular anatomy. In: Wright KW, ed. Textbook of ophthalmology. Baltimore: Williams & Wilkins, Chap 1, Fig 1.5a, b, 1997:7).

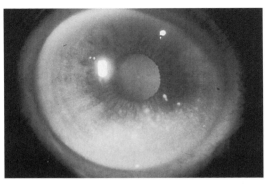

Figure 14.2. Dry eye syndrome demonstrating punctate staining of the cornea. Note the heavy fluorescein dye of the inferior cornea.

keratoconjunctivitis sicca include burning, ocular irritation, dryness, foreign body sensation, and occasionally blurred vision. Early in the disease and in milder forms of the disease, the irritation caused by the dry eye may actually lead to increased tearing and even epiphora (tears rolling down the face). This is secondary to a relative deficiency of the basal tear secretion causing ocular irritation. The reflex tearing is secondary to irritation of the highly innervated external surface of the eye and stimulation of tear production from the major lacrimal gland. In more severe cases of dry eye syndrome, chronic dryness of the mucus membranes, other than the conjunctiva (e.g., buccal and vaginal mucosa) may also be present. Patients may complain of both dry eyes and dry mouth.

Clinical signs associated with dry eyes include redness and irritation of the bulbar conjunctiva and a scant tear meniscus along the inferior eyelid margin. Ocular redness occurs from vascular injection and dilation secondary to chronic irritation. Excessive mucus secretion and accumulation may be seen in the lower fornix and along the lower lid line. The bulbar conjunctiva may lose its normal luster and appear edematous. Frequently, however, there are very few gross changes in the ocular appearance in patients with dry eye syndrome. With the magnified examination of the anterior surface of the eye provided by the slit lamp biomicroscope, fine punctate stippling may be seen using fluorescein staining (Fig. 14.2). Early signs may also include poor stability of the tear film. In normal individuals, the anterior surface of the eye should remain well-lubricated with tears for greater than 10 seconds without blinking. In patients with dry eyes, the tear film breaks up almost immediately upon cessation of blinking. In more severe cases, strands of mucous and dead epithelial cells (known as filaments) may form with strong attachments to the corneal epithelium. These strands, which can often be seen on gross examination, may cause considerable discomfort. Damaged corneal and conjunctival epithelium will stain with the vital dye, rose bengal, and frank defects in the epithelium can be detected with fluorescein dye. This usually can be seen with or without cobalt blue illumination. More sophisticated tests quantify the tear production (Schirmer's test), but these tests are generally performed only in an ophthalmologist's office.

Associated disorders which may be present in patients with dry eye syndrome include filamentary keratitis, recurrent corneal erosion syndrome, and contact lens

TABLE 14.1. Differential Diagnosis of Dry
Eye Syndrome

Blepharitis
External ocular foreign body (with chronic irritation)
Exposure keratopathy (lid abnormalities)
Nocturnal lagophthalmos

---

intolerance. As mentioned earlier, filaments are strands of mucous and dead epithelial cells with strong attachments to the corneal epithelium. With severe filamentary keratitis, multiple office visits for repetitive removal of the filaments are often necessary. Filaments are removed under topical anesthesia with smooth forceps with slitlamp or loupe magnification. Care should be taken to avoid creation of large corneal abrasions when removing the filaments.

Recurrent corneal erosion syndrome can develop and is characterized by acute attacks of severe ocular pain and foreign body sensation, photophobia, and epiphora due to repetitive sloughing of the corneal epithelium. Often this signifies significant corneal disease with alterations of the corneal epithelium, epithelial basement membranes, and even the deeper layers of the corneal stroma. Patients with recurrent corneal erosions should be evaluated by an ophthalmologist. Finally, many patients with dry eye syndrome become intolerant to contact lens wear. Initially, artificial tears and punctal occlusion may permit continued wear, but many individuals will eventually need to give up contact lens use with aging.

DIFFERENTIAL DIAGNOSIS

The differential diagnosis of keratoconjunctivitis sicca includes any external irritation of the ocular surface such as blepharitis or foreign bodies, and exposure keratopathies (Table 14.1) Because reflex tearing may occur whenever a patient experiences foreign body sensation, disorders such as blepharitis are often confused with dry eye syndrome. It is important to remember that early in the disease, patients with mild dry eyes may have reflex tearing. In addition to blepharitis, excessive exposure of the cornea and conjunctiva from insufficient blinking or poor eyelid closure (exposure keratopathy) may also result in insufficient distribution of tears and chronic ocular irritation. These problems may occur following a cranial nerve VII palsy and are frequently seen in patients with nocturnal lagophthalmos (incomplete closure of the eyelids while asleep).

The most common etiology of keratoconjunctivitis sicca is idiopathic (Table 14.2). Although many ocular and systemic diseases may result in poor tear quality or insufficient tear production, most patients with dry eyes have no other identifiable disorder. However, connective tissue diseases such as Sjögren's syndrome and systemic lupus erythematosus may result in dry eye syndrome. Multiple systemic medications are also associated with keratoconjunctivitis sicca, including antihistamines, antidepressants, oral contraceptives, and antispasmodics. Simple withdrawal of a suspicious medication may be simultaneously diagnostic and therapeutic. More unusual causes associated with decreased tear production include sarcoidosis or other infiltrative disorders of the lacrimal glands. Amyloidoses, lymphoma, and leukemia have all been identified as causes of decreased tear production. These disorders principally alter the watery tear layer production. Any infection or inflammatory syndrome which causes conjunctival

TABLE 14.2. Most Common Etiology
of Dry Eye Syndrome

Idiopathic
Meibomian gland disease
Ocular rosacea
Conjunctival scarring
Herpes zoster ophthalmicus
Stevens-Johnson's syndrome
Trachoma
Chemical burns
Ocular pemphigoid
Collagen Vascular Diseases
Sjögren's syndrome
Rheumatoid arthritis
Systemic lupus erythematosus
Drugs
Antispasmodics
Oral contraceptives
Antihistamines
Lacrimal gland disease
Inflammatory (i.e., sarcoidosis, etc.)
Infiltrative (i.e., tumors)
Vitamin A deficiency

scarring may also result in keratoconjunctivitis sicca. In the elderly, rheumatoid arthritis and herpes zoster ophthalmicus (see also Chapter 23, "Ocular Herpetic Infections") often result in severe dry eye syndrome with vision threatening complications. Diseases such as Stevens-Johnson syndrome and ocular cicatricial pemphigoid result in scarring of the conjunctiva and lids. This causes poor distribution of the tears and insufficient mucin production because of loss of goblet cells in the scarred conjunctiva. Ocular rosacea is a disease which affects the meibomian gland function resulting in an abnormal oil layer, rapid tear evaporation, and severe dry eye syndrome. Finally, Vitamin A deficiency also results in keratoconjunctivitis sicca and is most frequently seen in developing countries associated with poor dietary patterns.

TREATMENT

Although there are multiple causes of keratoconjunctivitis sicca, initial treatment is almost always artificial tear substitution (Table 14.3). If an underlying etiology can be identified or systemic abnormality diagnosed, these should be corrected when possible. Artificial tear preparations are available in preserved and nonpreserved formulations. Preserved artificial tears are provided in multiple use bottles and are less expensive. However, if the dosage needs to be more often than three times daily, artificial tear substitution is best provided with preservative-free and lanolin-free agents. In mild cases, short-term (several days to weeks), frequent lubrication (four to eight times daily) with tear substitutes often eradicates the epithelial changes and alleviates symptoms. In more severe cases, the need for prolonged lubrication may be evident. In these cases, lubricating ointment can be used, especially at bedtime. Again, preservative-free bland

● TABLE 14.3. Referral Guidelines: Dry Eye Syndrome

DIAGNOSIS (CODE)	TREATMENT	WHEN TO REFER
Mild keratoconjunctivitis sicca (370.33)	Artifical tear substitutes; night time ointments	Progressive/worsening symptoms; no improvement in 6–8 weeks
Moderate to severe keratoconjunctivitis sicca (370.33)	Artificial tear substitutes (nonpreserved); punctal occlusion; humidifiers; occlusive goggles	Need for punctal occlusion; development of associated disorders (i.e., filamentary keratitis, etc.)
Keratoconjunctivitis sicca associated with conjunctival scarring (370.33)	Artificial tear substitutes; night time ointments; lid/ conjunctival surgery	Always refer for initial evaluation
Filamentary keratitis (370.23)	Removal of filaments; artificial tear substitutes; night time ointments	Recurrence of filaments
Recurrent corneal erosion syndrome (918.1)	Artificial tear substitutes; night time ointments; pressure patching	Nonhealing abrasions; recurrent erosions

ointments are usually best. For severe cases, humidifiers and occlusive goggles (swim goggles) may be used to prevent excessive evaporation of the insufficient tear film. In cases with associated blepharitis, systemic and/or topical antibiotics may be required (see Chapter 12, "Blepharitis"). All artificial tears which are dispensed in multiuse bottles contain chemical preservatives, which may lead to corneal toxicity. In addition, many tear preparations contain vasoconstrictive agents to lessen the ocular hyperemia. These agents, when used chronically, may actually aggravate the ocular irritation associated with dry eye syndrome because of corneal toxicity. In any mild case of dry eye syndrome that is resistant to therapy, preservative toxicity should be suspected. A variety of artificial tears are provided in sterile, single use vials which often are better tolerated in patients needing chronic and frequent therapy.

Surgical treatment of chronic dry eyes includes occlusion of the nasolacrimal puncta, either permanent or temporary. Plugs can be placed into the puncta to test whether symptomatic relief is provided. If temporary punctal occlusion is beneficial, permanent closure can be achieved with thermal electrocautery or surgical treatment. In some patients, eyelid surgery may be required to partially close the palpebral fissure (tarsorrhaphy). This provides better apposition of the tears to the eyelid surface, as well as preventing evaporation. Patients with nocturnal lagophthalmos often benefit from forced eyelid closure and lubricating ointment at bedtime. The upper eyelids may be taped shut to the cheek with nonabrasive paper tape. Exposure keratopathy or lid abnormalities of any kind may result in poor lubrication of the ocular surface and may require surgical correction to alleviate symptoms (see Chapter 10, "Eyelid Malpositions").

Keratoconjunctivitis sicca secondary to conjunctival scarring from disorders such as Stevens-Johnson syndrome, ocular chemical burns and ocular pemphigoid, are often the most difficult to treat and the most devastating to visual function. Many of these patients require eyelid surgery and constant monitoring to prevent permanent visual loss from corneal scarring. Recent advances in conjunctival transplantation surgery offer new hope for these blinding conditions and all such patients should be evaluated by an ophthalmologist. Many collagen vascular diseases such as Sjögren's syndrome, rheumatoid arthritis, and systemic lupus erythematosus, are associated with dry eye syndrome and treatment should be determined by the severity of the ocular symptoms. Finally, lacrimal gland disease may result in inadequate tear production and dry eye symptoms. These include inflammatory disorders such as sarcoidosis, and infiltrative disorders such as metastatic tumors and lymphomas. The palpation of the lacrimal gland in the superior temporal region of the upper eyelid may reveal enlargement and tenderness. Any individual suspected of having lacrimal gland enlargement should be evaluated by an ophthalmologist for the consideration of a diagnostic biopsy and appropriate systemic therapy.

FREQUENCY OF VISITS

Frequency of ocular examination depends on the severity of the keratoconjunctivitis sicca. Patients with underlying systemic disease typically need to be monitored more closely. Often patients can help dictate their own follow-up schedule. When patients experience foreign body sensation and/or blurred vision, an increase in lubrication and reevaluation are necessary. Seasonal variations and associated symptoms may require more frequent follow-up during particular times of the year.

SUGGESTED READINGS

de Luise VP. Management of dry eye in focal points: clinical modules for ophthalmologist. San Francisco: American Academy of Ophthalmology, 1985.
Holly FJ, Lemp MA. Tear physiology and dry eye. Surv Ophthalmol 1977;22:69–80.

Chapter 15 ◖●◗

Ocular Trauma

M. A. Terry

INTRODUCTION

Trauma to the eyes and the surrounding tissue is quite common among all age groups. Each case of ocular trauma is unique and requires various levels of specialized care to optimize recovery. The initial evaluation and therapy of the injured eye may be the most critical factor in the final outcome. It is most important to first assess the vision and the severity of the injury, stabilize and protect the eye, and refer the patient to the appropriate level of care. Although some minor traumas, such as superficial foreign bodies, can be managed by the primary care physician, more severe trauma cases need to be referred after the initial assessment is completed. All patients with documented visual loss should be referred for a complete ophthalmologic evaluation.

ASSESSMENT OF THE SEVERITY OF INJURY

The assessment of injury begins with a detailed history of the circumstances surrounding the injury. The specific time and setting of the trauma should be recorded, as should the relative cleanliness of the injury, and the force of the injuring element (e.g., Was it the racquet or the racquetball that hit the eye?). The physical examination should be as complete as possible but should not endanger the integrity of the injured globe. For example, a ruptured globe may extrude the intraocular contents if excessive pressure is placed on the eye trying to open the swollen lids. Nonetheless, it is critical that all trauma patients have visual acuity tested and recorded at the time of initial examination. This vision assessment is important as it serves as baseline data against which to measure the success of therapy. Vision testing can be as simplified as testing the patient's ability to count the examiner's fingers at various distances, or, if the lids are swollen shut, a penlight can be turned off and on over the closed lids and the patient asked to identify the direction of incidence of the light. By shining the light from various directions, the gross function of the entire retina can be assessed. A general description of the eye and the lids should be recorded, as well as the movement of the eye in each direction of gaze. The pupillary response and a comparison of the pupil size to the uninjured eye should be assessed. The pupils should be tested for the presence of an afferent light defect (Marcus Gunn pupil; see Appendix B) to assure the integrity of the anterior visual pathways. The front of the eye is best assessed with a slitlamp examination, but if this is not available, magnifying loupes may be used. The integrity and clarity of the cornea and the anterior chamber should be recorded, as well as the presence of any blood or foreign body. A direct ophthalmoscope should be used to view the posterior segment of the eye and to assess the optic nerve and

◼ TABLE 15.1. Referral Guidelines: Blunt Trauma

DISEASE (CODE)	SIGNS AND SYMPTOMS	TREATMENT	WHEN TO REFER
Lid trauma (921.1)	Lid ecchymosis; subconjunctival hemorrhage	Assess globe damage; no pressure on the globe; cold compresses; shield if globe damage	Referral in 1 week if no globe damage; referral immediately if globe damage or unable to examine globe
Blowout fracture (802.6)	Lid edema; enophthalmos; diplopia; restricted movement	Assess globe damage; no pressure on globe; cold compresses; shield if globe damage	Referral in 72 hours if no globe damage; referral immediately if globe damage
Ocular contusion (921.3)	Lid edema; reduced vision ± hyphema ± pupil abnormality	Assess globe damage; shield and refer	Refer immediately if intraocular blood present or vision is decreased

retina. After the status of the anterior segment (cornea, iris, and anterior chamber) has been recorded, dilating drops can be applied to facilitate ophthalmoscopy (cyclopentolate 1% and neosynephrine 2.5%). The pupils should not be dilated if neurologic monitoring and evaluation requires periodic pupil checks. Once the pupils have been dilated, the "view-in," or ability of the physician to adequately see the retinal details with a direct ophthalmoscope, should be recorded. The inability to view the optic nerve and retinal vessels in the setting of reduced vision and a clear cornea indicates decreased clarity of the normally clear ocular media. The presence of blood in the vitreous cavity, a cataract of the lens, or blood in the anterior chamber (hyphema) may be responsible and signify a severe intraocular injury.

The systematic evaluation and meticulous documentation of the presenting history and physical at the initial examination by the primary care physician is critical to the successful management of the ocular trauma patient.

DIFFERENTIAL DIAGNOSIS

BLUNT TRAUMA

The eye is protected from blunt injury by the lids, the bony orbit, and by the surrounding soft tissues of the extraocular muscles and orbital fat (Table 15.1). One or more of these structures will usually show injury from blunt trauma. The level of injury is related to the size and kinetic force of the offending agent. Blunt objects such as fists or racquetballs, which have high kinetic energy and easily fit through the anterior orbital opening, may cause devastating injury to the globe and all the surrounding structures. Larger objects, such as a softball, may be blocked by the orbital rim, thereby preventing injury to the globe.

CLINICAL MANIFESTATIONS

The lids in blunt trauma are usually swollen, and, occasionally, examination of the globe is difficult. Gentle traction of the lids may be required to view the globe and

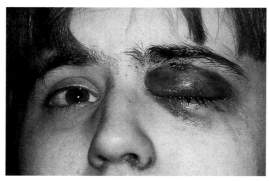

Figure 15.1. Blunt trauma with massively swollen lids and ecchymotic discoloration of the periorbital region.

assess the vision. If manipulation of the swollen lids will place undue pressure on the globe, then ophthalmic consultation is necessary (Fig. 15.1). If the examination reveals normal vision with normal movement of the eye and no apparent damage to the globe, then ice packs can be applied to reduce lid swelling and the patient reevaluated daily until full recovery occurs.

Blunt trauma may cause damage to the extraocular muscles, especially the inferior rectus muscle. This will be apparent as the patient may complain of double vision and the injured eye will not move in concert with the fellow eye (often a restriction in upgaze). An MRI scan of the orbit and extraocular muscles will usually demonstrate the damaged or entrapped muscle.

The bony orbit is especially susceptible to blunt trauma. The globe is a partially compressible structure that sits in a cushion of soft tissue composed of extraocular muscles and orbital fat. When a small blunt object strikes the globe directly, the force is transmitted by the compressed globe to the soft tissues, which in turn transmits the force to the walls of the bony orbit (Fig. 15.2). The thinnest bones of the walls of the orbit are the floor of the orbit, which separate the orbit from the underlying maxillary sinus, and the medial wall, which separates the orbit from the ethmoid sinus. Given enough force, the floor of the orbit will "blowout" into the underlying maxillary sinus and the orbital soft tissues will herniate inferiorly. If severe, the inferior rectus can become entrapped and restrict upward gaze of the eye, resulting in diplopia. The herniation of blood and orbital contents can easily be imaged by an MRI, a CAT scan, and even plain sinus x-rays. With severe "blowout" fractures, the eye can appear "sunken" (enophthalmos) with extensive restriction of movement in multiple fields of gaze (Fig. 15.3). As mentioned earlier, blunt trauma resulting from larger objects may have little contact with the globe. However, in these injuries the kinetic energy is directly transmitted to the bony orbital rim and extraocular injury can be significant. Fractures of the superior or inferior orbital rim may result, as well as posterior orbital fractures secondary to compression.

Ocular contusion should be assessed separately from the damage done to the lids and the bony orbit. The globe can sustain a surprising degree of blunt force without injury because of its cushion of orbital fat and the protection of the lids and bony orbit. However, whenever blunt trauma causes lid edema, a meticulous search for damage to the globe must be performed. If there is any question that the globe may

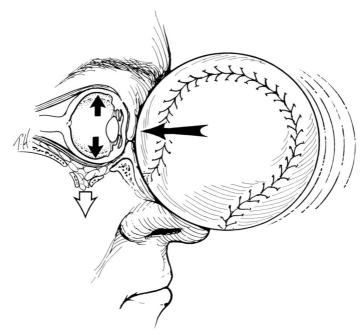

Figure 15.2. Orbital floor "blowout" fracture.

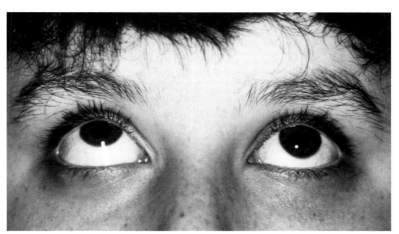

Figure 15.3. Patient with restricted gaze from blowout fracture of the left eye. (Reprinted by permission from Buus DR, Tse DT. Periorbital and orbital injuries. In: Wright KW, ed. Textbook of ophthalmology. Baltimore: Williams & Wilkins, Fig 26.11, 1997:424.)

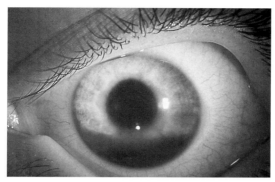

Figure 15.4.   Hyphema from blunt trauma (hockey puck). Note the blood layers inferiorly.

have sustained injury, then referral to an ophthalmologist for full and specialized evaluation is necessary.

As previously noted, the assessment of the visual acuity of the injured eye is critical. Multiple forms of ocular injury can result in the common symptom of reduced vision. A common cause of reduced vision after ocular contusion is blood in the interior of the globe. If the blood is in the front of the globe (the anterior chamber), it will scatter the light entering the pupil and reduce the vision. When this blood layers out in the inferior anterior chamber it can be seen with a penlight examination and is called a hyphema (Fig. 15.4). A hyphema which fills the entire chamber is called an "8-ball" hyphema, and completely blocks the visualization of the pupil and iris. Intraocular pressures can be dangerously high when a hyphema is present, and if therapy is delayed, permanent damage to the cornea and optic nerve may result. The source of bleeding in a hyphema is usually the iris or iris root (iris dialysis), and secondary glaucoma (angle recession glaucoma) is a common sequelae.

Another location of intraocular blood is in the vitreous cavity, and this can severely reduce vision. This posterior location of blood is more ominous and may represent a retinal tear, or detachment, or, often, a ruptured globe. Blood in the vitreous will obscure not only the patients vision, but also the physician's view of the retina.

TREATMENT

Blunt lid trauma without associated globe or orbit injury will usually resolve spontaneously. The lid ecchymosis should be treated with ice packs and the globe reassessed in several days when the lid edema is gone. When accompanied by globe damage or reduction in vision, a shield should be placed over the lids to protect against pressure on the globe and the patient referred to an ophthalmologist.

Blowout fractures of the orbit without associated globe injury can be treated conservatively with ice packs. Often the contused inferior or medial rectus muscles will recover spontaneously over several weeks. If muscle entrapment is confirmed by radiology and by examination, then a shield and ice packs should be used and the patient referred for management. Oculoplastic surgical repair of the blowout fracture is often delayed several weeks for optimal results and the prognosis for full visual recovery is quite good.

◑I TABLE 15.2. Referral Guidelines: Sharp Trauma

DISEASE (CODE)	SIGNS AND SYMPTOMS	TREATMENT	WHEN TO REFER
Lid lacerations (870.8)	Lid margin lacerations; lacrimal system lacerations	Protect globe from drying with ocular lubricant; ice packs; shield and refer	Refer within 12 hours if patient medically stable
Ocular lacerations (871.4)	Subconjunctival hemorrhage; corneal abrasion vs. laceration; chamber formed and no intraocular blood	Verify no perforation; ice packs; shield and refer; ofloxacin q2h if referral delayed	No referral for subconjunctival heme if no other damage; refer corneal lacerations in 8 hours if no perforation
Ocular perforations (871.7)	Stick or knife injury; "metal on metal hammering"; pupil distortion; intraocular blood; possible endophthalmitis	Shield and refer; no pressure on globe	Refer immediately

Ocular contusions should be treated as a ruptured globe until this diagnosis is excluded. Any patient with intraocular blood present and reduced vision should have a shield placed over the lids to prevent pressure on the globe and referred for an ophthalmic evaluation. The prognosis for ocular contusions is dependent upon the extent and location of the injury. Generally, injuries involving only the anterior regions of the eye have a better prognosis than injuries involving the retina and optic nerve.

REFERRAL GUIDELINES

Isolated blunt lid trauma cases can be referred for ophthalmic evaluation when the lid edema resolves and the globe can be thoroughly examined, usually about 3–7 days following the injury. Any patient with globe involvement, where intraocular blood is noted and/or vision is decreased should be referred immediately. Orbital blowout fractures without globe involvement can be referred in 72 hours for full assessment and treatment.

FREQUENCY OF VISITS

The frequency of visits for the ocular trauma patient is determined by the severity of the injury and the rate of healing. It is highly individualized and many of these patients require ophthalmic surgery for complete visual rehabilitation.

SHARP OR PENETRATING TRAUMA (LID AND OCULAR LACERATIONS)

Sharp or penetrating ocular trauma often accompanies other facial lacerations, especially in motor vehicle accidents, and a full inspection of the lids and eyes for lacerating injuries should be done in any facial trauma setting (Table 15.2). Sharp injuries to the globe can be trivial, producing only a corneal epithelial abrasion or subconjunctival hemorrhage; or sharp injuries can be devastating, producing corneal/scleral lacerations with prolapse and loss of intraocular contents.

The examination of the patient with an ocular laceration can be difficult and topical anesthetic drops should be placed at the start of the examination to immediately relieve pain and facilitate an adequate examination. Care should be taken not to place undue pressure on the globe when opening the lids, in case there is a perforation of the globe. Vision should be assessed immediately and recorded. The size, shape, and reactivity of the pupil should be recorded. Ideally, the slitlamp biomicroscope should be utilized to examine the cornea and anterior segment, but a penlight examination may suffice if the patient is going to be referred immediately. The ability to visualize the optic nerve and retina with the ophthalmoscope by the primary care physician should be noted, as well as the presence of any intraocular blood.

CLINICAL MANIFESTATIONS

Injury to the lids and brow may involve horizontal lacerations which do not involve the lid margin or lacrimal system, and which usually can be primarily repaired in the emergency room or primary care physician's office. These superficial lacerations usually do not result in deformation of the lid margin contour and they do not affect the globe. However, evidence of orbital fat herniation should alert the examiner to a deeper injury to the orbit or posterior globe. The presence of orbital fat in an eyelid laceration indicates that the orbital septum has been violated and injury to the extraocular muscles, posterior globe, and other retrobulbar structures are much more likely. Simple closure of such lacerations may result in retained orbital foreign bodies and may miss other more significant posterior injuries.

Eyelid lacerations which involve the lid margin (the portion of the upper or lower eyelid from which the lashes extend) are of a more serious nature. These patients may show profuse tearing and notching of the lid with exposure of the globe. In such injuries, specific attention must be given to the medial lid margins (medial canthal region). The medial canthal region contains the lacrimal drainage apparatus (the punctum, canaliculi, and nasal lacrimal sac). The punctum are two small openings in the upper and lower eyelids that drain tears away from the ocular surface. The punctum feed into a common canaliculi which subsequently drains into the nasal lacrimal sac. The nasal lacrimal sac empties into the nasal cavity via the nasal lacrimal duct. Lacerations of the tear drainage system will present as swelling of the tissue nasally with tearing. The exact extent of the damage can be deceptive and failure to recognize and correctly repair lacerations of the lacrimal drainage system will result in chronic tearing.

The majority of sharp injuries to the globe will present with some degree of pain, tearing, and redness. The degree of these symptoms varies with the severity of the injury. Superficial ocular lacerations of the conjunctiva will produce a bright red subconjunctival hemorrhage which usually pools under the inferior bulbar conjunctiva (the conjunctiva covering the globe), leaving other quadrants of the sclera normal and white. The bright blood-red appearance of a subconjunctival hemorrhage may be quite alarming to the patient, but as long as the injury did not perforate the underlying sclera, the injury is usually innocuous and self-limited. A thorough examination showing a normal vision, normal pupil, and no intraocular blood usually indicates only superficial injury.

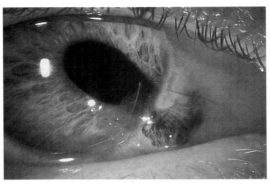

Figure 15.5.   Corneal laceration with perforation and iris plugging of wound. Note pupil distortion with "peaking" toward wound.

Corneal abrasions can be caused by sharp objects glancing off the corneal surface. The pain and tearing from a corneal abrasion can be quite intense and care must be taken to confirm the injury did not penetrate deeper (a laceration versus an abrasion) and that a perforation of the globe did not occur.

Corneal lacerations involve the deeper stromal tissue of the cornea. If not properly repaired, the resultant white and vascularized scar will cause reduced vision from irregular corneal topography even if the scar is not located over the pupil. Lacerations can be differentiated from abrasions by the hazy corneal swelling of the underlying tissue and by the fluorescein pattern seen with the slitlamp biomicroscope.

Corneal perforations represent an ocular emergency. The history accompanying a corneal perforation may be of a high velocity metal fragment hitting the eye or of a slow velocity sharp object lacerating the globe such as a stick or knife. Perforations from "metal on metal" hammering injuries can be quite small, but leave an intraocular foreign body which can be devastating to the eye. Any perforation, large or small, presents the potential for intraocular infection (endophthalmitis) and requires immediate ophthalmic evaluation. The pain, redness, and visual loss from small perforating injuries can be highly variable, so the history of the trauma and a meticulous slitlamp examination are critical. Larger perforating lacerations of the cornea allow aqueous fluid to drain from the eye, causing the iris tissue to come forward and plug the perforation site. In these cases, the pupil will not be perfectly round and will "point" to the quadrant of the perforation (Fig. 15.5). No attempt should be made by the primary care physician to remove or reposit the iris plug. The perforating agent may penetrate far enough to cause an iris laceration or crystalline lens laceration, severely reducing the vision with intraocular blood or lens opacification. The crystalline lens of the eye is surrounded by an ectodermal capsule which separates it from the aqueous fluid. This allows the lens material to remain clear in a relatively dehydrated state. Any perforating agent which disrupts the integrity of the lens capsule will allow water to enter the crystalline lens, and the resultant hydration of lens material turns the crystalline lens cloudy. This "traumatic cataract" formation may occur immediately or develop over several weeks or months until vision is sufficiently reduced to warrant surgery (Fig. 15.6). Additionally, hydrated lens proteins can incite acute inflammatory reactions (uveitis) and acute glaucoma which may necessitate early surgical intervention.

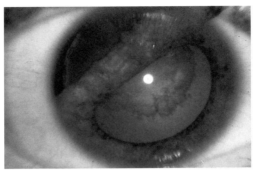

Figure 15.6. Traumatic cataract with iris dialysis. Note the iris is disinserted from its root and the central opacity in the lens.

TREATMENT

Lid lacerations without lid margin involvement or herniation of the orbital fat can usually be sutured by the primary care physician or emergency room physician. If exposure of the globe occurs from a margin or canthal laceration, the globe should be protected from drying with an ocular lubricant and an ice pack applied to reduce swelling prior to referral. Any laceration which involves the eyelid margin or lacrimal system should be evaluated and repaired by an ophthalmologist.

Corneal lacerations should be initially classified as nonperforating or perforating. All corneal lacerations should be evaluated by an ophthalmologist. Nonperforating lacerations may have ice applied to reduce lid swelling. The eye is then protected with a shield until referral. If referral is delayed, the patient should be started on antibiotic drops (not ointment) every 2 hours until seen by an ophthalmologist. Perforating corneal lacerations should have a Fox shield placed and pressure on the globe avoided. If referral is delayed more than 6 hours, the patient should be started on antibiotic drops every hour until seen by an ophthalmologist.

REFERRAL GUIDELINES

For lid lacerations involving the lid margin or lacrimal drainage system, the best results are attained if the primary repair by an ophthalmologist occurs within 12 hours of injury. Referral to an ophthalmologist for lid laceration repair can be delayed for up to 48 hours if other systemic medical conditions take precedence.

Superficial lacerations of the globe, which involve only the conjunctiva and show no signs of reduced vision or intraocular blood, can have ophthalmic referral delayed for a week or more and the patient treated with ice packs and gentamicin ointment four times a day.

If there is any question or concern for a deeper injury, then the patient should have a shield placed and be referred immediately. Any patient with a suspected ocular laceration with reduced vision should have a protective shield placed over the eye without pressure on the globe and sent immediately to an ophthalmologist for emergency intervention.

◖◗ TABLE 15.3. Referral Guidelines: Chemical Burns

DISEASE	SIGNS AND SYMPTOMS	TREATMENT	WHEN TO REFER
Acid burns (940.3)	Acute injury; redness, tearing, pain; less severe than alkali; photophobia	Anesthetic drops for examination only; assess degree of damage; irrigate with 500 cc of normal saline; remove residual particulate acids; patch, cycloplegia, gentamicin ointment; see each day until healed or referral needed	Refer only if vision down or cornea hazy; refer next day
Alkali burns (940.2)	Acute injury; redness, tearing, pain; very severe injury; corneal haze, necrosis; poor visibility of pupil	Anesthetic drops for examination only; assess degree of damage; irrigate with 500 cc of normal saline; remove residual particulate alkali; call ophthalmologist immediately if severe corneal and conjunctival necrosis; patch, cycloplegia, gentamicin ointment	Refer mild cornea hazy next day; refer severe corneal haze and conjunctival necrosis immediately

FREQUENCY OF VISITS

The patient with a conjunctival laceration or a simple corneal abrasion may need to be seen two or three times over a 2-week period to assess healing and prevent infection. Patients with globe lacerations often require surgical repair, and follow-up visits are highly variable as they are determined by the severity of injury.

CHEMICAL BURNS

Chemical burns to the eye can vary from a simple toxic conjunctivitis with no corneal involvement, to a devastating lye burn with necrosis of the lids and globe (Table 15.3). The degree of injury is most dependent on the acid or base characteristics (pH) of the chemical and the duration of contact. Although the initial emergency treatment of the injured eye should usually be done by the patient by flushing the eye with tap water, subsequent and immediate evaluation and therapy is often handled by the emergency room or primary care physician.

CLINICAL MANIFESTATIONS

The patient with a chemical burn will usually have a clear and distinct history of trauma, with knowledge of the time and setting of the injury. The patient will occasionally know the material causing the burn, but in cases of assault, this information may not always be available. The chemical burn may be associated with other forms of blunt or sharp injury (e.g., an automobile battery explosion to the face) and so other forms of injury must be looked for in addition.

Acid burns involve substances with a pH of less than 6.0. Common acids found with eye trauma include sulfuric acid from car batteries, sulfurous acid from bleaches and refrigerators, and hydrofluoric acid from metal refining work. When acid solution

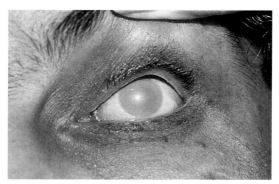

Figure 15.7.   Alkali burn with "cue ball" (totally white & necrotic) sclera and a "steamy" cornea.

or material comes in brief contact with tissue, the acid is neutralized by the surface tissue before it can penetrate to the deeper layers. Coagulation of surface tissue proteins acts as a barrier to further penetration. Acid injuries, therefore, tend to be more superficial and less destructive than alkali burns. However, the lower the pH, the more difficult the neutralizing process and the more extensive and severe the acid burn. Most acid burns will produce a conjunctival and/or a corneal epithelial defect, resulting in the symptoms of redness, profuse watery tearing, photophobia, and pain. Lid edema and a protective ptosis are also frequently associated. Anesthetic drops at the time of examination will relieve the patient's symptoms and allow a full examination. If the deeper cornea is uninvolved, the cornea will be clear and the vision nearly normal. Reduced vision and abnormal pupil, or a poor view of the interior structures of the globe, should alert the primary care physician to the possibility of deeper injury.

Alkali burns involve substances of a pH usually higher than 8.0. The most common alkali found in eye trauma are ammonia (NH_3), lye (NaOH), caustic potash (KOH), and lime [$Ca(OH)_2$]. An alkali substance penetrates tissue immediately, and the surface tissues are not as protective as in acid burns. The higher the pH, the deeper the tissue injury. With high pH, there is a saponification of fatty components of the cell membrane, resulting in immediate cell disruption and death. In addition to the general signs and symptoms of pain, redness, tearing, and photophobia, the coagulative necrosis caused by severe alkali injuries can present with more ominous signs. The appearance of an avascular, white "cue ball" conjunctiva and sclera with a hazy cornea is a grave prognostic sign (Fig. 15.7). The vision will be very poor and evaluation of pupillary response difficult. The relative absence of pain may indicate that the corneal nerves have been destroyed. Fluorescein staining for an epithelial defect may not be effective because there is total absence of any viable corneal or conjunctiva epithelium to create the contrasting edge for a recognizable staining pattern. Finally, facial skin and lid injuries may show blistering and necrosis which present other challenges to full evaluation of the globe.

The key to evaluating the chemically injured eye is to determine the pH of the chemical and the length of contact with the offending agent. The patient's family or coworkers should be encouraged to bring in the chemical and any descriptive product literature regarding the chemical to the initial examination. Although the initial emergency treatment is the same for acid or alkali injuries, the prognosis and secondary treatment will vary with the extent of injury. Finally, the physician must do a thorough examination to be certain that there are no other injuries to the globe (e.g. lacerations, intraocular foreign bodies, etc.) in addition to the chemical injury.

TREATMENT

The initial management of chemical burn trauma should follow the steps outlined for any trauma. Anesthetic drops should be applied and the vision, pupillary response, corneal clarity, and conjunctival redness all recorded. The pH of the tear film can be tested with a litmus test strip. If there is no sign of any perforations or lacerations, the eye should be irrigated with at least 500 cc of normal saline after anesthetic drops have been applied. Any particulate matter should be swabbed or flushed from beneath the lids. Irrigation should continue until the pH of the tears is neutralized. Patients with superficial burns can be treated as with a corneal abrasion, including application of gentamicin ointment, a drop of cycloplegic agent, and pressure patching until healed. Patients with deeper tissue damage (e.g., reduced vision or cloudy cornea) may be patched until seen by an ophthalmologist.

The prognosis of chemical burns is dependent upon the extent and depth of the injury. Patients with burns which destroy less than 75% of the surface tissue and do not involve the corneal endothelial layer and anterior chamber will generally recover full visual function with medical management. Eyes which suffer total surface coagulation or complete corneal opacification have a much worse prognosis. However, after primary healing occurs, unilateral injuries can be surgically rehabilitated with surface tissue transplanted from a fellow uninjured eye initially, followed by cadaveric corneal transplantation. Improved surgical techniques are increasingly successful in restoring vision to these severely burned eyes. However, even with primary healing and surgical visual rehabilitation, patients with severe chemical burns may have long-term disability from chronic dry eye, recurrent corneal erosion, glaucoma, uveitis, and a host of other vision threatening sequelae.

REFERRAL GUIDELINES

The severity of the injury should initially be assessed by the primary care physician and emergency or urgent treatment administered. If the vision is normal and the cornea is crystal clear, then only superficial damage has resulted and the patient can be treated with patching until full recovery. If deeper or more extensive injury is suspected in acid burns, then the patient should be patched and referred by the next day. In alkali burns, mild corneal haze from weak alkalis can be patched and referred within 24 hours. Patients with severe corneal haze and extensive conjunctival necrosis should be referred immediately.

FREQUENCY OF VISITS

Patients with superficial burns will require two or three visits in the first week until the chemical epithelial abrasion heals with a final visit 3–4 weeks after the injury to evaluate any long-term sequelae. Patients with extensive or deeper burns (usually alkali) may require hospitalization and surgical intervention to save the eye, with frequent visits necessary after discharge to assess and treat the myriad of complications resulting from this devastating injury.

SUGGESTED READINGS

Asbury T, Tabbara K. Initial examination of ocular trauma. In: Vaughan D, Asbury T, Tabbara K, eds. General ophthalmology. San Mateo, CA: Appleton & Lange, 1989:343–344.

Asbury T, Tabbara K. Abrasions and lacerations of the lids. In: Vaughan D, Asbury T, Tabbara K, eds. General ophthalmology. San Mateo, CA: Appleton & Lange, 1989:343–344.

Eagling E, Roper-Hall M. Fractures of the orbit. In: Eye injuries: an illustrated guide. Philadelphia: JB Lippincott, 1986:32–36.

Herman D. Evaluation and care of injuries to the eye and ocular adnexa. In: Bartley G, Liesengang T, eds. Essentials of ophthalmology. Philadelphia: JB Lippincott, 1992:275–283.

Wagoner M, Kenyon K. Chemical injuries. In: Shingleton B, Hersh P, Kenyon K, eds. Eye trauma. St Louis: Mosby-Year Book, 1991:79–94.

PART B
Orbital Disorders

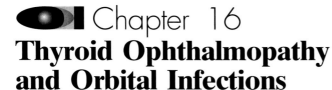 Chapter 16
Thyroid Ophthalmopathy and Orbital Infections

W. T. Shults

INTRODUCTION

The orbit contains an amazing variety of tissues with a correspondingly large number of clinical disorders thereof. This chapter deals with the more common of these clinical problems, including thyroid ophthalmopathy, orbital cellulitis, mucormycosis, and idiopathic orbital inflammatory pseudotumor. Before discussing these individual disorders, the reader may wish to review the basics of orbital anatomy described in Appendix A, "Basic Orbital and Ocular Anatomy."

PATIENT EXAMINATION

Much can be learned by examination of a patient with orbital pathology. The presence of proptosis, the sine qua non of orbital mischief, is often best determined by viewing the patient from above and behind judging the relative position of each cornea. While there are a variety of instruments devised for performing this measurement, the "bird's-eye" view afforded by this technique (Fig. 16.1) is probably as reliable as any other method, though it does not afford the ability to reproducibly quantify the degree of proptosis. Viewing old photos can be of great help in defining the duration of an orbital problem. Resistance to retrocession of the globe may signal a retrobulbar mass. This is easily accomplished by simultaneously applying gentle pressure on the globes though closed lids and sensing differential resistance to backward movement of one globe into the orbit. A firm mass lesion such as an orbital tumor will be relatively noncompressible, thus impeding posterior movement of the globe, while proptosis produced by a vascular lesion such as an orbital varix will recede in the face of such gentle pressure. Pain on palpation regularly accompanies orbital inflammatory disorders, while it is rare in orbital tumors and endocrine exophthalmos.

Inspection readily reveals lid edema, conjunctival injection, conjunctival edema (chemosis), lid retraction, lid lag, and limitation of ocular movement, all features characteristic of thyroid ophthalmopathy. These signs should be looked for in every

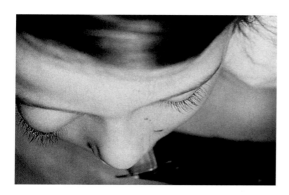

Figure 16.1. Viewing the patient from above facilitates appreciation of relative proptosis as this picture of a child with unilateral proptosis from optic nerve glioma illustrates.

proptotic patient given the frequency with which thyroid ophthalmopathy produces such a clinical picture.

Examination of the fundus in patients with orbital disease may be helpful. Orbital tumors may produce visible (usually transverse) folds in the retina and choroid seen when viewing the posterior pole of the eye (Fig. 16.5). An occasional patient with an enlarged globe due to high myopia will present with longstanding proptosis. This outpouching of the highly myopic globe (known as a staphyloma) may be suspected from the fundus appearance showing retinal thinning in the affected area. Optic nerve sheath meningiomas, while relatively uncommon tumors, can be predicted with high reliability in a proptotic patient with optic atrophy and the presence of optociliary shunt vessels on the optic disc (Fig. 16.2). The presence of unusual vessels on the surface of an atrophic optic nerve head should prompt referral to an ophthalmologist for further assessment. In addition to optic nerve sheath meningiomas, such vessels may occasionally herald the presence of optic nerve glioma, arachnoid sheath cyst, or orbital apex meningioma, as well as a compensated central retinal vein occlusion.

The orbit lends itself very nicely to neuroimaging with ultrasound, computed tomography (CT), and magnetic resonance imaging (MRI). The use of these techniques is discussed in Section III, "Specialized Ophthalmic Tests."

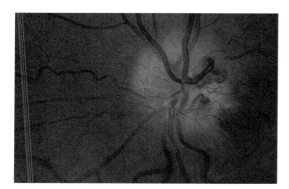

Figure 16.2. Optociliary shunts, optic atrophy, and slowly progressive vision loss strongly imply a compressive optic neuropathy such as an optic nerve sheath meningioma which impedes egress of blood from the eye through the central retinal vein causing shunt vessels to form to reroute blood from the retina to the choroidal circulation.

◼︎◼︎ TABLE 16.1. Referral Guidelines: Thyroid Ophthalmopathy

SYMPTOM OR SIGN (CODE)	TREATMENT	WHEN TO REFER
Lid retraction (374.41)	Topical lubricants (gtts or ointments), air-tight shield taped over orbits at night; surgery if corneal exposure	If corneal epithelium is compromised despite conservative measures
Lid lag (374.41)	Surgery if cosmetic problem	If patient troubled by cosmetic appearance
Conjunctival chemosis (372.73)	Same as for lid retraction above; may respond to systemic steroids; rarely requires surgical excision	If patient troubled by cosmetic appearance
Conjunctival injection (372.71)	Same as for lid retraction above; may respond to systemic steroids	Not an indication for referral unless diagnosis in doubt, then referral appropriate
Proptosis (376.30)	Nothing, steroids, radiation, or surgery depending on associated findings	If associated with diplopia or evidence of optic neuropathy
Diplopia (368.2)	Monocular patching, systemic steroids, radiation, or surgery on the ocular muscles	Diplopia should prompt referral for at least a baseline evaluation even if conservative treatment is elected
Blurred vision, decreased light brightness sense or decreased peripheral visual field (368.8)	Depends on the cause	Should be referred to allow definition of which of the many possible causes of vision loss is operative

DIFFERENTIAL DIAGNOSIS

THYROID OPHTHALMOPATHY

Though known by a variety of names (Graves' ophthalmopathy, infiltrative ophthalmopathy, congestive orbitopathy, thyroid eye disease, the eye changes of Graves' disease, malignant exophthalmos, endocrine exophthalmos, dysthyroid ophthalmopathy, dysthyroid restrictive myopathy), thyroid ophthalmopathy is universally recognized as the most common cause of orbital pathology in adults (Table 16.1). Glaser states it is the most common cause of spontaneous diplopia in middle age and early senescence. Involvement before age 20 is uncommon. Though the signs and symptoms of well-established thyroid eye disease generally present no diagnostic problems, the early presentation of this condition can be less obvious. Not uncommonly, patients with early motility dysfunction are thought to have various ocular motor nerve palsies prompting a fruitless and expensive neuroimaging search for intracranial pathology. It should be remembered that thyroid ophthalmopathy is a clinical diagnosis and is not dependent upon the presence of any abnormal thyroid function studies. Failure to appreciate this fact has delayed diagnosis in countless patients whose presentation, while typical of thyroid ophthalmopathy, did not prompt consideration of this diagnosis because the laboratory tests were negative for a thyroid metabolic disturbance.

The ocular muscle enlargement which characterizes thyroid ophthalmopathy results from the deposition of mucopolysaccharide and infiltration by lymphocytes and plasma cells in the muscle tissue. Histochemical staining suggests that the mucopolysaccharide derives from fibroblastic activation, which in turn causes progressive fibrosis of the muscle with consequential restrictive ophthalmoplegia.

CLINICAL MANIFESTATIONS

Patients with Graves' orbitopathy often voice complaints of scratchiness and irritation of the eyes, generally worse upon awakening. They may also complain of a pulling or tightness in their orbits especially when attempting to look in an upward direction. Transient diplopia may give way to more constant double vision as restrictive changes affect the ocular muscles. Both vertical and horizontal diplopia may be present in combination or in isolation depending upon the direction of gaze and the pattern of muscle involvement. The inferior rectus muscles are most often affected with the medial rectus muscles being the next most commonly involved. Increased light sensitivity and tearing are frequent accompaniments of endocrine ophthalmopathy. Blurred vision may connote superficial changes in the corneal epithelium secondary to exposure from a reduction in the patient's blink rate, or it may portend the more ominous onset of compressive optic neuropathy stemming from enlargement of the ocular muscles in the orbital apex.

A very important early clue to the diagnosis of thyroid eye disease is the presence of unilateral or bilateral lid retraction. Often the lid signs antedate the appearance of other manifestations of Graves' orbitopathy by a considerable period so attention to their presence permits prompt diagnosis of otherwise cryptic symptoms. It is best to look at the resting position of the lids when taking the history, as many patients will unknowingly widen their palpebral fissures once the formal "examination" commences. Normally, the resting position of the open upper lid is about 1.0 mm below the corneoscleral junction (limbus), obscuring the uppermost portion of the iris. Lid retraction exists if one can see the superior limbus (i.e., if one is able to see sclera above the upper corneoscleral junction). While there is some interpatient variability in the resting position of the lid, the presence of "scleral show" coupled with lid lag implies pathologic lid positioning (Fig. 16.3). Lid lag is tested by asking the patient to fixate a relatively rapidly moving descending target. Normally the upper lid descends with the globe, but in the patient with lid lag, the lid will lag behind the descending globe. The degree of lid retraction is often enhanced when the patient gazes in a downward direction. It is important to take into account any redundant upper lid skin (dermatochalasis) which may be hanging over the upper lid margin and obscuring the presence of otherwise apparent lid retraction. Patients will sometimes complain of the normal lid drooping when, in fact, the opposite lid is pathologically retracted.

Conjunctival vascular injection is common particularly overlying the points of insertion of the medial and lateral rectus muscles but may also be rather generalized.

Conjunctival chemosis is a common early sign most apparent as a clear, fluid-filled roll of conjunctiva extending over the temporal lower lid to a variable degree.

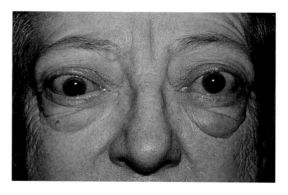

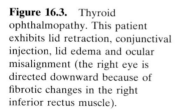

Figure 16.3. Thyroid ophthalmopathy. This patient exhibits lid retraction, conjunctival injection, lid edema and ocular misalignment (the right eye is directed downward because of fibrotic changes in the right inferior rectus muscle).

Often, this finding is greatest when the patient arises and gradually diminishes as the day progresses. Conjunctival injection often accompanies chemosis and is especially apparent overlying the insertions of the medial and lateral rectus muscles, which may be more apparent because of the muscle enlargement seen in thyroid eye disease. Edema may also affect the upper and lower lids and is often the concern which brings the patient to the physician. The degree of edema can vary from barely detectable to extreme, though the latter is relatively uncommon. It, too, tends to be most noticeable when the patient first awakens in the morning after a night with the orbits in a relatively dependent position, and improves with the assumption of a more upright posture.

In those patients complaining of diplopia, the most common limitation of ocular motility is a reduction in elevation of one or both eyes resulting from involvement of the inferior rectus muscles with a restrictive myopathic process. Fibrotic change within the muscle belly permits relatively normal muscle contraction, but impairs relaxation with a resultant tethering of the globe on attempted upgaze. Though most often bilateral, the degree of ocular muscle involvement is commonly asymmetrical. In some patients, the degree of functional motility impairment seemingly affects only a single muscle in one orbit with diplopia restricted to only one field of gaze, while in others, all of the ocular muscles are affected with resultant severe limitation of eye movement in all planes. In more advanced cases, hypotropia (one eye fixing lower than the other) or esotropia (one eye crossing relative to the other) may arise from progressive fibrosis in the inferior rectus or medial rectus muscles respectively. A clue to the presence of a restrictive myopathy is an intraocular pressure which rises dramatically (>7 mm Hg) in upgaze during which the globe's intraocular pressure is affected by an actively contracting superior rectus and a relatively unyielding inferior rectus. Intraocular pressure is commonly elevated in thyroid eye disease, even in the absence of restrictive myopathy or proptosis. As mentioned earlier, motility disturbances are usually preceded by the signs of congestive orbitopathy previously discussed.

Complaints of blurred vision are relatively common in patients with thyroid ophthalmopathy and may stem from increased tearing, superficial corneal changes resulting from incomplete blinking of retracted lids, minimal diplopia, or from compressive optic neuropathy. The latter is accompanied by signs of afferent pathway dysfunction such as decreased visual acuity, color vision, contrast sensitivity, pupillary function, and visual field. Vision loss due to optic nerve compression in thyroid eye disease is usually of gradual onset and characterized by greater central than peripheral depres-

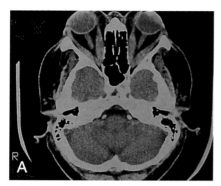
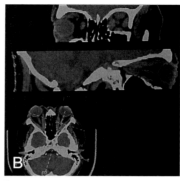

Figure 16.4.   Axial (**A**) and coronal and sagittal (**B**) CT images of orbits in patient with thyroid ophthalmopathy. Note enlargement of muscle bellies in the posterior and mid-orbit and relative preservation of tendinous insertions. Coronal and sagittal views are particularly suited to defining impingement of ocular muscles on apical optic nerve.

sion. Rarely, arcuate visual field defects occur. Because the detection and quantification of these deficits requires special testing techniques and follow-up, referral to an ophthalmologist is appropriate for any thyroid eye disease patient who voices complaints of blurred vision.

Muscle enlargement in thyroid ophthalmopathy tends to be most apparent in the apical portions of the muscle bellies with relatively less enlargement in the more anterior portion of the muscle and sparing of the tendinous insertions of the muscle to the globe. This pattern provides a useful neuroimaging differential diagnostic clue for distinguishing the myopathy of Graves' disease from that of idiopathic inflammatory orbital pseudotumor in which the tendinous muscle insertions are characteristically enlarged (Fig. 16.4). Apical muscle enlargement in thyroid eye disease impinges upon the optic nerve passing through the annulus of Zinn. This compression may be associated with optic disc edema presumably due to interruption of axoplasmic transport in the compressed nerve fibers. However, the fundus may also be completely normal in a patient with compressive optic neuropathy so the absence of funduscopic abnormalities should not dissuade one from the diagnosis in the face of other evidence of afferent pathway dysfunction. Though patients with thyroid ophthalmopathy often exhibit proptosis, those who develop compressive optic neuropathy often are *not* those with the most profound degree of globe protrusion. Rather, they may have little or no proptosis, presumably because their muscle enlargement is more isolated to the apex with a lesser degree in the main portion of the muscle bellies. Funduscopy may also demonstrate choroidal folds in some patients with endocrine exophthalmos (Fig. 16.5). Surprisingly, their presence does not seem to correlate with the degree of proptosis.

Proptosis in patients with thyroid ophthalmopathy is common, particularly in those with extensive ocular muscle enlargement. The boney confines of the orbit permit only one route of exit for expanding orbital tissues–forward. While the direction of displacement is generally straight-ahead, isolated enlargement of one or more muscles can divert the direction of the globe downward or inward, potentially providing a false localization for the problem (i.e., a downwardly directed globe in a patient with thyroid ophthalmopathy implies restrictive myopathy of the inferior rectus muscle, not a superior orbital tumor).

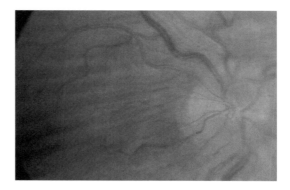

Figure 16.5. Choroidal folds in a patient with thyroid ophthalmopathy. Such horizontal ripples in the choroid may occur without associated disc edema or visual loss. (See also color section.)

Neuroimaging, particularly CT scanning, provides elegant depictions of the orbital contents in axial and coronal planes. In the infancy of CT scanning, inferior rectus enlargement in patients with thyroid optic neuropathy was mistaken for orbital tumor, but the use of coronal and reconstructed off-axis sagittal images in the plane of the optic nerve has eliminated this confusion. In addition to revealing the location and extent of ocular muscle enlargement in a clinically involved orbit, CT scanning often discloses subclinical muscle enlargement in the clinically "uninvolved" orbit.

While thyroid ophthalmopathy is the most common cause of proptosis and diplopia in the adult population, idiopathic inflammatory orbital pseudotumor, orbital cellulitis, and orbital tumors all share certain features that mimic thyroid eye disease and can cause confusion as to the correct diagnosis. However, these conditions are usually differentiable on clinical and neuroradiologic grounds. While the clinical picture of thyroid ophthalmopathy is often unmistakable, confusion can arise in patients with early symptoms and signs or in those with atypical presentations.

Idiopathic inflammatory orbital pseudotumor shares a number of features with thyroid ophthalmopathy in that both can produce proptosis, periorbital edema, conjunctival injection, diplopia with impaired ocular motility, and optic neuropathy. While exceptions do occur, orbital pseudotumor is most often unilateral, usually more abrupt in onset and quite painful. The pain is generally exacerbated by eye movement and is exquisitely sensitive to systemic corticosteroid therapy. Orbital pseudotumor often causes a CT picture of scleral thickening and ill-defined infiltration of orbital fat surrounding the ocular muscles and optic nerve. Muscle insertions are thickened rather than spared.

Orbital cellulitis, an acute bacterial infection of the orbital contents, can mimic thyroid ophthalmopathy but is more abrupt in onset and is accompanied by such systemic signs as fever and elevated white count. A superficial skin lesion or evidence of coexistent sinusitis is generally present. Orbital cellulitis is distinctly more common in children than thyroid ophthalmopathy which, as noted earlier, is quite rare before the age of 20. It is generally more difficult to separate idiopathic orbital pseudotumor from orbital cellulitis than to differentiate either from thyroid eye disease.

Orbital tumors can also mimic thyroid ophthalmopathy, but are not accompanied by lid retraction and lid lag, and have a distinctively different neuroimaging picture from the ocular muscle enlargement so typical of Graves' orbitopathy.

It cannot be overemphasized that the diagnosis of thyroid eye disease is a clinical one and is not dependent upon the demonstration of any abnormalities of thyroid function with even the most sophisticated laboratory tests. Thus, if the clinical signs are compatible with a diagnosis of thyroid ophthalmopathy the clinician should not discard it in the absence of abnormal thyroid function studies. Only 40% of patients with euthyroid Graves' disease in some studies have had a positive thyrotropin-releasing hormone (TRH) test.

TREATMENT

Thyroid orbitopathy is ultimately a self-limited disease; however, the clinical course may extend over years before activity subsides. Given the unpredictable course, it seems reasonable to begin with symptomatic therapy for signs of mild congestive orbitopathy consisting of elevating the head of the bed at night, use of ointments and drops for symptoms of exposure keratopathy, and use of a mild diuretic for relief of periorbital edema. Worsening symptoms can be treated with systemic steroid therapy in doses up to 120 mg of prednisone daily, which is generally effective within 3 weeks. If no improvement is evident after that period of time, another therapeutic approach should be tried. In such patients, orbital radiation may be beneficial, though not risk-free. Thyroid optic neuropathy may respond to such treatment, but if ineffective, orbital decompression is warranted to relieve pressure on the apical optic nerve. Many would skip the radiation step and move directly to surgical intervention, though opinion is divided on this point. Many methods of orbital decompression have been proposed, but authorities now agree that the key to a successful outcome is to adequately decompress the apex of the orbit as that is where optic nerve impingement is greatest. Removal of the medial and inferior orbital wall provides as much as an additional 15 cc of orbital volume and produces excellent results in the hands of experienced surgeons. Fixed ocular motility deficits secondary to restrictive myopathy require ocular muscle (strabismus) surgery to restore some semblance of normal motility. While results are usually excellent, in some patients residual motility problems persist. Lid retraction can be of sufficient magnitude that corneal protection is compromised. Less dramatic degrees of retraction are a common cosmetic complaint of patients with dysthyroid ophthalmopathy. Plastic surgery procedures on the retractors of the upper lid afford relief and improve the patient's appearance.

The most difficult aspect of caring for patients with Graves' orbitopathy is making the patient comfortable with the notion that they have a condition for which there is palliative, but not curative, treatment. Graves' patients often have a difficult time accepting that their physician knows their diagnosis, but seems, at times, powerless to completely relieve their complaints. Assisting the patient in arriving at an accommodation with their disease is one of the most time consuming, yet rewarding, aspects of caring for patients with this disorder. Since thyroid ophthalmopathy is ultimately a self-limited disease, a good rule of thumb is to "do as little as possible for as long as possible." The patient's clinical course may force the physician's hand, but temporizing is often the best approach. Glaser said it best: "sometimes with regard to thyroid ophthalmopathy it's better to just stand there, don't do something."

FREQUENCY OF VISITS

How often one follows a patient with thyroid ophthalmopathy depends entirely upon the severity of the patient's symptoms. For a patient with mild lid retraction and

◼▮ TABLE 16.2. Referral Guidelines: Idiopathic Inflammatory Pseudotumor

SYMPTOM OR SIGN (CODE)	TREATMENT	WHEN TO REFER
Painful proptosis with periorbital edema and chemosis (372.73/ 376.33)	Systemic steroids in dose range of 60–80 mg/day	Failure of symptoms to resolve, or recurrence of symptoms as steroids decreased, or if uncertain about diagnosis
Diplopia (368.2)	Systemic steroids in dose range of 60–80 mg/day	Failure of symptoms to resolve, or recurrence of symptoms as steroids decreased, or if uncertain about diagnosis
Blurred vision (368.8)	Systemic steroids in dose range of 60–80 mg/day	Failure of symptoms to resolve, or recurrence of symptoms as steroids decreased, or if uncertain about diagnosis

minimal periorbital edema which is nonprogressive, follow-up at 6 month intervals or longer may suffice as long as the patient knows to come in promptly in the face of progressive symptoms. Given the obtrusive nature of such symptoms as diplopia and visual loss, most patients can be relied upon to seek medical attention in a timely manner. For patients whose symptoms warrant systemic steroid therapy because of diplopia, or compressive optic neuropathy, weekly, or even daily, follow-up may be necessary. While compressive optic neuropathy in dysthyroid ophthalmopathy generally evolves gradually, more rapid decline can occur and the patient may require urgent orbital decompression to avert permanent visual loss. The approach must be individualized to the patient.

IDIOPATHIC INFLAMMATORY ORBITAL PSEUDOTUMOR

A variety of space-occupying inflammatory conditions involving one or more orbital structures are subsumed under the rubric of idiopathic inflammatory orbital pseudotumor (Table 16.2). The process may involve one or several types of orbital tissues and may be acute or subacute in presentation. When the involvement is localized to a single tissue it is named accordingly; for example, myositis (ocular muscle), dacryoadenitis (lacrimal gland), perineuritis (optic nerve), and so on. The clinical manifestations vary according to the structures involved and whether the onset is acute or subacute. All age groups are affected. Involvement is usually unilateral, though sequential and bilateral simultaneous cases have occurred. The latter may be a harbinger of a systemic disorder such as Wegener's granulomatosis. Collagen vascular diseases may also manifest as orbital pseudotumor. The inflammatory infiltrate in orbital pseudotumor consists variably of lymphocytes, plasma cells, reticulum cells, macrophages, giant cells, fibroblasts, and, occasionally, polymorphonuclear neutrophils and eosinophils.

CLINICAL MANIFESTATIONS

Periorbital pain, proptosis, lid swelling (sometimes with reddish discoloration), periorbital edema, chemosis, and diplopia are the cardinal symptoms and signs of orbital pseudotumor, though not all are found in every patient and the evolution varies from acute to indolent. As implied earlier, the presentation depends upon whether the orbital involvement is localized or diffuse—orbital myositis will produce motility disturbance while dacryoadenitis will cause more focal swelling in the lacrimal fossa and surrounding tissues. Optic nerve involvement with concomitant vision loss is not as common a complaint. As in thyroid ophthalmopathy, conjunctival vascular engorgement over the insertions of the ocular muscles is typical. Some patients experience generalized malaise.

Thyroid ophthalmopathy shares many of the clinical features of orbital pseudotumor. Both tend to involve the inferior rectus muscle preferentially though this propensity is less regular in pseudotumor than in thyroid eye disease. Pain is a more prominent feature of orbital pseudotumor and tends to be a predominant complaint, whereas pain is not prominent in thyroid ophthalmopathy and, when present, is most often related to either corneal exposure or eye movement in directions restricted by myopathy. Neuroimaging features are often helpful in distinguishing one from the other. As mentioned in the section on thyroid eye disease, orbital muscle involvement in Graves' orbitopathy generally spares the muscle tendons, while that in orbital pseudotumor produces enlargement of the tendinous insertions. Scleral thickening is another distinguishing feature not found in the typical thyroid ophthalmopathy patient (Fig. 16.4). Inflammatory infiltration of the orbital fat can often be identified in orbital pseudotumor cases. Despite these differentiating features, it may not be possible to define which clinical entity one is dealing with on the basis of neuroimaging studies alone. Diplopia arises earlier in the clinical course of orbital pseudotumor than in thyroid ophthalmopathy. Orbital pseudotumor tends to be much more responsive to systemic steroid therapy than thyroid orbitopathy which, though improved by steroids, tends to require higher doses to produce a favorable response. Lastly, orbital pseudotumor is much more often unilateral than is thyroid ophthalmopathy which is regularly bilateral, though not uncommonly asymmetrical in its involvement.

Spontaneous dural cavernous sinus fistulas may produce clinical signs which mimic those of inflammatory orbital pseudotumor, though the arterialized vessels of the former are a very helpful clue not found in pseudotumor patients. Metastatic neoplasms to the orbit may present with rather fulminant proptosis and pain, but the CT picture clarifies the diagnosis. Systemic lymphoma may arise in the orbit. Biopsy of the orbital mass coupled with a systemic evaluation (physical examination, serum protein electrophoresis, bone marrow aspiration) is usually necessary in such cases.

TREATMENT

Dramatic steroid sensitivity is a regular feature of orbital pseudotumor. It is not uncommon for pain to diminish within the first 24 hours of treatment with rather rapid subsidence of proptosis and periorbital edema following. Sixty to 80 mg of prednisone daily for 2–4 weeks followed by a gradual taper will be sufficient in the majority of patients. Unfortunately, recrudescence of symptoms may develop with reduction in the steroid dosage. Recurrences, either in the same or opposite orbit, can occur and some patients have a chronic course which is suppressed but not cured by systemic

●I TABLE 16.3. Referral Guidelines: Mucormycosis		
SYMPTOM OR SIGN	**TREATMENT**	**WHEN TO REFER**
Periorbital pain, proptosis, periorbital edema, sudden ophthalmoplegia, blindness in a diabetic or immunosuppressed patient	Immediate biopsy of sinus to establish diagnosis and begin amphotericin B therapy when broad, nonseptate hyphae seen in tissue; consider surgical debridement in all cases	Such cases are best approached by a multidisciplinary team including ophthalmologists, rhinologist, infectious disease specialist, and orbital/neurosurgeon

steroid therapy. Orbital radiation and immunosuppressive therapies are reserved for such recalcitrant orbitopathies. Despite our best efforts, rare patients fail to respond to all therapeutic modalities and develop a blind, immobile, painful globe requiring orbital exenteration for relief.

FREQUENCY OF VISITS

The patient's pain and periorbital edema should begin to respond within 24–48 hours. Failure to see such improvement casts doubt upon the diagnosis of orbital pseudotumor. Thus, the patient should be seen within a day or so of initiating steroid therapy to insure that a favorable response has occurred. If the patient is a reliable observer, such a determination could be made by phone, but it is always more prudent to personally observe the expected reduction in periorbital inflammatory response. A return visit after 10–14 days is appropriate to assess the extent of continued improvement, with telephone contact thereafter as long as improvement continues. Thereafter, the patient can be seen as dictated by symptoms. If pain and edema recur, or if the improvement engendered by higher dose corticosteroids ceases as the dose is diminished, then a return visit will be necessary to reassess the therapeutic options. Vision loss requires an urgent visit, as the decrease in vision can be rapid and is best dealt with sooner rather than later (usually with a boost of the corticosteroid dosage). Recurrence of symptoms as corticosteroids are tapered can often be ameliorated by increasing the dose slightly and tapering more slowly. A prolonged taper (over 6 months or more) may be necessary in some patients. As in thyroid ophthalmopathy, the approach must be individualized to the patient.

MUCORMYCOSIS

Mucormycosis (phycomycosis, zygomycosis) is one of the most feared and acutely fatal fungus infections of man (Table 16.3). This ubiquitous organism is probably inhaled daily by most humans. Neuro-ophthalmic symptoms in mucor infections most often occur through tissue infarction engendered by the propensity of the organism to invade and occlude blood vessels as it spreads from the nose to orbit and cavernous sinus. Symptoms progress rapidly, and if diagnosis is delayed, or treatment ineffective, the clinical course to death is measured in days to weeks. Patients are often diabetics with or without ketoacidosis, or immunocompromised by systemic disease or corticosteroid therapy. Rarely, the infection can arise in a host who seemingly has no risk factors.

Interestingly, acquired immune deficiency syndrome (AIDS) patients are not often infected with this organism because they usually have adequate circulating polymorphonuclear neutrophils (PMNs).

CLINICAL MANIFESTATIONS

Given the predominantly vaso-occlusive nature of the pathogenesis of the orbital pathology in rhinocerebral mucormycosis, it is not surprising that sudden painful visual loss may herald the onset of this disease. Orbital swelling in an acutely ill, immunocompromised patient with an immobile, proptotic blind eye and evidence of sinusitis, should instantly prompt consideration of this fungal infection. Evidence of central retinal artery occlusion (cloudy retinal swelling with a "cherry-red" spot present in the macula) may also be present, as might a black eschar involving the palate, nasal mucosa, or periorbital skin. In addition to orbital/facial pain, facial numbness and weakness may follow as the organisms spread rapidly across the skull base to involve the fifth and seventh cranial nerves. Even corneal ulceration and gangrene of the eye have been reported. Though initially unilateral, if undiagnosed and untreated, the infection may spread to involve the contralateral orbit within days. Involvement of the internal carotid artery within the cavernous sinus may lead to cerebral infarction and hemiparesis, aphasia, or seizures. Given the often precipitous onset and magnitude of the clinical dysfunction seen in mucormycosis, the neuroimaging findings are often surprisingly modest. Sinusitis (often mild) with evidence of subtle boney destruction is commonly present. Though MRI fails to define these bony defects as well as CT, it is able to define the vascular occlusive process involving the internal carotid artery which so often accompanies this condition.

A diagnosis of mucormycosis must be considered in any patient with acute onset of periorbital/facial pain, proptosis, ophthalmoplegia, and blindness, particularly if they are diabetic or immunocompromised. Confirmation with a tissue diagnosis is crucial and should be obtained on an emergency basis. The demonstration of broad, nonseptate branching hyphae in the removed tissue, given this clinical setting, should prompt initiation of amphotericin B therapy while awaiting final mycologic identification of the organism. Aspergillus infections in the sinuses can also produce orbital apex syndromes (ophthalmoplegia and visual loss), but the course is far more indolent and less apt to be associated with a debilitated or diabetic patient. Orbital cellulitis patients may mimic the clinical findings of patients with mucormycosis; however, the infarctive nature of the latter with such signs as central retinal artery occlusion and eschar formation are not part of the picture in orbital cellulitis which more often affects a younger age group.

TREATMENT

The ultimate therapeutic outcome in patients with mucormycosis is as dependent upon appropriate management of the underlying condition as it is upon timely diagnosis and treatment of the fungal infection. Diabetic hyperglycemia and acidosis must be promptly controlled and corticosteroids or immunosuppression therapy reduced or discontinued if possible. Amphotericin B in liposomal or colloidal form should be instituted immediately (1.0–1.5 mg/kg/day). Prognosis may be improved through the use of the liposomal delivery system for amphotericin B which allows for higher

TABLE 16.4. Referral Guidelines: Preseptal and Orbital Cellulitis

SYMPTOM OR SIGN (CODE)	TREATMENT	WHEN TO REFER
Preseptal cellulitis: edema and erythema of lids with minimal signs of orbital involvement (such as impaired ocular motility) (373.13)	In infants and small children I.V. antibiotics (penicillinase-resistant penicillins if suspect staphylococcus or streptococcus [most common] or amoxicillin or 2nd or 3rd generation cephalosporins if suspect haemophillus)	Infectious disease input extremely valuable in determining optimum choice of antibiotic; such input is essential if response to initial therapy is inadequate (progressive symptoms or signs of extension of preseptal process into orbit while patient on treatment)
Orbital cellulitis: pain on eye movement, proptosis, ophthalmoplegia, chemosis, visual loss, pupillary abnormality (376.01)	I.V. antibiotics based initially upon empiric choice and subsequently upon results of cultures; penicillinase-resistant penicillins reasonable first choice as staphylococcus and streptococcus are most common organisms in adults while H. flu (amoxicillin) common in infants and small children	As with preseptal cellulitis, input from an infectious disease consultant may be invaluable in selecting the optimum antibiotic; this is imperative in patients with cavernous sinus thrombosis and/or meningitis; orbital abscess formation will require the services of an orbital surgeon for drainage while persistent paranasal sinus infection may require otolaryngolic consultation for possible drainage

doses. Treatment is best carried out in concert with an infectious disease consultant. Aggressive tissue debridement is usually necessary to provide the best chance of cure. Repeated surgery, including orbital exenteration, may be necessary to save the patient's life. Adjunctive therapy with hyperbaric oxygen may improve the prognosis.

Even with these measures, the prognosis for recovery is only about 50%. The prognosis is worse when the central nervous system is affected, or if the internal carotid artery or cavernous sinus are occluded. Blindness is permanent and the recovery of neurologic deficits unpredictable.

FREQUENCY OF VISITS

Mucormycosis should be managed in an in-patient setting.

ORBITAL CELLULITIS

Orbital cellulitis results from an acute bacterial infection of the orbital tissues, usually spreading from the paranasal sinuses or the skin of the lid (Table 16.4). Infections in this region are usually divided into two types: those affecting tissues anterior to the orbital septum (preseptal cellulitis) and those arising in tissues posterior to the septum (orbital cellulitis). If not diagnosed and treated promptly, extension into the cavernous sinus with consequent cavernous sinus thrombosis is possible.

CLINICAL MANIFESTATIONS
PRESEPTAL CELLULITIS

Infection of the preseptal tissues often results from introduction of bacteria from lid trauma or a superficial skin lesion. Edema and erythema of the lid may be severe, but the globe is uninvolved and there is minimal chemosis, and no ocular motility disturbance or pupillary involvement. Visual acuity is unaffected. If proptosis, reduced acuity, altered motility, or pupillary abnormalities arise, then the infection has likely spread into the orbit proper. Particulary in younger children, bacteremia, septicemia, and even meningitis may occur, emphasizing the need for prompt diagnosis and treatment. Even with preseptal infection, the child may be febrile and a peripheral leukocytosis may exist with either a preseptal or an orbital cellulitis.

ORBITAL CELLULITIS

Infection posterior to the orbital septum may arise from the paranasal sinuses, extend from a preseptal infection (discussed earlier), arise from septic embolization, or result from extension of an infection of the lacrimal gland (dacryoadenitis), or even from the globe itself (endophthalmitis). The patient is usually systemically ill with fever and leukocytosis. Pain on eye movement, proptosis, chemosis, ocular motility disturbance, reduced vision, and presence of an afferent pupillary defect all characterize infection of the retroseptal space and alert the clinician to the risk of abscess formation or extension of the orbital infection to involve the cavernous sinus. Prompt and aggressive therapy is essential to avoid these complications. Computerized tomography may reveal paranasal sinus infection and orbital infiltration, as well as abscess formation. Failure to respond to antibiotic therapy and the presence of orbital fluctuance signify the formation of an orbital abscess requiring surgical drainage.

It may be difficult to define whether a preseptal infection has extended into the orbital space, as even in the absence of infection there is often substantial inflammation of the orbital tissues in response to a preseptal cellulitis. CT scanning may be of some help in deciding if the orbit is involved, but may not be diagnostic. The clinical differentiation of orbital cellulitis from cavernous sinus thrombosis is difficult to impossible. In cavernous sinus thrombosis, there is usually a cellular reaction in the cerebrospinal fluid and cultures of spinal fluid are often positive for the causative organism. The appearance of ocular motility impairment of the contralateral eye signals extension of the thrombotic process across the midline through anastomotic connections into the other cavernous sinus (Fig. 16.6).

TREATMENT

Early treatment of orbital cellulitis is empirical while awaiting culture results from skin, conjunctiva, nasopharynx and perhaps cerebrospinal fluid. The most common

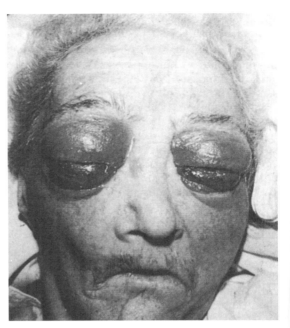

Figure 16.6. Septic cavernous sinus thrombosis causing massive bilateral proptosis, eyelid swelling, and hemorrhagic conjunctival chemosis in an 82-year-old woman with bacterial sinusitis. The patient was blind and had bilateral complete ophthalmoplegia. (Reprinted with permission from Daxecker F, Bichler E. Beidseitiger Exophthalmus Be: Sinus-cavernosus-Thrombose. Klin. Monatsbl. Augenheilkd 182:235–236, 1983).

organisms are *Staphylococcus aureus* and *Streptococcus.* Treatment with a penicillinase-resistant penicillin in either intravenous (usually indicated in infants and young children) or oral form is the initial treatment of choice. Some young children with a history of a recent upper respiratory infection, fever, and coryza will develop a preseptal or orbital cellulitis secondary to *Haemophilus influenzae* requiring treatment with amoxicillin or one of the cephalosporins. The ultimate drug chosen will depend upon the results of cultures and smears (and perhaps biopsy in the case of fungal infections) and should be determined in consultation with an infectious disease specialist given the profusion of therapeutic agents available today and the importance of aggressive treatment to prevent complications of abscess formation or cavernous sinus thrombosis. Should an abscess form, then surgical drainage will need to be accomplished, the best route being determined on the basis of neuroimaging studies and clinical signs such as localized fluctuance in a lid. If sinusitis accompanies orbital cellulitis, then the services of an otolaryngologist will likely be necessary to surgically drain the affected paranasal sinuses. If cavernous sinus thrombosis has developed, then heparinization may be indicated (in the absence of evidence of intracranial hemorrhage) to limit the extension of thrombosis to other sites.

FREQUENCY OF VISITS

The frequency with which one sees a patient with preseptal or orbital cellulitis is determined on an individual basis and is entirely dependent upon the severity of the patient's infection and the response to therapy. Given the potential for serious systemic consequences should orbital cellulitis produce cavernous sinus thrombosis, intense and aggressive treatment is required early in the patient's course. In children, this will likely require hospitalization for intravenous antibiotics, while adolescents and adults with milder infections may respond well to oral antibiotics. Daily follow-up should be employed until it is clear that the patient is exhibiting a favorable response.

SUGGESTED READINGS

Apers R, Oosterhuis J, Bierlaagh J. Indications and results of prednisone treatment in thyroid ophthalmopathy. Ophthalmologica 1976;173:163–167.

Armstrong D. Treatment of opportunistic fungal infections. Clin Infect Dis 1993;16:1–9.

Bernardino M, Zimmerman R, Citrin C, Davis D. Scleral thickening: a CT sign of orbital pseudotumor. AJR 1977;129:703–706.

Bhattacharyya A, Deshpande A, Nayak S, et al. Rhinocerebral mucormycosis: an unusual case presentation. J Laryngol Otol 1992;106:48–49.

Blatt S, Lucey D, DeHoff D, Zellmer R. Rhinocerebral zygomycosis in a patient with AIDS. J Infect Dis 1991;164:215–216.

Brennan M, Leone C, Janaki L. Radiation therapy for Graves' disease. Am J Ophthalmol 1983;96:195–199.

Brismar J, Davis K, Dallow R, Brismar G. Unilateral endocrine exophthalmos. Diagnostic problems in association with computed tomography. Neuroradiology 1976;12:21–24.

Burns R. Mucormycosis of the sinuses, orbit and central nervous system. Trans Pac Coast Otoophthalmol Soc 1959;40:83–101.

De La Paz M, Patrinely J, Marines H, Appling W. Adjunctive hyperbaric oxygen in the treatment of bilateral cerebro-rhino-orbital mucormycosis. Am J Ophthalmol 1992;114:208–211.

Ellie E, Houang B, Louail C, et al. CT and high field MRI in septic thrombosis of the cavernous sinuses. Neuroradiology 1992;34:22–24.

Enzmann D, Donaldson S, Kriss J. Appearance of Graves' disease on orbital computed tomography. J Comp Assist Tomogr 1979;3:815–819.

Evans D, Kennerdell J. Extraocular muscle surgery for dysthyroid myopathy. Am J Ophthalmol 1983;95:767–771.

Feldon S, Wiener J. Clinical significance of extraocular volumes in Graves' ophthalmopathy. A quantitative computed tomography study. Arch Ophthalmol 1982;100;1266–1269.

Ferry A, Abedi S. Diagnosis and management of rhino-orbito-cerebral mucormycosis (phycomycosis): a report of 16 personally observed cases. Ophthalmology 1983;103:1096–1104.

Galetta S, Wule A, Goldberg H, Nichols C, Glaser J. Rhinocerebral mucormycosis: management and survival after carotid occlusion. Ann Neurol 1990;28:103–107.

Gamblin G, Harper D, Galentine P, et al. Prevalence of increased intraocular pressure in Graves' disease: evidence of subclinical ophthalmopathy. N Engl J Med 1983;308:420.

Glaser J. Graves' ophthalmopathy. Arch Ophthalmol 1984;102:1448–1449.

Glaser JS. Infranuclear disorders of eye movement. In: Neuro-ophthalmology. Philadelphia: JB Lippincott, 1990:398.

Gorman C. Ophthalmopathy of Graves' disease. N Engl J Med 1983;308:453–454.

Gorman C. Temporal relationship between onset of Graves' ophthalmopathy and the diagnosis of thyrotoxicosis. Mayo Clinic Proc 1983;58:515–519.

Grimson B, Simmons K. Orbital inflammation, myositis and systemic lupus erythematosus. Arch Ophthalmol 1983;101:736–738.

Grove A. Upper eyelid retraction and Graves' disease. Ophthalmology 1981;88:499–506.

Hartness A, Doughty D, Hirst A, et al. Radiotherapy in benign orbital disease: II. Ophthalmic Graves' disease and orbital histiocytosis X. Br J Ophthalmol 1988;72:289.

Harvey J, Anderson R. The aponeurotic approach to eyelid retraction. Ophthalmology 1981;88:513–524.

Hufnagel T, Hickey W, Cobbs W, et al. Immunohistochemical and ultrastructural studies on the exenterated orbital tissues of a patient with Graves' disease. Ophthalmology 1984;91:1411–1419.

Imes R, Schatz H, Hoyt W, Monteiro M, Narahara M. Evolution of optociliary veins in optic nerve sheath meningioma. Arch Ophthalmol 1985;103:59–60.

Jakobiec F, Jones I. Orbital inflammations. In: Jones IS, Jakobiec FA, eds. Diseases of the orbit. Hagerstown, MD: Harper & Row, 1979:197–204.

Jellinek E. The orbital pseudotumor syndrome and its differentiation from endocrine exophthalmos. Brain 1969;92:35–58.

Kennerdell J, Dresner S. The nonspecific orbital inflammatory syndromes. Surv Ophthalmol 1984;29:93–103.

Kennerdell J, Maroon J. An orbital decompression for severe dysthyroid exophthalmos. Ophthalmology 1989;89:467–472.

Kinyoun J, Kalina R, Brower S, Mills R, Johnson R. Radiation retinopathy after orbital irradiation for Graves' ophthalmopathy. Arch Ophthalmol 1984;102:1473–1476.

Klingele T, Hart W, Burde R. Management of dysthyroid optic neuropathy. Ophthalmologica 1977;174:327–335.

Lim K, Potts M, Warnock D, et al. Another case report of rhinocerebral mucormycosis treated with liposomal amphotericin B and surgery. Clin Infect Dis 1994;18:653–654.

Linberg J, Anderson R. Transorbital decompression. Indication and results. Arch Ophthalmol 1981;99:113–119.

Miller N. Fungi and mycotic diseases. In: Miller NR, ed. Clinical neuro-ophthalmology. Baltimore: Williams & Wilkins, 1995;5:3194–3195.

Mottow L, Jakobiec F. Idiopathic inflammatory orbital pseudotumor in childhood. I. Clinical characteristics. Arch Ophthalmol 1978;96:1410–1417.

Mottow-Lipp L, Jakobiec F, Smith M. Idiopathic inflammatory orbital pseudotumor in childhood. II. Results of diagnostic tests and biopsies. Ophthalmology 1981;88:565–574.

Olivotto I, Ludgate C, Allen L, et al. Supervoltage radiotherapy for Graves' ophthalmopathy: CCABC technique and results. Int J Radiat Oncol Biol Phys 1985;11:2085–2090.

Perlmutter J, Burde R, Gado M, Roper-Hall GL. Endocrine ophthalmopathy: a disease wearing many masks. In: Glaser JS, ed. Neuro-ophthalmology. St Louis: CV Mosby, 1977:160–176.

Pinchoff B, Spahlinger D, Bergstrom T, Sandall G. Extraocular muscle involvement in Wegener's granulomatosis. J Clin Neuro Ophthalmol 1983;3:163–168.

Price C, Hameroff S, Richards R. Cavernous sinus thrombosis and orbital cellulitis. South Med J 1971;64:1243–1247.

Putterman A. Surgical treatment of thyroid-related lid retraction: graded Müller's muscle and levator resection. Ophthalmology 1981;88:507–512.

Reader A. Normal variations of intraocular pressure on vertical gaze. Ophthalmology 1982;89:1084–1087.

Rootman J, Nugent R. The classification and management of acute orbital pseudotumors. Ophthalmology 1982;89:1040–1048.

Sanders M, Brown P. Acute presentation of thyroid ophthalmopathy. Trans Ophthalmol Soc UK 1986;105:720–722.

Scott W, Thalacker J. Diagnosis and treatment of thyroid myopathy. Ophthalmology 1981;88:493–498.

Slavin M, Glaser J. Idiopathic orbital myositis. Report of six cases. Arch Ophthalmol 1982;100:1261–1265.

Solomon D, Chopra I, Chopra U, Smith F. Identification of subgroups of euthyroid Graves' ophthalmopathy. N Engl J Med 1977;2986:181–186.

Spoor T, Kennerdell J. Thyrotropic-releasing hormone test and the diagnosis of dysthyroid ophthalmopathy. Ann Ophthalmol 1981;13:443–445.

Stabile J, Trokel S. Increase in orbital volume obtained by decompression in dried skulls. Am J Ophthalmol 1983;95:327–331.

Susac J, Martins A, Robinson B, Corrigan D. False diagnosis of orbital apex tumor by CAT scan in thyroid disease. Ann Neurol 1977;1:397–398.

Trobe J, Glaser J, Laflamme P. Dysthyroid optic neuropathy: clinical profile and rationale for management. Arch Ophthalmol 1978;96:1199–1209.

Trokel S, Hilal S. Recognition and differential diagnosis of enlarged extraocular muscles in computed tomography. Am J Ophthalmol 1979;87:503–512.

Weiss A, Friendly D, Eglin K, et al. Bacterial periorbital and orbital cellulitis in childhood. Ophthalmology 1983;90:195–203.

PART C
Ocular Movement Disorders

⬤❚ Chapter 17
Pediatric and Adult Strabismus

A. C. Tongue

INTRODUCTION

Strabismus is an abnormal ocular alignment resulting in disruption of binocular vision and fusion of the two eyes. Strabismus has a motor and sensory component. The motor component is the physical alignment of the eyes; the sensory component is the way the brain handles the information it receives from the two eyes.

In acquired strabismus, the abnormal sensory consequences are confusion of images (different visual images falling on corresponding retinal areas in the two eyes) and diplopia (same visual image falling on different, noncorresponding retinal areas in the two eyes). Adults with acquired strabismus may therefore complain of seeing different images in the same place (confusion of images), or, more commonly, of seeing the same image in two different places (diplopia). Infants and young children generally do not suffer these consequences for any length of time, but quickly suppress both the confusing image and the diplopic visual signals from the nonfixing eye. The child's brain ignores the second image.

Unfortunately, this adaptive mechanism in children may also lead to permanent loss of vision, or amblyopia, if the strabismus occurs before age 5–7 years. The younger the child, the more rapidly the suppression and adaptation to the strabismic state. In infants and toddlers, it may be hours to days. The time period for development of amblyopia is also quite short in young infants. In those under 1 year of age, it may only be a matter of days to weeks. Children under age 7–9 years are susceptible to developing amblyopia secondary to strabismus. Strabismus in children may therefore lead to permanent loss of fusion of the images from both eyes (binocular vision) and to permanent loss of eyesight in the suppressed eye.

CLINICAL MANIFESTATIONS

Classification of strabismus is by (a) age of onset, (b) direction of deviation, (c) eye fixation preference, (d) constancy or change of angle as measured in different directions of gaze, and (e) underlying cause.

By definition, congenital strabismus is a deviation which occurs before age 6

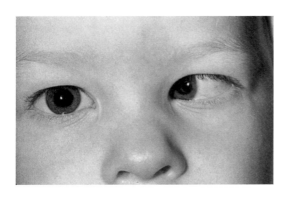

Figure 17.1. Left esotropia. (Courtesy of A. Tongue, M.D.)

months. Congenital esotropia is the most common congenital strabismus. Other forms of strabismus, which may not be noted by parents or physicians alike during the first year of life, but which are congenital, are congenital fourth cranial nerve (superior oblique) paralysis, Duane syndrome, Brown tendon sheath syndrome, and, rarely, exotropia.

Acquired strabismus occurs after 6 months of age. The most common acquired strabismus in the pediatric age group is accommodative esotropia. Intermittent exotropia is usually not evident until after 6 months. Some children with cosmetically inapparent microtropia (very small deviation) may become more strabismic as they get older. Acquired strabismus, if not of the accommodative or intermittent exotropia variety, requires careful scrutiny to rule out possible underlying neurologic or ophthalmologic disorders. Trauma, central nervous system tumors and disorders, and blind eyes may cause acquired strabismus.

Children with vision loss can develop strabismus. Strabismus is the second most common presenting sign of retinoblastoma. Optic nerve hypoplasia, cataract, and other congenital malformations leading to uniocular vision loss may present clinically as strabismus. Increased intracranial pressure may cause esotropia. Tumors may cause third, fourth, or sixth cranial nerve palsies. Ocular myasthenia gravis occurs in children and presents with a variable strabismus and ptosis.

Strabismus is further categorized by the type of deviation. In relation to the fixing eye the deviated eye turns inward in esotropia (Fig. 17.1), outward in exotropia (Fig. 17.2), upward in hypertropia (Fig. 17.3), and downward in hypotropia. Alternating strabismus refers to the spontaneous alternation of the fixing eye. The strabismic individual will fix on a visual target with one or the other eye at different times. Alternation may occur readily during the examination period, or may not be observed by the physician, but may be historically present (i.e., parents or patient states that either eye deviates). If the patient is noted to have a strong fixation preference for one eye and always is strabismic with the same eye, then decreased vision in that eye is suspected. In the infant and young child, unilateral strabismus will also lead to amblyopia.

If the angle of deviation changes in magnitude with direction of gaze, paralysis or malfunction of one or more extraocular muscles is suspected (Fig. 17.4). In paretic strabismus, the deviation will be greater with the paretic eye fixing. However, in

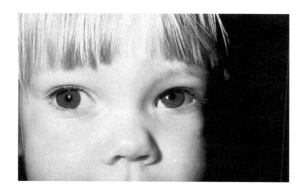

Figure 17.2. Left exotropia
secondary to retinoblastoma.
(See also color section.)
(Courtesy of A. Tongue, M.D.)

infantile or congenital nonparetic strabismus, the angle may change between up- and downgaze. These types of patterns are referred to as A or V pattern strabismus and occur in both esotropia and exotropia. In some patients, the eyes may be esotropic in one direction or exotropic in the other (Fig. 17.5). Orbital and craniofacial anatomy or innervation abnormalities may be responsible for these patterns. A pattern strabismus is more common in hydrocephalus and in Down syndrome. These patterns are, at times, associated with oblique muscle malfunction, such as bilateral inferior oblique overaction in V patterns and bilateral superior oblique overaction in A patterns. Unlike in paretic strabismus, limited movement secondary to weakness or paralysis of individual muscles is absent. Thorough neurologic evaluation is indicated in patients who have a clear-cut acquired, nontraumatic incomitant deviation at any age.

It is to be noted that accommodative strabismus secondary to uncorrected hyperopia in children will be variable in its angle of presentation. The angle of deviation is dependent on the accommodative effort of the child. When a child looks at a target such as a penlight, no accommodation is necessary to see the light. However, when the child looks at a picture or small detail a large esotropia may become evident, secondary to accommodative convergence. Patients with accommodative esotropia often have straight eyes as they look into the distance, and crossed eyes as they look

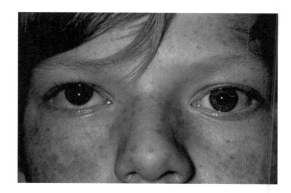

Figure 17.3. Right hypertropia.
(Courtesy of A. Tongue, M.D.)

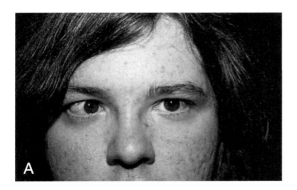

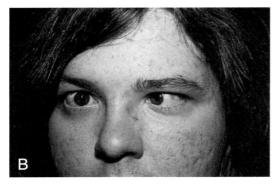

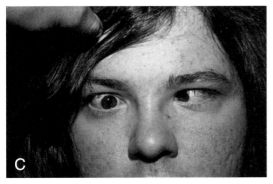

Figure 17.4. Right sixth cranial nerve paralysis. **A.** Primary gaze fixing with nonparetic eye. **B.** Fixing with paretic eye. Note increased deviation. **C.** Attempted right gaze. Note total abduction deficit of right eye. (Courtesy of A. Tongue, M.D.)

at visual targets at near. However, the angle of deviation is the same in all directions of gaze; it is not incomitant, it is just not constant.

Intermittent exotropia is also a deviation which is not constantly noted and the amount of deviation is often much greater at distance than near. Patients who focus on a visual target accommodate and thereby exert accommodative convergence. This accommodative convergence may keep their exotropic deviation in check at near. These patients often are exotropic when daydreaming, looking far out of a window,

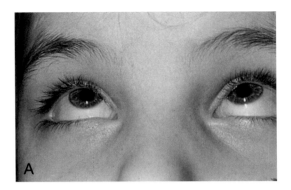

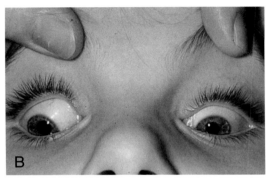

Figure 17.5. "A" pattern strabismus. **A.** Esotropia in upgaze. **B.** Exotropia in downgaze. (Courtesy of A. Tongue, M.D.)

down the hallway, and so forth, but have totally straight eyes when focusing on near objects.

DIFFERENTIAL DIAGNOSIS

STRABISMUS IN INFANTS AND CHILDREN

Many infants under 3 months of age will show disconjugate eye movement or eye position for fleeting moments, often as they are going to sleep (Table 17.1). However, when they are alert and clearly making eye contact with the parent, their eyes should be straight. The intermittent exotropic or esotropic eye positions should decrease in frequency during the first 3 months and essentially be gone by 4 months of age. Tonic downgaze, especially when associated with lid retraction, may be a sign of hydrocephalus. Some premature infants with ventricular hemorrhages may also show tonic downgaze.

Any strabismus in an infant, regardless of the age, that is constant or manifest for more than just fleeting moments should be investigated and should be referred to an ophthalmologist (Table 17.2). This is particularly to be emphasized in the case of unilateral (i.e., child does not alternate fixation) strabismus, since the strabismus may be a sign of underlying disease such as a cataract, retinoblastoma, coloboma of choroid, optic nerve hypoplasia, or other sight-impairing disease. Alternating strabismus should

TABLE 17.1. Congenital Strabismus in Pediatric Age Group

Esotropia	Usually apparent by 6 months of age
	Associated with
	Overt (on abduction) or latent nystagmus
	Cross-fixation
	Reluctance to abduct eyes
	Inferior oblique overaction
	Alternating hypertropia
	May be secondary
	To poor vision in one eye
	Lateral rectus malfunction
Exotropia	Less frequent than esotropia
	May be secondary to
	Poor vision in one eye
	Orbital mass lesions such as hemangioma
	Total or partial third cranial nerve paralysis
	Abnormal innervation such as Duane syndrome
	Congenital extraocular muscle fibrosis
Duane syndrome	Due to abnormal innervation of extraocular muscles
	Clinical picture dependent on extent of innervation anomaly
	Unilateral more common than bilateral
	Most commonly affects
	Abduction more than adduction
	Left eye more than right
	May be
	Familial
	Associated with other anomalies
Fourth cranial nerve paralysis	Hypertropia of involved eye
	Deviation worse an adduction of involved eye
	Torticollis or head tilt common (tilt to opposite shoulder)
	Usually have straight eyes in primary gaze
	Involved eye elevates
	On attempted adduction
	On head tilt to same side
Superior rectus paralysis	Usually associated with ptosis
	Hypotropia of involved eye
	Rare as isolated lesion
Double elevator palsy	Involved eye cannot be elevated normally, often not above horizontal midline
	May be due to
	Aberrant innervation
	Fibrosis of inferior rectus
	Eyes may be aligned in downgaze and in primary gaze
Tonic downgaze	Occurs in neonatal hydrocephalus, ventricular hemorrhage
	Occasionally normal transient occurrence in neonates

also be referred when it is detected since early surgical alignment may have a better prognosis for fusion and binocularity than alignment at an older age.

Some infants with epicanthal folds or broad nasal bridge have the appearance of esotropia (pseudostrabismus; Fig. 17.6A). Parents usually state that one eye looks crossed. The crossing does not last, is more apparent when the child looks to the side or the parent looks at the child from an angle, and may be most noticed in photos.

◐▮ TABLE 17.2. Referral Guidelines for Congenital Strabismus

| Congenital strabismus (378.9) | Strabismus which manifests during first 6–12 months of life. Newborn infants may have some intermittent, short-lived (seconds to minutes) of strabismus or convergent or divergent eye movements. Constant strabismus, however, is not normal. | Refer when diagnosis is established even if under 6 months of age. Early eye alignment is desirable for improved fusion and binocularity. Unilateral strabismus may be a sign of poor vision in the strabismic eye. Incomitant strabismus may be a sign of underlying neurologic disorder or congenital extraocular abnormalities (see Table 17.1). Fundus examination and refraction are essential in evaluation of strabismus and should be performed as soon as diagnosis is made. Urgent referral is recommended in case of unilateral strabismus. |
| | History of strabismus per mother's observation, intermittent strabismus | Refer for comprehensive eye evaluation including cycloplegic refraction. Pseudoesotropia may be a possibility. |

The pseudoesotropia may also be more noticeable when the child is tired. Most of the time the parents feel that the apparent esotropia is less noticeable as the child gets older. Evaluation of the Hirschberg (corneal reflex) and the Bruckner (red reflex) test (see Appendix C, "Special Pediatric Examination Techniques"), in conjunction with a cover test, should identify whether a true esotropia is present. In some infants, a small angle esotropia can be missed if the infant is not really fixing or is uninterested in the testing situation. Parents should be asked if it is primarily the lack of sclera showing (white part of eye) that they interpret as esotropia. When any question remains as to whether a true esotropia is present, the child should have an evaluation by an ophthalmologist. A subsequent careful visual acuity evaluation at age 3 is to be recommended for any child suspected of pseudostrabismus at an earlier age because of the potential of a missed microtropia with amblyopia.

Congenital cranial sixth nerve paralysis occurs rarely secondary to birth trauma. These infants are esotropic and the esotropia generally disappears by age 3 months. They require ophthalmologic follow-up to monitor for microtropias and amblyopia until they are verbal and can cooperate for optotype acuity testing.

Duane syndrome is a congenital eye muscle disorder which can mimic a cranial sixth nerve paralysis on attempted abduction. Patients with this condition usually present because a parent has noted that one eye does not move laterally. Often it is not noticed until the child is old enough to look around and follow objects with his or her eyes. In the primary gaze position, the involved eye may look slightly smaller

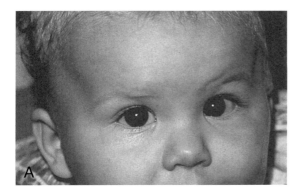

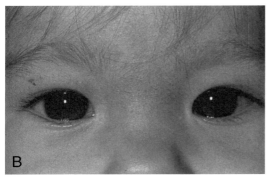

Figure 17.6. **A.** Pseudostrabismus secondary to epicanthal folds. Note symmetrically placed corneal reflexes. (See also color section.) **B.** True strabismus with right esotropia of approximately 8–10°. Note asymmetric corneal reflexes. (Courtesy of A. Tongue, M.D.)

because of a narrower palpebral fissure (Fig. 17.7*A*). The eyes are usually straight in the primary gaze position, unlike a cranial sixth nerve paralysis in which esotropia is present in straight-ahead gaze (Fig. 17.4). On attempted abduction of the involved eye, the palpebral fissure widens (Fig. 17.7*B*) and the eye does not fully abduct (Fig. 17.7*C*). It is most often a unilateral condition, but may be bilateral. Some patients are esotropic in primary gaze and have a head turn to keep the involved eye in an adducted position for fusion. In this case, it may mimic a cranial sixth nerve paralysis. Some patients with Duane syndrome have adduction limitation and exotropia in primary gaze, others have vertical eye movement abnormalities. Duane syndrome is secondary to abnormal innervation of the extraocular muscles. In the typical Duane patient, there is abnormal innervation to the lateral and medial rectus muscle. The condition is one of a spectrum of cocontraction or abnormal innervation syndromes. It may be dominantly inherited, has variable penetrance and expressivity, and may be associated in some families with other systemic abnormalities. These children should have an initial evaluation by an ophthalmologist whenever the condition is noted and should be monitored by an ophthalmologist for amblyopia, anisometropia, and fusion until age 5 or 6 years.

Brown tendon sheath syndrome involves the superior oblique muscle of one or both eyes. The involved eye does not elevate when in the adducted position (Fig. 17.8). It is a mechanical problem involving the superior oblique tendon sheath, tendon, and/or trochlea. Most are congenital and idiopathic. It may look like an inferior oblique

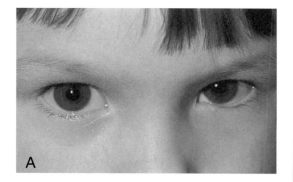

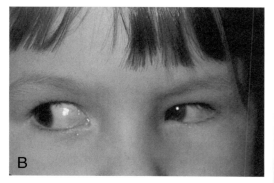

Figure 17.7. Duane syndrome, left side. **A.** Mild palpebral asymmetry with left eye lid fissure narrower than right. **B.** Narrowing of fissure on adduction of left eye. **C.** Esotropia secondary to abduction deficit of left eye on left gaze, widening of palpebral fissure of left eye on attempted abduction. (Courtesy of A. Tongue, M.D.)

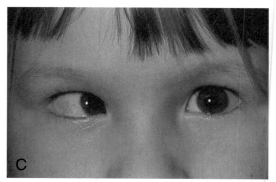

paralysis, but the latter is quite rare in children. Forced ductions (using a forceps to rotate the eye in the field of limited movement) differentiates between a Brown tendon sheath syndrome, which is a mechanical abnormality, and an inferior oblique paralysis. Some Brown tendon sheath syndromes are acquired. They may be secondary to involvement of the trochlea or tendon sheath such as in rheumatoid disease, local granuloma formation, tumors, or trauma and hematomas. A number of these spontaneously resolve over a period of months to years. If the patient is symptomatic and the vertical deviation affects primary gaze, surgical intervention may be required. Children with Brown tendon sheath syndrome also need to be monitored during the first 5–6 years

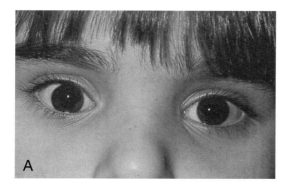

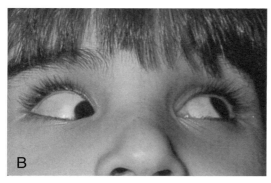

Figure 17.8. Brown tendon sheath syndrome, right eye. **A.** No deviation in primary gaze. **B.** Elevation deficit of right eye in adduction (left gaze). (Courtesy of A. Tongue, M.D.)

of life because of the risk of developing a breakdown of fusion, strabismus in primary gaze position, and amblyopia.

Patients with congenital ptosis often have superior rectus weakness on the involved side with elevation difficulty. Acquired infantile strabismus may be secondary to orbital involvement with hemangioma. The strabismus is due to mechanical restriction caused by the tumor or to amblyopia secondary to induced refractive errors. Early intervention and treatment are required to avoid severe vision loss in these children.

Accommodative esotropia is the single most common type of acquired strabismus in childhood (Table 17.3). Its onset is usually after age 1, often between 2 and 4 years. Patients are generally significantly hyperopic (over +3.00 diopters, sometimes as much as +6.00 to +8.00). In most, normal ocular alignment is achieved by wearing the hyperopic correction (Fig. 17.9). Some, however, have a normal or even myopic refractive error with a large amount of convergence for each diopter of accommodation (accommodative convergence). Bifocals may be required to eliminate the near esotropia. Topical anticholinesterase agents (i.e., phospholine iodide solution) may decrease accommodative effort and, thereby, accommodative convergence. Anticholinesterase agents can have side effects such as asthma, gastrointestinal disturbance (diarrhea, stomachaches), headaches, and lens opacities. Ingestion of the contents of a bottle may be fatal.

Most patients with accommodative esotropia outgrow their condition, becoming less hyperopic as they reach their teens. However, a number do not and require glasses

TABLE 17.3. Etiology of Nonparalytic (Comitant)
Acquired Strabismus

I. Child	Accommodative esotropia
	Partially accommodative esotropia
	Intermittent exotropia
	Blind eye, visually impaired eye
	Breakdown of microtropia, phoria
	Idiopathic
	Intracranial tumor (rare but reported)
	Arnold-Chiari (rare but reported)
II. Adult	Consecutive strabismus (prior eye muscle surgery)
	Blind or visually impaired eye
	Breakdown of microtropia or phoria
	Idiopathic
	Arnold-Chiari (rare but reported)
	Intracranial tumor (rare but reported)

or contact lenses to control the deviation and correction of vision for the rest of their life. A family history of high hyperopia or accommodative esotropia is not uncommon. Siblings and offspring of accommodative esotropia patients or high hyperopia patients should also be evaluated during infancy and at 3 years of age.

Rare cases of accommodative or partially accommodative esotropia present in teenagers who receive contact lenses to correct myopia. These patients have a high accommodative convergence ratio. Without the myopic correction, little or no accommodation is needed to focus at near. With a myopic spectacle refraction, the patient has to accommodate to focus at near. An even greater amount of accommodation is needed when contact lenses are worn. This extra accommodative effort can convert a precariously balanced myopic accommodative esotropia into a constant esotropia.

Intermittent exotropia usually presents after 6 months of age. Most parents note an intermittent deviation when the child is tired, sick, daydreaming, or looking into

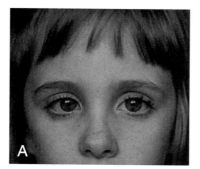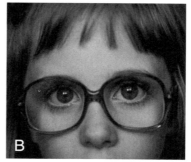

Figure 17.9.   Accommodative right esotropia and hyperopia. **A.** Esotropia without refractive correction. **B.** Straight eyes with refractive correction. (Courtesy of A. Tongue, M.D.)

TABLE 17.4. Etiology of Noncomitant Acquired Strabismus (Child)

CAUSE	SIGNS
Trauma	See Table 17.1
Tumors and masses of orbit	Depending on size and location of lesion orbital tumors associated with proptosis and if near apex or involving optic nerve with vision loss.
Central nervous system Posterior fossa tumors Astrocytoma Medulloblastoma Glioma Increased intracranial pressure Inflammatory	Intracranial tumors may be associated with isolated or multiple cranial nerve paralysis. 6th nerve paralysis may be secondary to increased intracranial pressure. Gaze paralysis, jerky eye movements, nystagmus, convergence, and divergence weakness may be present with intracranial tumors.
Postviral	Isolated unilateral cranial nerve paralysis, especially 6th nerve occurs in children after benign viral disease (upper respiratory illness) usually resolves within weeks to 3–6 months. No other signs of neurologic and systemic deficit present. Guillain-Barré may cause multiple cranial nerve paralysis.
Bacterial	Petrositis, postotitis media, may manifest with facial pain, hearing loss, and 6th nerve paralysis.
Pseudotumor of orbit	Pseudotumor of orbit associated with pain on eye movement, appearance of cellulitis.
Demyelinating—multiple sclerosis (MS)	Strabismus rare as presenting sign of MS in children
Neurodegenerative diseases Vascular	Usually associated or preceded by other signs and symptoms.
Ophthalmoplegic migraine	3rd cranial nerve most common, usually preceded by severe hemicranial headache. Paralysis may last 3–4 days, recur. Requires neuroimaging to rule out other etiologies such as aneurysm. Rare in infants and young children.
Arteriovenous malformations	Usually associated with other signs of CNS impairment.
Myaesthenia gravis	Usually associated with ptosis, variable incomitant strabismus. Responds to edrophonium or neostigmine.

the distance. Intermittent exotropia patients usually maintain good vision and usually are not amblyopic as long as the deviation is latent a good part of the time. About one-third spontaneously improve, one-third deteriorate. If the deviation becomes more frequent, amblyopia and loss of fusion are possible. These children should be monitored every 6 months by an ophthalmologist, even if the parents feel there is no change in their status. Microexotropia can occur and suppression and vision loss can result. Deterioration of the fusion status requires intervention which may be nonsurgical. Adults with well-controlled intermittent exotropia during childhood sometimes become symptomatic as they reach presbyopia and wear bifocals.

It is rare for a child to acquire strabismus other than the above mentioned (Table 17.4). Paretic or incomitant strabismus may be due to trauma, tumors and masses of the orbit or central nervous system, inflammatory disease, neurodegenerative diseases, vascular disease, and myopathies (see Tables 17.3 and 17.4). Children can develop isolated cranial sixth nerve paralysis secondary to viral infections. Usually a history of a preceding upper respiratory infection can be elicited and there are no other associated signs or symptoms. The palsy should improve within 8–12 weeks, but in some patients, may take up to 6 months to resolve. Rarely, central nervous system tumors can cause isolated cranial sixth nerve paralysis and it is not unreasonable to obtain neuroimaging studies early, rather than to wait until 8 or 10 weeks go by. If neuroimaging is not performed at the onset of the palsy, then careful monitoring by an ophthalmologist is certainly in order to rule out the existence or emergence of any other signs or symptoms. Other causes of paretic strabismus are essentially the same in childhood as they are in the adult.

ADULT STRABISMUS (ACQUIRED)

The most common causes of acquired strabismus are trauma, thyroid ophthalmopathy, local orbital or intracranial central nervous system masses, vascular accidents, and neurologic disorders such as myasthenia gravis (Tables 17.3 and 17.5–17.7). In older patients, localized vascular accidents and diabetes may cause isolated cranial nerve damage with resultant strabismus. Myasthenia gravis generally is associated with ptosis. The deviation and the ptosis are variable and may not always be present. A Tensilon test is performed while the deviation is present to see if it resolves. Strabismus may occur after cataract surgery and after other ocular or orbital surgical procedures.

Extraocular muscle involvement in Graves' disease is not uncommon (see Chapter 16, "Thyroid Ophthalmopathy and Orbital Infections"). Most often the inferior rectus and medial rectus muscles are involved. However, any extraocular muscle can be affected, and in some unfortunate patients, multiple muscles are affected at the same time. Extraocular muscle involvement may not become evident until years after the initial diagnosis and may be recurrent over a number of years. Different muscles may be involved at different times. CT and MRI scans show enlarged muscles. Patients usually develop strabismus secondary to mechanical restriction caused by the inelastic muscles. Occasionally, the involved muscle may be paretic. In patients with isolated or only a few muscles involved, surgical correction is highly successful. Simultaneous multiple muscle involvement carries a more guarded prognosis for attainment of single vision with surgery.

If neurologic and systemic evaluation are negative, or the etiology established and treated, acquired paretic and traumatic strabismus in both children and adults should be followed conservatively for about 6 months before surgery is contemplated. Traumatic cranial sixth nerve palsies often resolve spontaneously. Traumatic cranial third nerve palsies tend not to have the same prognosis, and often aberrant regeneration occurs. (In infants and young children, amblyopia may develop, and patching to avoid amblyopia should be instituted). Glasses with prism to align the images help some patients when the deviation in primary gaze is not large. Oculinum (botulinum) injection into the medial rectus muscle of the involved eye may also eliminate the esotropia temporarily and allow for single vision. Patients with bilateral cranial sixth nerve paralysis often develop significant contracture of the medial rectus over a 3–4 month period. Patients whose cranial sixth nerve paralysis does not resolve usually have a very good prognosis with surgery for single vision in the primary field of gaze. Generally, however, they are left with abduction weakness.

TABLE 17.5. Acquired Noncomitant Strabismus (Adult)

CAUSE	SIGNS
Trauma	See Table 17.1
Tumors	
Orbit	Usually associated with proptosis, restrictive and/or paretic strabismus. Rarely isolated cranial nerve paralysis.
CNS	
may arise anywhere in CNS	Signs depend on location, size of tumor. May cause isolated extracranial nerve lesions, but more likely to have multiple involvement and other signs and symptoms. Increased intracranial pressure may cause 6th nerve paralysis.
Inflammatory/immune	Rare to present as isolated extraocular muscle paralysis in adults. May be associated with herpes zoster, particularly in HIV-positive patients.
Thyroid ophthalmopathy	Usually restrictive strabismus with abnormal traction test. Most often presents in patients who are euthyroid; may occur long after episode of hyperthyroidism and treatment for this. Isolated or multiple muscle involvement. Inferior rectus most commonly involved. Lateral rectus least commonly involved. Neuroimaging reveals characteristic appearance of enlarged affected muscles. Proptosis and lid retraction may be present. Thyroid ophthalmopathy is one of the most common causes of acquired vertical muscle deviation other than trauma in adult patients.
Demyelinating—MS	Bilateral internuclear ophthalmoplegia with nystagmus on abduction and adduction deficit is most frequently secondary to MS.
Vascular	
Small vessel disease	Most common etiology is diabetes mellitus and hypertension. May cause isolated cranial nerve paralysis with pupil sparing in 3rd nerve paralysis. Resolution of the paralysis within a few months is common.
AV malformations and aneurysms	May cause 3rd nerve paralysis or multiple cranial nerve palsies depending on location. Pupil involvement is almost always present.
Ophthalmoplegic migraine	Neuroimaging required to rule out other etiology.
Myaesthenia gravis	Usually associated with ptosis and a variable incomitant strabismus. Responds to edrophonium or neostigmine. Some patients may develop constant strabismus that responds well to surgery.

The exception to conservative management are orbital blowout fractures which may require early intervention to avoid permanent scarring and fibrosis of the entrapped muscle (see Chapter 15, "Ocular Trauma") (Table 17.7). Fat atrophy and enophthalmos also may result. Blowout fractures may at times be followed for a few days to 2 weeks after the initial injury to see if there is any improvement in eye movement since hematomas may also cause restriction of movement. As these resolve, eye movement is restored.

◼▮ TABLE 17.6. Referral Guidelines for Acquired Strabismus in Adults and Children

Acquired strabismus childhood	Most common between ages 2 and 4 is accomodative strabismus. Deviation usually intermittent at first, greater at near than at distance. Usually secondary to high hyperopia.	Refer when diagnosis is established. Most patients with accommodative esotropia respond well to glasses and will regain normal fusion and stereopsis if treated early and amblyopia is avoided. Deferred treatment may result in amblyopia and loss of fusion capacity.
	Unilateral strabismus which is comitant may be result of poor vision in one eye or amblyopia.	Refer when diagnosis is established.
	Incomitant strabismus.	Refer to ophthalmologist if no other signs or symptoms. Refer for immediate neurologic evaluation if patient has associated systemic findings suggestive of intracranial or neurologic disease and no known etiology for strabismus (i.e., trauma).
	Incomitant strabismus secondary to trauma.	Refer patient when stable. Trauma isolated to orbit resulting in diplopia should be evaluated acutely.
Acquired strabismus adult	Incomitant strabimus.	Referral guidelines as above for children. If associated signs or symptoms point to systemic disease or neurologic etiology this should be evaluated on urgent basis. If no associated signs or symptoms and patient in good health, refer to ophthalmologist.
	Comitant strabismus.	Refer to ophthalmologist.

EXAMINATION OF THE PATIENT WITH STRABISMUS

A careful personal and family history may be helpful in establishing the diagnosis and etiology of strabismus.

The examination of strabismic patients includes measuring vision in each eye. In infants, this is done by qualitative evaluation of fixation. Forced preferential looking tests (most commonly Teller Preferential Looking; see Appendix C, "Special Pediatric Examination Techniques") may be used to quantify visual acuities. In older children, visual acuities should be measured with optotypes (pictures, tumbling E, letters, num-

TABLE 17.7. Strabismus Secondary to Trauma

SITE OF INJURY	TYPE OF INJURY	CLINICAL SIGNS
Orbit	Direct injury and avulsion of muscle(s)	Incomitant strabismus
	Entrapment of muscle(s) in fracture site	Isolated muscle involvement
	Injury to orbital portion of nerve(s)	Multiple muscle involvement
	Injury to trochlea of 4th cranial nerve	Posterior orbital lesions more likely to cause multiple muscle involvement and associated ptosis associated vision loss
	Mechanical restriction due to Mass effect from hematomas and edema Scar tissue involving tenon's capsule and/or muscle	Mechanical restriction associated with abnormal forceps traction test
Brainstem	6th cranial nerve(s) most common	Esotropia, abduction deficit
	4th cranial nerve often bilateral	Subjective torsion of images Hypertropia
	3rd nerve, total or partial, usually involves pupil	Exotropia, adduction deficit, hypertropia, hypotropia, mid-dilated unreactive pupil
Pontine area	Gaze paralysis horizontal vertical	Inability to look right or left, up or down
	Skew deviation	One eye up, other down
	Convergence paralysis	Exotropia/phoria at near
	Divergence paralysis	Esotropia/phoria at distance
	Accommodation weakness	Unable to focus on small print at near like a presbyopic patient
Cerebellum	Dysmetric saccades	Jerky eye movements as patient looks from one object to another
Cerebrum	Conjugate gaze paralysis	Exotropia/phoria at near
	Abnormal pursuit movements	Unable to follow an object smoothly
	Absent voluntary horizontal saccades, preserved pursuit movements	Unable to look from one object to another, but able to follow an object

bers). Pupils should be checked for direct and consensual light reaction. When a Marcus Gunn or consensual afferent pupillary defect is present, pathology of that eye or the optic nerve is highly likely.

Anterior inspection of the ocular media and eye should also be performed. Particular attention is paid to clarity of the media. The red reflex test is an excellent way to look for media opacities as well as for determination of the strabismic eye (see Appendix C, "Special Pediatric Examination Techniques"). In strabismus, the nonfixing eye is the brighter eye unless that eye is severely hyperopic, or myopic, or if some media abnormality is present.

Eye movement is then assessed. Patients who do not have full eye rotations or movements are suspect of having neurologic or mechanical causes underlying their strabismus. Some of these may be congenital such as in Duane and Brown syndrome,

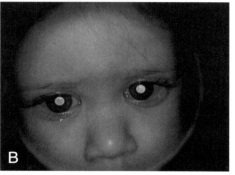
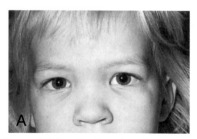

Figure 17.10.   Small angle left exotropia. **A.** Small left exotropia or small right esotropia. (See also color section.) **B.** Same patient with brighter red reflex from left eye indicating that right eye is fixing eye and therefore patient has left exotropia. (See also color section.) (Courtesy of A. Tongue, M.D.)

while others may be acquired secondary to intracranial tumors, intracranial hypertension (usually cranial sixth nerve paralysis), tumors of the orbit, thyroid ophthalmopathy, myasthenia gravis, trauma, orbital blowout fractures, and so forth. Obviously, history will often be helpful in pinpointing the diagnosis. At other times, cranial nerve paralysis may be the only indication of a malignancy, or tumor, or disease. In a subgroup of congenital esotropia patients, nystagmus on abduction of the eye occurs. These patients keep their eyes adducted. They do not look laterally and they vigorously resist every attempt to get them to do so. Most cross-fixate (use right eye for left gaze viewing and left eye for right gaze viewing). They are often difficult to differentiate from congenital sixth nerve paralysis.

An estimate of the deviation can be made by looking at the corneal reflex (Hirschberg test) (Fig. 17.6*B*). Normally, the corneal reflex is slightly nasal to the center of the pupil in each eye. If the light reflex is displaced to the pupil margin, the deviation is about 15° or 25–30 diopters. In esotropia, the reflex will be temporal, in exotropia, nasal, in hypertropia, inferior, and in hypotropia, superior to the normal position of the light reflex or in comparison to the fixing eye.

The Hirschberg test can be performed in conjunction or simultaneously with the red reflex (Bruckner test; see Appendix C, "Special Pediatric Examination Techniques"). Even small angles of strabismus can be detected by the red reflex test. Figure 17.10 shows a patient with a small angle exotropia. The deviated eye has the brighter red reflex. Detection of the small angle strabismus is instantaneous and easier with the red reflex test than with external inspection and Hirschberg test.

In cooperative patients, a cover test can be utilized to elicit the deviation and to evaluate the fixing eye (see Appendix C, "Special Pediatric Examination Techniques"). Ophthalmologists use the alternate cover test in association with prism to measure the angle of deviation in strabismus patients.

Slitlamp examination and funduscopy are performed. In children, cycloplegic drops are utilized to determine the refractive error. Unequal refractive errors are corrected, as are significant hyperopia and myopia. In general, all children with esotropia and a hyperopia of +3.00 should get glasses before surgery. Some children will have a partial correction of the angle of deviation with plus lenses and this needs to be taken into account when planning surgery. Surgery is aimed for correction of the deviation which occurs with the glasses. Many children become less hyperopic with age (usually by age 12–16), and the convergence which is secondary to accommodation will disappear along with the hyperopia. If this is not taken into account when doing surgery, overcorrection and consecutive exotropia are more likely to occur. Children who have a purely accommodative esotropia straighten completely with glasses and do not require surgery. Some accommodative esotropia patients need bifocals to keep the near deviation controlled.

Unequal refractive errors in children need correction to treat and/or avoid amblyopia. Correction of refractive errors is a major part of the medical treatment of strabismus in children. Neurologic evaluation and consultation, neuroimaging studies, and genetic and metabolic consultation may be required for some patients who have suspected underlying identifiable causes for their strabismus. Many of these patients will have acquired paretic type of strabismus.

TREATMENT

Prior to strabismus surgery the patient is treated with optical correction when significant refractive errors exist. Hyperopia is almost always corrected if greater than 3 diopters. Anisometropia (unequal refractive errors) is also corrected prior to strabismus surgery to eliminate, avoid, or treat amblyopia. Amblyopia, or nonalternating strabismus, is treated with patching. Surgical alignment of the eyes does not necessarily result in sufficient fusion to eliminate the risk of amblyopia. Infants and young children who undergo strabismus surgery need careful follow-up, until they are at least 6 or 7 years old, to monitor and manage amblyopia and strabismus. Unfortunately, some children do not get appropriate follow-up because the eyes are straight and the child appears to be seeing well. Several years later a school vision exam may detect severe amblyopia of 20/200 or 20/400. It is therefore important that children get ophthalmologic follow-up during the first 5–6 years of life even if their postsurgical eye alignment appears to be normal.

In general, strabismus surgery for congenital and infantile strabismus is performed as soon as the deviation is stable (i.e., angle of strabismus is not changing), amblyopia is eliminated, glasses are worn when indicated, and the patient is not at undue risk for undergoing general anesthesia. There may be a slight increased risk for anesthesia complications in infants under 6 months of age.

It is well-accepted that surgery for strabismus is ideally performed in patients when other management does not eliminate the strabismus before age 2 years. Only a very small number of infants with congenital esotropia operated on before age 2 achieve totally normal stereopsis and binocularity. However, the quality of fusion appears to be better in those operated on before age 2 than those operated on after age 2 for congenital esotropia. A number of strabismologists are advocating operating at a very early age, that is, 6 months or before, in select patients in hopes of achieving even better binocularity.

The surgical procedure for esotropia entails weakening one or both medial rectus muscles by moving them from their original insertion into the sclera further posteriorly (recession). The lateral rectus of one or both eyes may be resected (removing a piece of muscle), thereby shortening the muscle. The amount of muscle recession or resection is guided by well-known and accepted formulas, and depends on the angle of strabismus to be corrected. Some surgeons prefer to perform bilateral medial rectus recessions as the primary procedure for esotropia or lateral rectus recessions for exotropia; others prefer to do a uniocular recession/resection operation if the strabismus is of a moderate amount only. In very large angles, both eyes may require surgery. In general, if one eye has poor vision, a uniocular surgery will be performed on that eye.

In exotropia, the lateral rectus muscles are recessed and the medial recti resected. Again, the amount and the choice of doing one or both eyes depend on vision, the amount of deviation, and the surgeon's personal preference.

Hypertropias are a greater diagnostic and treatment challenge than eso- and exotropia. The reason for this is that there are two muscles responsible for elevation in each eye (superior rectus and inferior oblique) and two for depression (inferior rectus and superior oblique). A paresis of any one of the four muscles in either eye can be responsible for a vertical deviation. The clinician needs to determine which muscle of the eight verticals it is. In childhood, paresis of the fourth cranial nerve is the most common cause of an isolated vertical deviation. Patients often present with torticollis tilting their head to the shoulder opposite to the involved eye. In this position, they can often control the deviation and remain binocular. If the head is tilted to the shoulder on the side of the involved eye, a hypertropia of that eye often becomes evident.

Congenital esotropia patients often have associated vertical deviations which may not become apparent until after correction of esotropia. Often, the vertical deviation is of an alternating type with either eye going upward when it is not used for fixation or if an alternate cover test is performed. This condition is called alternating sursumduction or dissociated vertical deviation. Eye muscle weakness or paralysis is not the cause. In a paretic vertical deviation, the nonfixing eye either goes up or down, both eyes do not go up. For example, in a superior oblique paralysis the eye with the paralysis goes up under cover. The nonparetic eye (i.e., opposite eye) goes down under cover. In alternating sursumduction, the eye under the cover, regardless of which one it is, drifts upward. Often this condition is associated with upshoot of the eye on attempted adduction (inferior oblique overaction).

Approximately 20% of congenital or infantile esotropia require more than one surgical procedure for correction of their strabismus. Every attempt should be made to align the eyes early in life. Postoperative glasses or miotics may be used to eliminate a small residual esotropia in children who are hyperopic. Correction of the hyperopia decreases convergence secondary to accommodation. The use of miotic agents (anticholinesterase drops) also decreases accommodative convergence. If a significant undercorrection exists, further surgery may be advisable at that time. Some patients who have good surgical alignment postoperatively may become exotropic several years after the initial procedure. Reoperation to correct secondary exotropia is indicated if the patient is diplopic or the deviation is sufficiently large to be bothersome to the patient.

Children with acquired nonaccommodative strabismus not secondary to neurologic problems or progressive systemic disease should have surgical realignment as soon as possible. Most of these children have fusion and binocular vision potential and will demonstrate it once the eyes are aligned again.

Children with intermittent exotropia may be followed as long as they show evidence of fusion and binocularity. However, if their deviation becomes manifest, the majority of the time surgical intervention may be required. Nonsurgical treatment for intermittent exotropia consists of patching the dominant eye for a period of weeks full-time and/or the use of minus lenses to stimulate accommodation. Patching is

◗▌ TABLE 18.1. Referral Guidelines: Corneal Abrasions and Corneal Ulcers

DISEASE (CODE)	SIGNS AND SYMPTOMS	TREATMENT	WHEN TO REFER
Abrasion (918.1)	Distinct trauma history; pain, redness + fluorescein; underlying stroma clear	Verify no stroma involved; pressure patch over cycloplegia + antibiotic ointment; recheck each day	If epithelium not healed in 72 hours, then refer in 24 hours; if abrasion associated with contact lens wear, refer within 24 hours
Ulcer (370.0)	History of epithelial breakdown/defect; history of contact lens wear; white spot on cornea	Examine patient (include VA); verify ulcer	Refer immediately

DIFFERENTIAL DIAGNOSIS

Corneal abrasions are usually easily diagnosed and are not confused with other entities (Table 18.1). However, corneal abrasions can be associated with more serious conditions such as corneal ulceration and infectious keratitis, corneal edema secondary to extremely elevated intraocular pressure (see Chapter 29, "Glaucoma"), recurrent epithelial erosion syndrome (see Chapter 14, "Dry Eye Syndrome"), neurotrophic cornea and herpes simplex (see Chapter 23, "Ocular Herpetic Infections"). A detailed history and examination will usually differentiate the common abrasion from these other entities.

TREATMENT

The treatment of a simple corneal abrasion is straightforward. If a foreign body is present on the surface, it should be removed in its entirety before treatment of the abrasion. A foreign body may be embedded in the superficial cornea, or may be located under the upper or lower eyelids. To remove a corneal foreign body, a topical anesthetic drop (proparacaine or tetracaine) should be administered. An attempt to remove the foreign body with a cotton-tipped applicator can be tried, but often is unsuccessful. Frequently, a 25-gauge needle is needed to gently remove the foreign body from the corneal surface, making sure not to damage the underlying corneal stroma. Any corneal foreign body located within the central visual axis (within the central 2 mm), should be removed with slitlamp magnification to avoid central corneal stromal injury with secondary scarring and permanent vision loss. The upper and lower eyelids should be everted and examined in any case of corneal abrasion (see Appendix B: General Examination Techniques). Often, a foreign body will be embedded within the conjunctiva covering the inner surface of the eyelid and a corneal abrasion will result from blinking. In the case of multiple small, particulate, ocular foreign bodies, irrigation of the upper and lower lid cul-de-sac will assure complete removal of the debris.

The eye should be dressed with an antibiotic ointment (such as gentamicin or tobramycin) that does not contain corticosteroids. Corticosteroids are not needed in the setting of a corneal abrasion and may inhibit the normal anti-infectious activities of the external ocular surface. The eye is patched with firm pressure to prevent blinking and lid margin movement over the abrasion. Prevention of lid movement serves two purposes; it aids in epithelial cell migration over the abrasion and it relieves pain for the patient. An ocular pressure patch is correctly applied by placing the antibiotic in the lower lid fornix, the patient gently closes the upper lid and then two round gauze eyepads are applied over the closed lids. The patch is very firmly taped into position by placing multiple strips of adhesive paper tape diagonally from the medial forehead to the lower cheek. The taping should be tight enough to place enough pressure on the lids to prevent blinking by the patient (Fig. 18.2). Pressure patching should only be performed for corneal abrasions with an intact globe and any injury that might suggest a perforation or laceration of the globe should not be pressure patched.

A cycloplegic agent such as Scopolamine 0.25% or Homatropine 5% will dilate the pupil, relax the internal ciliary muscle, and relieve the aching pain of ciliary spasm often associated with corneal abrasions. The patch should be replaced each morning and evening with reapplication of ointment by the patient each time. The patient should be seen every day until the abrasion is completely healed. Most abrasions will heal and symptoms will subside within 72 hours of treatment. If the patient does not respond to treatment within 72 hours, the diagnosis of corneal abrasion should be questioned and other more serious, vision-threatening problems considered for prompt evaluation and treatment.

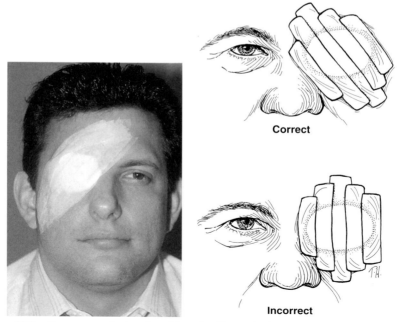

Correct

Incorrect

Figure 18.2.   Pressure patched patient. Note the diagonal orientation of the tape.

REFERRAL GUIDELINES

Corneal abrasions do not need to be referred to an ophthalmologist unless one of the following applies: (a) the abrasion is not fully healed within 72 hours; (b) the abrasion is associated with contact lens wear; or (c) corneal ulcer or infection is suspected.

CORNEAL ULCERATION

Corneal ulceration is a condition where trauma or disease has created sufficient injury to the deeper layers of the corneal tissue to cause stromal loss and corneal thinning. Frequently, corneal ulcerations involve an infectious etiology. In situations of active corneal ulceration, the overlying epithelium is missing and fluorescein staining will help delineate the area of involvement. The primary goal of medical therapy of corneal ulcers is to aid the epithelium to heal over the ulcerative site and prevent further loss of stromal tissue. The treatment of corneal ulcers is difficult and requires specialized equipment and an experienced ophthalmologist. Therefore, the primary care physician must recognize the early corneal ulcer and refer the patient immediately for treatment before blindness or loss of the eye occurs.

CLINICAL MANIFESTATIONS

The setting for corneal ulceration can be quite varied. The patient will usually have a history of corneal epithelial compromise, since the epithelium is the primary barrier to stromal infection and injury. A history of corneal abrasion, ocular trauma, dry eye syndrome, excessive ocular exposure from lid abnormalities, diabetes mellitus, and rheumatoid arthritis are all possible reasons for epithelial compromise leading to corneal ulcers. However, in the United States, the most common cause of infectious corneal ulceration is the use of cosmetic contact lenses, especially lenses worn overnight. Any patient with a history of contact lens wear and an epithelial corneal defect or abrasion should be suspected of having a corneal ulcer until proven otherwise.

The symptoms of a corneal ulcer are the same as an epithelial abrasion: pain, redness, and tearing. In addition to the epithelial defect found on fluorescein staining, the stromal tissue beneath the epithelial defect will be swollen and have a characteristic white infiltrate of the white blood cells concentrated in the ulcerative tissue center. This "white spot on the cornea" in the setting of an epithelial defect should be a red flag for the primary care physician to refer the patient for immediate evaluation and treatment (Fig. 18.3).

The most common organisms in corneal ulceration are staphylococcus, streptococcus, and pseudomonas, although other bacteria, fungi, and protozoa are also seen.

TREATMENT

Corneal ulcers are an ocular emergency and treatment is best done by an ophthalmologist. Therapy involves an initial corneal diagnostic scraping for specific culture and sensitivity, followed by intensive application of topical broad spectrum antibiotics every 15–30 minutes around the clock. Aggressive therapy is necessary as many ulcerations can progress within 24 hours to perforation, blindness, and loss of the eye. With aggressive early treatment, the offending organism can be eradicated and perforation

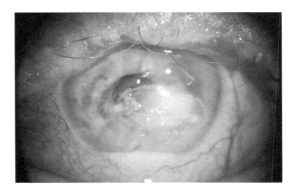

Figure 18.3. Corneal ulcer showing white infiltrate. The white infiltration indicates stromal involvement and the presence of white blood cells.

of the globe prevented. The cornea will heal with a white, often vascularized scar. If the scar is near the visual axis of the central cornea, vision will be permanently impaired and surgical treatment with a corneal transplant will be necessary to restore vision.

REFERRAL GUIDELINES

The success of preserving vision and avoiding surgery for the patient with a corneal ulcer is largely dependent upon early treatment (see Table 18.1) The primary care physician's recognition and prompt referral of the patient within 8 hours of the diagnosis is critical to a successful outcome.

FREQUENCY OF VISITS

Patients with an epithelial abrasion should be examined every day until the abrasion is healed. The ophthalmologist will see the referred patient with a frequency appropriate to the severity of the disease. A neurotrophic corneal erosion may be evaluated once a week, while a bacterial corneal ulcer patient may be hospitalized and seen twice a day until stabilized and surgery averted.

SUGGESTED READINGS

Dart J. Predisposing factors in microbial keratitis: the significance of contact lens wear. Br J Ophthalmol 1988;72:926–930.

Kenyon K, Wagoner M. Conjunctival and corneal injuries. In: Shingleton B, Heash P, Kenyon K, eds. Eye trauma. St Louis: Mosby-Year Book, 1991:63–78.

Matoba A. Infectious keratitis. In: Focal points: clinical modules for ophthalmologists. San Francisco: American Academy of Ophthalmology, 1992;10:6–12.

Schein O, Glynn R, Poggio E, et al. The relative risk of ulcerative keratitis among users of daily-wear and extended-wear soft contact lenses. N Engl J Med 1989;321:773–778.

Schein O, Buehler P, Stamler J, Verdier D, Katz J. The impact of overnight wear on the risk of contact lens-associated ulcerative keratitis. Arch Ophthalmol 1994;112:186–190.

Terry A, Lemp M, Margolis T, et al. Bacterial keratitis: preferred practice pattern. San Francisco: American Academy of Ophthalmology, 1995:1–19.

◖◗◗ Chapter 19
Refractive Errors and Their Correction

M. A. Terry

INTRODUCTION

A refractive error is a defect in the focusing of light by the cornea and lens onto the retina. In normal vision (emmetropia), light enters the eye through the cornea and is focused perfectly onto the retina at the back of the eye (Fig. 19.1). The central region of the retina, the macula, is the point of focus for the light in the normal eye. Although the entire retina can detect a light stimulus, the macular region is responsible for the most defined perception such as reading. The retina transmits the light information via the optic nerve to the brain. Light must be perfectly focused on the macula for normal vision. With a refractive error, the light rays are focused in front of the retina (myopia), or behind the retina (hyperopia), or even simultaneously at two different points (astigmatism). All of these refractive or focusing errors result in abnormal retinal detection of the light stimulus and are perceived as blurry vision. Usually the refractive error occurs because there is a defect in the length of the eyeball; however, abnormalities of the cornea or intraocular crystalline lens may also produce a refractive error.

Accommodation (focusing ability) is the term used to describe the voluntary physiologic process whereby the curvature of the crystalline lens increases and the focus of the eye shifts from a distant object to an object closer to the eye. The accommodative effort is inversely proportional to the distance of the object from the eye and is measured in diopters, with 1 diopter of accommodation required for an object 1 meter away, 2 diopters required for an object 0.5 meter away and so on.

The crystalline lens is supported, just posterior to the iris and pupil and anterior to the vitreous space, by hundreds of fibers known as zonules, which attach to the equator of the lens and the muscular ciliary body within the wall of the eye. In youth and young adulthood, the crystalline lens is pliable and its shape can be changed by altering the tension on the zonules. Muscular tension exerted on the zonules by the ciliary body alters the curvature of the anterior and posterior surface of the lens. This change of shape allows for a variable focus and the clear viewing of objects both close to the individual and in the distance. With age, the composition of the lens changes, and the lens becomes less pliable. This limits its ability to focus on close objects (accommodation). Less accommodative effort is required for the normal (emmetropic) eye to read a newspaper at 18 inches away than at 8 inches away from the eye, and relatively no accommodation is necessary for the normal eye to see objects greater than 20 feet away. Accommodative amplitude begins to decline after the age of 18,

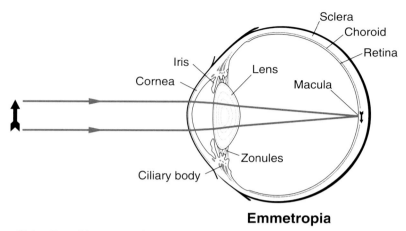

Emmetropia

Figure 19.1.   Eye with emmetropia.

but it generally does not become an impediment until the fifth decade of life when accommodation amplitude is so reduced that reading becomes difficult (presbyopia).

Myopia (nearsightedness) is a condition in which close objects can be seen clearly without glasses, while distant objects appear blurred. Without correction, distance objects cannot be brought into focus on the retina, despite accommodative effort by the individual. Usually, myopia occurs because the eye is too long and the light rays are focused in front of the macula. The rays of light then diverge and are out of focus before they intercept the retina (Fig. 19.2).

Hyperopia (farsightedness) is a condition in which, without correction, some accommodative effort is required to bring distant objects into focus and a large amount of accommodative effort is needed to view close objects clearly. This condition usually

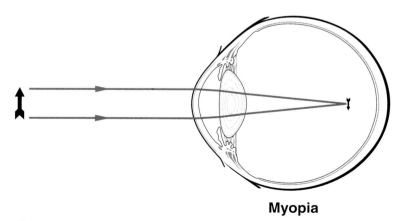

Myopia

Figure 19.2.   Eye with myopia.

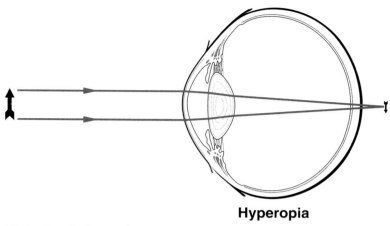

Hyperopia

Figure 19.3. Eye with hyperopia.

occurs because the eyeball is too short and the light rays are not fully focused when they hit the retina (Fig. 19.3).

Astigmatism is a condition in which both near and distant objects appear somewhat indistinct and distorted without correction, and no amount of accommodation by the individual can make them sharp and clear. This condition usually results from an irregularity of the corneal curvature which causes the light rays to be focused at two different distances from the retina (Fig. 19.4). The normal cornea is approximately spherical in shape. The astigmatic cornea is not spherical and therefore focuses light rays irregularly. Astigmatism is common, and vision is usually fully correctable with spectacles or contact lenses. Astigmatism can occur alone or associated with myopia or hyperopia. Astigmatism may also result from pathologic conditions of the cornea (such as scarring), and vision may not be fully correctable.

Presbyopia (trouble reading up close after the age of 40) is an aging change of

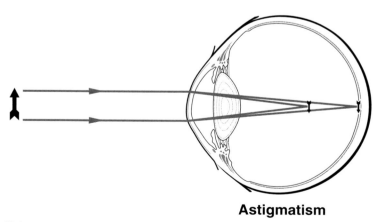

Astigmatism

Figure 19.4. Eye with astigmatism.

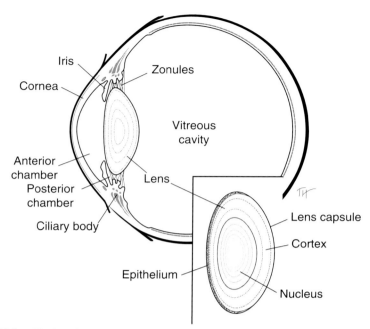

Figure 20.1. The location and components of the lens of the eye.

largely on age (Table 20.1). Between 18% and 28.5% of patients over the age of 65 experience significant cataracts, and as many as 12% of patients over the age of 45 have some lens opacification which may or may not be visually significant.

CLINICAL MANIFESTATIONS

Cataracts can be subclassified by the extent, characteristics, and location of the opacities within the lens. The most common types of age-related cataracts are nuclear, cortical,

TABLE 20.1. Percent of Individuals with Lens Opacities and Visually Significant Cataracts by Age

STUDY	45–54	55–64	65–74	75–84	>85
Framingham					
Lens opacities	—	41.7	73.2	91.1	—
Cataract	—	4.5	18.0	45.9	—
NHANES					
Lens opacities	12.2	27.6	57.6	—	—
Cataract	2.6	10.0	28.5	—	—
Watermen					
Lens opacities	5.7	37.0	72.1	94.2	100.0
Cataract	—	5.0	25.0	59.0	—

Adapted from Cataract Management Guideline Panel. Clinical practice guidelines (4): cataracts in adults: management of functional impairment. AHCPR publication no. 93-0542. Rockville, MD: U.S. Department of Health & Human Services, Table 1.1, 1993;Feb:14.

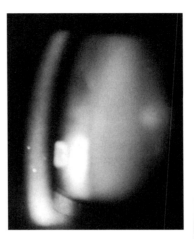

Figure 20.2. Slitlamp photograph of a nuclear sclerotic cataract. Note the yellow-brown color of the nucleus. (See also color section.) (Reprinted by permission from Deutsch TA. Lens and cataract. In: Wright KW, ed. Textbook of ophthalmology. Baltimore: Williams & Wilkins, Fig. 53.3, 1997:780.)

and subcapsular. With age, the central nucleus of the crystalline lens becomes harder and more pigmented, a condition known as nuclear sclerosis. Initially, these changes may actually enhance the near vision by causing thickening of the central lens and a resulting myopic shift. This phenomenon is known as second sight and results from central thickening of the lens, which, in turn, provides increased magnification for the individual and an enhanced ability to read at close range. With time, these sclerotic changes (brownish discoloration and hardening) of the nucleus result in a generalized opacification of the nucleus and decreased vision (Fig. 20.2). In addition to nuclear sclerosis, the lens cortex may also become opacified. Cortical cataracts appear as clefts or opacified radiations within the cortical material surrounding the lens nucleus (Fig. 20.3). Focal cataracts may also occur just anterior to the posterior capsule and are known as posterior subcapsular cataracts. Posterior subcapsular cataracts occur more commonly in middle-aged adults than do nuclear cataracts. These focal lenticular opacities most often occur centrally within the visual axis and are granular in clinical appearance. Posterior subcapsular cataracts are frequently associated with corticosteroid use, or previous trauma, and often progress more rapidly than other types of

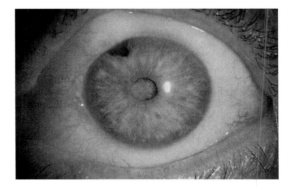

Figure 20.3. Cortical cataract. The white lens can be seen through the miotic pupil. Note the triangular surgical iridectomy (*top left* of the iris) at the site of a previous glaucoma surgery. (See also color section.)

◼❚ TABLE 20.2. Referral Guidelines: Adult Cataract		
SIGNS AND SYMPTOMS	**TREATMENT**	**WHEN TO REFER**
Early: Patient complains of generalized visual difficulties. Initial problems may include trouble reading, driving (especially at night) and close work. Physician may note blurring of retinal detail and dulling of the red reflex on direct ophthalmoscopy.	Early: Provide best refractive correction. Chronic dilation of the pupil may enhance vision in some cataract patients.	Referral is based primarily on the extent of visual disability experienced by the patient. In the absence of other ocular disease, visual complaints comprise the primary indication for cataract surgery. For most patients, this occurs at visual acuities of 20/50 or less.
Late: Increased trouble in performing activities of daily living. Fundoscopic examination may become impossible. The cataract ultimately obscures the pupil and can be seen without special examination techniques.	Late: Cataract extraction with posterior chamber intraocular lens placement.	

cataracts. Because of the central location of posterior subcapsular cataracts, small opacities may result in significant vision loss.

The functional visual impairment which results from these various lens opacities is highly individualized. Patients with early cataracts often have nonspecific complaints of generalized visual difficulties. They may note more difficulty with tasks which place high demands on the visual system, such as driving, reading or close work. As the cataracts progress, activities of daily living may become impossible. However, each patient's visual needs are different. Some patients with a visual acuity of 20/40 or worse on Snellen chart testing may report no functional disability, while others who measure visual acuities better than 20/40 may have multiple visual complaints, and may even curtail activities of daily living and/or work activities. Snellen visual acuity is the most accepted method of assessing visual function; however, this visual function measurement may not reflect every patient's true visual loss. Patients with specific types of opacities such as posterior subcapsular cataracts, may have only a mild decrease in their visual acuity when measured in a dimly lit room. However, the visual decrease associated with glare can be quite disabling in daylight conditions or with nighttime driving from oncoming headlights. Reading may become difficult early in the development of a posterior subcapsular cataract, due to the pupillary constriction which occurs with near vision. This prevents the individual from looking around the central opacity.

DIFFERENTIAL DIAGNOSIS

The diagnosis of cataracts is made by clinical examination of the eye using the illumination and magnification of the slitlamp biomicroscope (Table 20.2). However, the functional significance of the cataract can only be made by interviewing the patient and establishing his or her visual needs. Since cataract extraction is almost always an elective procedure, the functional impairment of the patient far outweighs the anatomic presence of lens opacities seen on clinical examination. A complete eye examination should be performed to rule out other ocular morbidity which may account for the symptom of decreased vision. Particular attention should be paid to the presence of other opacities in the visual axis (such as corneal scarring or vitreous opacities) and to the relative health of the neurosensory portions of the eye (the retina and optic nerve). Removing the opacified, cataractous lens will be of no functional benefit if the macula or optic nerve are diseased to such an extent that visual information cannot be processed.

PREVENTION AND RISK FACTORS

Many studies have shown a higher prevalence of cataracts in geographic regions with high ultraviolet B (UVB) radiation levels. This data suggest the potential benefit of wearing sunglasses which reduce ocular exposure to UVB. Diabetes mellitus is also a risk factor associated with the development of cataracts. Many drugs are considered to be cataractogenic, including corticosteroids, some major tranquilizers (particularly phenothiazines), and possibly diuretics. Cigarette smoking, as well as heavy alcohol consumption, may increase the risk of cataract development. Although many attempts have been made to identify particular dietary components that may increase the risk of cataract development or may be beneficial in the prevention of cataracts, none have been identified.

TREATMENT
SURGICAL INDICATIONS

The decision to perform cataract surgery is generally made after assessing the effect of the cataract on the individual's visual function and visual needs. Nonsurgical management of cataracts includes providing the optimal refractive correction. Also, chronically dilating the pupil with mydriatic drops to allow light to enter the eye around central opacities within the lens can be attempted in early cataracts. As cataracts progress, these interventions become inadequate. Visual decrease to a Snellen acuity of 20/50 or worse is commonly accepted as sufficient visual loss to justify cataract extraction. A decrease to this level of vision prevents the individual from reading most printed material. As well, 20/40 or better vision in at least one eye is needed to obtain a drivers license in most states. If the Snellen acuity is 20/40 or better, an individual may still have sufficient visual complaints to warrant consideration of cataract extraction, if the visual needs are higher than normal or other factors are involved. In general, patients with 20/40 or better vision must be additionally disabled by glare in bright light situations, visual disparity between the eyes, or monocular diplopia (double vision) resulting from the lens opacifications. Other, much less common, indications for cataract extraction include rare lens-induced diseases (such as uveitis or glaucoma) and the need to visualize the fundus for adequate diagnosis and treatment of other eye disorders such as diabetic retinopathy, requiring laser therapy that is prevented by the lens opacification.

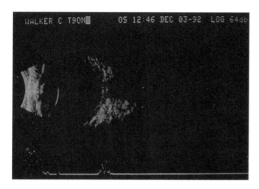

Figure 20.4. Combined A-scan and B-scan ultrasound of the eye. The B-scan (*top*) shows the round contour of the globe, while the A-scan (*bottom*) is used to measure the length of the eye. The spikes along the A-scan represent reflective interfaces of the various tissues of the eye.

PREOPERATIVE OPHTHALMIC TESTING

As mentioned earlier, the most critical preoperative ophthalmic procedure is a complete eye exam to rule out the possibility of concurrent ocular disease. In addition, all individuals in whom an intraocular lens will be placed at the time of surgery must undergo ultrasonic eye length measurements. An A-scan ophthalmic ultrasound is used to measure the axial length of the eye. This measurement is used to approximate the appropriate power of the lens to be implanted (Fig. 20.4).

Glare testing may be used in an effort to establish the true functional impairment of an individual. Glare testing may be performed in an office setting by a variety of techniques that simulate bright light situations. Many individuals complain of a severe vision decrease which cannot be duplicated in routine vision testing. Glare testing methods aim to reproduce situations such as oncoming headlights or bright sunshine,

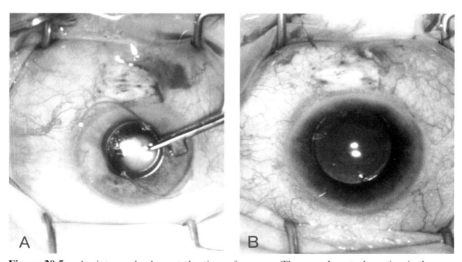

Figure 20.5. An intraocular lens at the time of surgery. The round central portion is the optical component of the lens and the two side haptics are for stabilization within the eye.

which have minimal effect on vision in a normal eye, but significant adverse effects in the cataractous eye.

In some individuals, it is difficult to predict the relative health of the eye and the potential for visual rehabilitation following cataract extraction. This is especially true in an eye with concomitant disease such as glaucoma, diabetic retinopathy, or macular degeneration. In these cases, potential vision testing may also be performed prior to surgery. A variety of potential acuity meters have been developed which try to assess the visual potential of the retina. Although not infallible, these tests aid the clinician in giving the patient the best estimate of the ultimate visual result following cataract surgery.

PREOPERATIVE MEDICAL EXAMINATION

A preoperative medical examination should be performed for all individuals undergoing cataract surgery, whether in the hospital or outpatient surgical facility and regardless of the type of anesthesia to be administered. The preoperative medical assessment is guided by the patient's age and concurrent medical illnesses.

ANESTHESIA

Anesthesia for cataract surgery can be either general or local. Local anesthesia is often preferred to general anesthesia by both the patient and the surgeon. In most settings where local anesthesia is used, concurrent oral or intravenous sedation is provided to the patient. Local anesthesia includes a regional block to the retrobulbar space which provides akinesia and anesthesia of the eye. Often an additional block of the facial nerve is performed to prevent eyelid squeezing during the surgery. Recently, cataract surgery has even been performed using topical anesthetics alone in very cooperative patients.

SURGICAL TECHNIQUES

Over the past two decades a revolution has occurred in the microsurgical techniques used for the removal of cataracts. In the 1970s, there was a transition from traditional intracapsular cataract surgery to extracapsular cataract extraction. In extracapsular cataract extraction, the anterior capsule of the crystalline lens is opened and the lens nucleus removed intact through a 10–14 mm incision at the corneoscleral junction. The remaining cortical material is then aspirated leaving the lens capsule (specifically the posterior capsule) to support the placement of an artificial intraocular lens. Unlike the old intracapsular surgical technique in which the entire lens and its capsule were removed, extracapsular cataract surgery allowed the development of improved artificial intraocular lenses, virtually eliminating the need for thick cataract glasses or uncomfortable aphakic contact lens for the elderly patient. In the 1980s, rapid development of a new surgical technique, termed phacoemulsification cataract extraction, occurred. In phacoemulsification cataract extraction, the lens nucleus is fractured into small pieces and removed with an aspiration instrument through a 3–4 mm incision. This technique employs ultrasound power, which fractures the lens into smaller pieces prior to removal. Because a smaller ocular incision is used with phacoemulsification cataract extraction, smaller and even foldable intraocular lenses have been developed. A smaller

TABLE 20.3. Visual Acuity Following Cataract Surgery*

PERCENT OF EYES 20/40 OR BETTER	NUMBER (PERCENT) OF STUDIES
≥80	33 (100%)
≥90	31 (94%)
≥95	23 (70%)
≥98	12 (36%)
100	6 (18%)

* This compilation of multiple studies confirms the excellent visual prognosis following cataract surgery in eyes without other significant ocular disease.

incision site allows for a safer, more controlled cataract extraction with quicker postoperative visual rehabilitation. With both extracapsular cataract extraction and phacoemulsification cataract extraction, the integrity of the posterior capsule is important for the stability of the intraocular lens. Both techniques are still in common practice, although phacoemulsification is preferred by most surgeons. The choice between these two techniques for the removal of cataracts depends largely on the experience level of the surgeon and the type of cataract being removed.

Intraocular lenses are routinely placed at the time of cataract extraction in most individuals (Fig. 20.5). Over the past several decades, a variety of synthetic materials have been developed to manufacture intraocular lenses, including plastics such as polymethylmethacrylate, silicone, and acrylics. Intraocular lenses are well-tolerated and should be used in most surgeries to enhance the visual outcome. The visual results achieved with contact lenses and spectacle correction in patients without an intraocular lens are generally felt to be inferior. In selected cases, intraocular lens placement may be avoided. In eyes with severe uveitis (intraocular inflammation), and in eyes in which the support of the posterior capsule is insufficient to hold an intraocular lens, lens placement may be omitted. Surgical techniques have been recently developed which allow placement of an intraocular lens even in the absence of a posterior capsule and may be done even years after the original cataract removal.

VISUAL OUTCOME FOLLOWING CATARACT EXTRACTION

Cataract extraction is one of the safest surgical procedures performed. Most patients can expect recovery of excellent vision (Table 20.3); however, as with any surgical procedure, adverse events may occur (Table 20.4). Well over 90% of patients can expect a final postoperative visual acuity of between 20/15 and 20/40 following cataract removal. The majority of postoperative patients require some spectacle correction.

TABLE 20.4. Complications of Cataract Surgery

COMPLICATION	RATE (PERCENT)
Bullous keratopathy	<0.3
Intraocular lens malposition	<1.0
Endophthalmitis	<0.3
Retinal detachment	<1.0
Significant macular edema	<3.0

POSTERIOR CAPSULE OPACIFICATION

Posterior capsule opacification (also known as a secondary cataract) occurs in many individuals after cataract surgery. The posterior capsule of the crystalline lens is purposely preserved at the time of cataract surgery in both extracapsular or phacoemulsification cataract extraction. Preservation of the posterior capsule maintains the normal anatomic structure of the eye and prevents the vitreous humor from entering the anterior segment of the eye and surgical wound. Rupture of the posterior capsule at the time of cataract extraction is considered an undesirable complication which may prevent immediate intraocular lens placement and limit visual outcome. However, long-term vision is largely dependent on maintaining the clarity of the posterior capsule. Gradual opacification of the posterior capsule occurs in between 15–20% of eyes within the first postoperative year and in as many as 50% of patients by the fifth postoperative year. Prior to the development of modern laser technologies, an invasive procedure was required to open the opacified capsule with a surgical knife. More recently, with the advent of the neodymium-YAG laser, it is possible to perform a posterior capsulotomy in the office setting. This minimally invasive, low-risk procedure is frequently required following cataract extraction. The laser is used to create a small central opening in the capsule allowing for a clear visual axis. Most patients do not require posterior capsulotomy prior to 6 weeks following a surgical cataract extraction, but may require a capsulotomy at any time following the procedure. The very small risk of intraocular lens damage or displacement, uveitis, glaucoma, and retinal detachment must be considered prior to capsulotomy.

COMPLICATIONS OF CATARACT SURGERY

As with any surgical procedure, adverse outcomes may occur. Table 20.4 lists the most frequent complications seen following cataract extraction surgery.

Glaucoma, ptosis, and small intraocular hemorrhages may all occur following an otherwise uncomplicated cataract extraction. Often these problems are self-limited or responsive to medical therapeutic intervention. Endophthalmitis (intraocular infection), retinal detachment, and bullous keratopathy (corneal decompensation with edema) are of greater concern, because of the increased likelihood of permanent visual loss. Fortunately, these complications occur rarely (<1%). Significant macular edema (postoperative swelling of the central retina) may occur following cataract surgery and may decrease the best corrected visual acuity. This abnormality most often occurs between 4 and 12 weeks after surgery. Leakage of fluid into the macular region results from a breakdown of the vascular blood/retinal barrier. Macular edema is thought to be related to postoperative intraocular inflammation and usually can be successfully treated with short-term corticosteroid therapy. Expulsive choroidal hemorrhage is a ominous complication which often results in the complete loss of vision and/or the eye. This complication is estimated to occur in approximately 1 in 10,000 cases. All patients should be informed of the possibilities of these complications during the preoperative period to allow them to weigh the relative risks against the expected benefits of cataract surgery.

FREQUENCY OF VISITS

Preoperative assessment of a patient with cataracts should involve an initial complete ophthalmic examination and discussion of the risks and benefits of the procedure.

Following cataract extraction, the patient's eye is typically patched for 24 hours. The patch is removed on the first postoperative day. Most patients are treated with a topical corticosteroid anti-inflammatory and an antibiotic during the immediate postoperative period. Patients are usually seen the day after the surgery and then 1 and 4 weeks following cataract extraction. Visual rehabilitation with a new corrective lens prescription is usually achieved within 4–6 weeks following the cataract extraction, and often sooner. Variations in the timing of the final refractive correction depend largely on the healing response of the individual patient.

SUGGESTED READINGS

Burrows J, Briggs RS, Elkington AR. Cataract extraction and confusion in elderly patients. J Clin Exp Gerontol 1985;(10):51–70.

Cataract Management Guideline Panel. Clinical practice guidelines (4): cataracts in adults: management of functional impairment. AHCPR publication no. 93–0542. Rockville, MD: U.S. Department of Health & Human Services, 1993;Feb.

Elliott J. Poor vision and the elderly–a domiciliary study. Eye 1989;3:365–369.

Taylor HR, Sommer A. Cataract surgery: a global perspective. Arch Ophthalmol 1990;108(6):797–798.

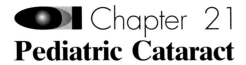 Chapter 21
Pediatric Cataract

A. C. Tongue

INTRODUCTION

An opacity of the lens is referred to as a cataract. Slitlamp examination may reveal minor opacities, particularly of the nucleus of the lens, which do not interfere with vision. Significant opacities of the lens can be identified by the Bruckner or red reflex test (Fig. 21.1). Total opacities will obscure the red reflex or markedly dampen its quality. Partial opacities show up as darker areas within the red reflex. Other media opacities, including corneal and vitreous opacities, may produce an abnormal darker red reflex. A white or grey reflex, as seen with total cataracts (Fig. 21.2), may also be secondary to retrolental membranes such as in retinopathy of prematurity, total retinal detachments, or organized vitreous (see Table 31.1 in Chapter 31, "Pediatric Intraocular Tumor: Retinoblastoma"). Retinoblastoma usually has a slightly yellow, rather than stark white or grey, reflex. Blood vessels or a reddish hue may also be visible on the surface However, a previously undiagnosed white or grey reflex in the pupil should be considered an extremely urgent clinical sign which needs immediate further evaluation by an ophthalmologist.

CLINICAL MANIFESTATIONS

Unilateral lens opacities which can cause significant vision loss if not treated early in life are generally larger than 3 mm in diameter, interfere with funduscopy with the direct ophthalmoscope, and are readily identifiable with the red reflex test. The examiner will note a dark opacity or a darker reflex on the side of the lens opacity. Total opacification of the lens or large dense opacities may be seen by direct inspection and may give rise to a white or grey pupil (Fig. 21.3). Lens opacities which are readily detected by the primary care physician in the newborn or young infant should be considered an urgent problem and be referred immediately to an ophthalmologist. Early surgical removal of cataracts, which if left alone would cause severe amblyopia and essentially blind eyes, can result in good visual outcome. There is a definite correlation between visual outcome and the timing of surgery in congenital cataracts–the earlier the surgery (in terms of days to a few weeks), the better the result. Visual acuities of 20/40 or better can be achieved. Children who have surgery for significant congenital lens opacities after 2–4 months of age have a poorer visual prognosis.

Some cataracts may progress or develop during the first year or two of life. Even though some of these may be present during the newborn period, they may not become of significant size and density to be visually impairing until the child is a few months or a year old (Fig. 21.3). Children with this type of cataract may have a relatively good

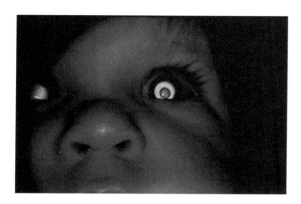

Figure 21.1. Central lens opacity in infant noticeable with red reflex test. (See also color section.) (Courtesy of A. Tongue, M.D.)

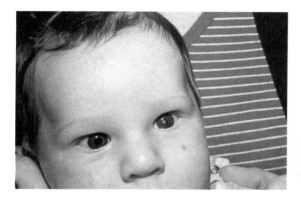

Figure 21.2. Leukocoria (white reflex) left eye, secondary to cataract. (See also color section.) (Courtesy of A. Tongue, M.D.)

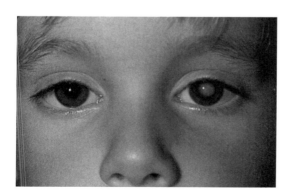

Figure 21.3. Total cataract. Same eye as in Figure 21.1, but 1 year later. Opacification occurred over a period of a week, probably secondary to rupture of posterior lens capsule. Visual acuity after cataract surgery 20/40. (See also color section.) (Courtesy of A. Tongue, M.D.)

prognosis with later surgery (i.e., after 4 months). Information about the quality of the red reflex test during the newborn period can be very helpful to the ophthalmologist in making a decision as to the visual prognosis for a dense cataract in a child older than 4 months.

Bilateral congenital cataracts should be surgically removed as soon as they are noted to be of sufficient density to interfere with good vision development. Sometimes the cataracts are asymmetric in density and size, and amblyopia develops rapidly in the more involved eye.

Cataracts which are small and compatible with a visual acuity of 20/60 to 20/70 or better may not be operated and may be treated by patching of the uninvolved eye, or, in case of bilateral cataracts, of the less involved eye. Infants with small lens opacities noted by the parents or physician need referral for amblyopia treatment and follow-up.

Evaluation of the family's ability to comply with postoperative management of unilateral aphakia is important in the decision-making process of whether to operate or not.

Differential Diagnosis

Small cataracts which do not impede vision can be amblyogenic (Table 21.1). The most common of these is the anterior polar cataract. It is usually visible by direct examination and may be noted by the parent (often by the mother as she breast feeds) as a small grey fleck in the pupil. The opacity is small (usually 1 mm or less), does not progress, and is compatible with normal vision (20/20 to 20/30). However, about one-third of these small opacities are associated with significant refractive errors which can lead to amblyopia as dense as 20/200 to 20/400. Children with these opacities need to be closely monitored by an ophthalmologist until they are 5–7 years old, even if during the first year or two of life good fixation and following are noted. Amblyopia treatment and refractive correction are instituted when visual acuity and refractive changes are suspected or identified. The author has had personal experience with children with small unilateral anterior polar opacities, who had excellent fixation and following as infants, but were lost to follow-up between ages 2 and 4, and subsequently presented with 20/400 acuity in the involved eye secondary to refractive amblyopia.

It should be pointed out here that small posterior lens opacities slightly eccentric to the visual axis (usually nasal) are caused by tiny remnants of the hyaloid system and are referred to as Mittendorf dots. These opacities are never seen with the naked eye and require visualization with the ophthalmoscope. Because of their posterior location, they move opposite to eye movement (if the eye moves nasally, the opacity will appear to move temporally; if the eye moves up, the opacity moves down). Anterior opacities will move in the direction of the eye; that is, eye up, opacity up. Noticeable Mittendorf dots (only notable with the ophthalmoscope) are seen in about 2% of the population.

Posterior lenticonus (outpouching of posterior lens capsule) is a unilateral lens change, which early in life may not be cataractous, but causes a significant refractive error. These children require refractive correction and amblyopia treatment. With time the lens may become cataractous and may rapidly opacify when the lens capsule ruptures. Good visual results can be obtained in this group of children if treatment for amblyopia is instituted early. Early posterior lenticonus may appear as a darker

⬤◗ TABLE 21.1. Referral Guidelines: Pediatric Cataracts (366.00)

SYMPTOMS OR SIGNS	TREATMENT	WHEN TO REFER
Leukocoria (360.44) Media opacity noted with red reflex test Unable to visualize fundus Family history Unilateral strabismus Poor vision, one or both eyes Systemic disease or syndrome at high risk for cataract	For small lens opacities nonsurgical management with correction of amblyogenic refractive errors and amblyopia treatment as indicated during first 5–7 years of life. Prompt surgical removal of cataract if dense or large and vision impairing. Immediate refractive correction and amblyopia treatment. Monitor refractive status, visual acuity and complications such as glaucoma, retinal detachments, and strabismus. Treat as indicated. Examine parents and siblings and obtain family history in absence of specific etiology for cataract. Initiate appropriate laboratory tests and referrals as indicated by type of cataract and systemic findings. Minimum annual lifetime comprehensive eye evaluation once amblyopia treatment and observation is terminated.	If large opacity immediate referral. Total cataract in neonates and infants less than 4 months should be considered very urgent (i.e., 1 to a few days). Small (1 mm or less) anterior polar opacities or 3 mm or less posterior opacities are less urgent, but should receive comprehensive eye evaluation within 1–2 weeks in preverbal age group (i.e., can't test visual acuity). Genetic counseling and evaluation in all cases of bilateral cataracts unless nongenetic etiology securely established. Genetic evaluation and counseling for unilateral cataracts if indicated. Referral to diagnostic centers may be appropriate if suspicion of systemic, metabolic disease, developmental delay, or other nonspecific abnormalities arise. Refer for low vision aids and community support services when appropriate.

circle within the red reflex. The outpouching of the lens capsule, and therefore also the lens, usually occurs centrally.

Persistent hyperplastic primary vitreous (PHPV) is a common cause of unilateral cataracts. The involved eye is usually smaller than the uninvolved eye. The abnormality is due to persistence of the primitive hyaloid vascular system which extends from the disc to the posterior lens capsule. In severe cases, the anterior chamber may be very shallow due to the anterior displacement of the lens. In some patients, retinal involvement with a thick vascular stalk and anatomic distortion of the disc and macula may preclude a good visual outcome. Surgical removal of the lens in some severe cases is indicated (even if the visual prognosis is not good) to avoid angle closure glaucoma which may occur during the first year or two of life. Anterior persistent hyperplastic primary vitreous, which involves primarily the lens only and causes a significant lens opacity, can have excellent visual results if operated early.

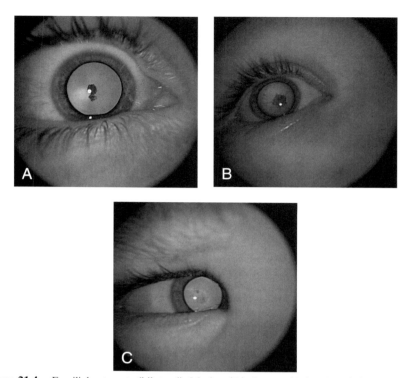

Figure 21.4.   Familial cataracts (bilateral). Mother (**A**), 3-year-old daughter (**B**), and 1-year-old daughter (**C**). Note lens opacity in youngest child is less dense than in older child and mother. These lens opacities did not require removal but, because of asymmetry, required amblyopia treatment. (Courtesy of A. Tongue, M.D.)

The etiology of congenital cataracts is often not established. In bilateral cases, hereditary cataract is common (40%) (Fig. 21.4). Parents and siblings should be examined with a slitlamp. Dominantly inherited cataracts are more common than autosomal recessive or X-linked. About 25% of bilateral hereditary cataracts represent a new autosomal dominant mutation.

Cataracts may be associated with systemic diseases or syndromes (5%). In a pediatric practice, the most common is probably Down syndrome. Visually significant cataracts are often posterior in the lens (posterior subcapsular) and may show progressive opacification during the first year or two of life. Down syndrome patients should therefore have their red reflex monitored at every well-baby checkup. Visually insignificant cataracts, which are usually only noted by slitlamp, are scattered cortical opacities (snowflake or cerulean cataract) and are common in Down patients. They usually do not require treatment and are generally not seen with the ophthalmoscope or red reflex test.

Metabolic cataracts are uncommon in infants and young children unless associated with systemic clinical manifestations of the metabolic disease, such as Lowe syndrome.

Galactokinase deficiency is the exception, and the cataract may be reversible if the condition is identified. The cataract of galactosemia is usually posterior and is

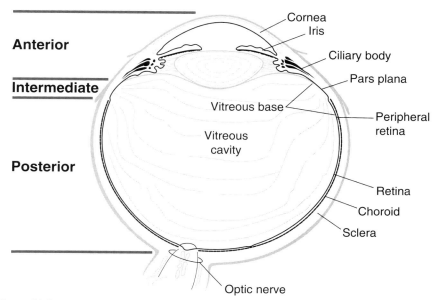

Anterior

Intermediate

Posterior

Cornea
Iris
Ciliary body
Pars plana
Vitreous base
Peripheral retina
Vitreous cavity
Retina
Choroid
Sclera
Optic nerve

Figure 22.1. Uveal tract composes the middle layer of the eye (the iris, the ciliary body, and the choroid). The eye can be divided into three anatomic zones: anterior, intermediate, and posterior. Uveitis (intraocular inflammation) may be isolated to one of these three regions or may simultaneously involve multiple segments of the eye.

The underlying etiologies of intraocular inflammation are quite varied and may be isolated to the eye or associated with a variety of systemic disorders (Table 22.1). The etiology of uveitis may be genetically predispositioned (e.g., HLA-B27 associated anterior uveitis), may be secondary to an infectious agent (e.g., syphilis or cytomegalovirus retinitis), may be associated with a systemic autoimmune disorder (e.g., inflammatory bowel syndrome), may be the result of ocular trauma, or may be idiopathic. This chapter focuses on the most common forms of uveitis and their diagnosis and treatment. Ocular disorders associated with the human immune deficiency virus (HIV) and acquired immune deficiency syndrome (AIDS) are reviewed at the conclusion of this chapter.

CLINICAL MANIFESTATIONS

The clinical signs and symptoms of intraocular inflammation are dependent primarily on the site of the inflammation. The most common signs of uveitis are summarized in Table 22.2.

Anterior Uveitis

Individuals with acute anterior uveitis present with photophobia (light sensitivity), epiphora (tearing), ocular pain (deep-seated aching), redness, and variably decreased

TABLE 22.1. Most Common
Etiologies of Ocular
Inflammation—Separated
by Location

Anterior Uveitis
  Granulomatous
    Sarcoidosis
    Syphilis
    Tuberculosis
  Nongranulomatous
    HLA-B27 associated
    Idiopathic
    Traumatic
    Ocular herpetic infections
    Inflammatory bowel syndrome
Intermediate Uveitis
  Pars planitis
Posterior Uveitis
  Retinitis
    Toxoplasmosis
    Syphilis
    Cytomegalovirus (CMV)
  Choroiditis
    Tuberculosis
    Toxocariasis
    Ocular histoplasmosis
Panuveitis
  Sarcoidosis
  Behçet's syndrome
  Lyme disease
  Vogt-Koyanagi-Harada syndrome
Episcleritis
  Idiopathic
Scleritis
  Idiopathic
  Ankylosing spondylitis
  Rheumatoid arthritis
  Wegner's granulomatosis
  Systemic lupus erythematosus

vision. In comparison, patients with chronic anterior uveitis often present with nonspecific blurring of vision and very few other ocular symptoms.

Anterior uveitis is generally separated into two broad categories, nongranulomatous and granulomatous, based upon the inflammatory reaction within the eye. Nongranulomatous uveitis is much more common. In nongranulomatous anterior uveitis, the onset is typically acute, with marked ocular pain, photophobia, and circumcorneal redness from vascular engorgement. Ocular pain and photophobia result from inflammation of the muscular portions of the uvea, primarily the iris. Complaints of a deep-seated ache within the eye are frequent. Normal room lights may be sufficiently bright to induce ciliary spasm and intense photophobia. The vision may be blurred or severely

TABLE 22.2. Common Signs of Ocular Inflammation

Eyelid and Skin
    Vitiligo
    Skin nodules
Conjunctiva
    Perilimbal vascular injection
    Inflammatory nodules
Cornea
    Keratic precipitates*
Anterior Chamber
    Inflammatory cells*
    Flare (proteinaceous influx into aqueous
        humor)*
Iris
    Nodules*
    Posterior synechiae with pupil distortion
    Atrophy
Intraocular Pressure
    Hypotony (very low)
    Elevation
Retina
    Whitening of the retina
    Retinal ischemia
    Inflammatory cuffing of blood vessels
    Inflammatory cell aggregates
    Pigment clumping
    Neovascularization
Choroid
    Inflammatory infiltrates
    Atrophy
    Neovascularization
Optic Nerve
    Edema
    Neovascularization

* Require slitlamp biomicroscope to identify

altered, but is often only minimally decreased. In cases of prolonged uveitis, cataract formation and subsequent vision loss are frequent.

Nongranulomatous uveitis is characterized by acute episodes with frequent recurrences. However, between episodes, the patient may be without symptoms, and the examination may be totally normal. Pupillary response is often sluggish, and the shape of the pupil may be irregular due to adherence of the iris to the anterior lens capsule (posterior synechiae). Pupil irregularities typically occur later in the disease, following multiple episodes of inflammation. Inflammation within the trabecular meshwork, the drainage site for aqueous humor from the anterior segment of the eye, may cause obstruction and the intraocular pressure may become markedly elevated (inflammatory glaucoma) (see Chapter 29, "Glaucoma"). Conversely, inflammation of the ciliary body, the site of aqueous humor formation, may result in decreased production and

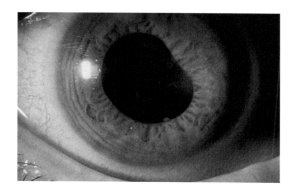

Figure 22.2. Pupil irregularity secondary to uveitis. Distortion of the pupil and lack of response to light stimulation frequently occur from adhesion of the iris to the crystalline lens.

abnormally low intraocular pressure (hypotony). In most cases of mild-to-moderate uveitis, intraocular pressure remains unchanged.

With a handheld light, signs such as decreased pupillary responses and irregularly shaped pupils can be noted (Fig. 22.2). However, a slitlamp biomicroscope is needed to visualize the inflammatory reaction within the anterior chamber. The slitlamp allows the examiner to evaluate the eye for the presence of "flare," or inflammatory turbidity of the aqueous humor, and for the presence of inflammatory cells floating within the aqueous humor. Aqueous "cell" and "flare" usually occur together. Flare is described as "a headlight shining through fog," when the turbidity of the aqueous is seen with the illumination of the slitlamp. Aqueous cells appear as "dust particles" floating in the anterior chamber. The hallmark of nongranulomatous uveitis is very fine inflammatory precipitates on the posterior surface of the cornea. These can be seen with slitlamp magnification. These inflammatory precipitates are aggregates of lymphocytes and plasma cells, and are also known as keratic precipitates (KPs). These three clinical signs (keratic precipitates, aqueous humor flare, and aqueous humor cells) are used as markers to grade the severity of disease and the efficacy of therapeutic intervention. If the inflammation is severe, accumulation of white blood cells may layer out in the inferior anterior chamber, known as a hypopyon (Fig. 22.3). With resolution of the acute episode, either spontaneously or with treatment, the keratic precipitates, the aqueous cells, and the flare disappear.

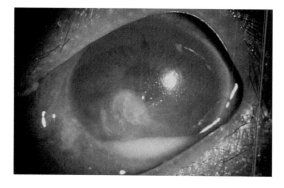

Figure 22.3. Hypopyon. A collection of inflammatory white blood cells in the anterior chamber of the eye may occur in severe intraocular inflammatory disorders.

In the granulomatous form of anterior uveitis, there is generally an insidious onset with minimal ocular pain and redness; however, moderate-to-marked vision loss is common, even early in the disease process. This form of uveitis is most often chronic and characterized by long periods of intraocular inflammation (months to years), punctuated by intervals of increased inflammation and adverse sequelae. Photophobia may be present but is often minimal. Because the ocular discomfort can be slight and the vision loss gradual, the patient may not notice significant changes. In light of this, patients with chronic granulomatous uveitis should be prophylactically monitored on an ongoing basis to minimize vision loss. Many clinical findings are similar to nongranulomatous uveitis with sluggish pupillary reactions and irregularly shaped pupil due to adhesions between the iris and the lens. Cataract formation and glaucoma secondary to the inflammation are more frequent with granulomatous uveitis. Slitlamp examination is needed to identify the hallmark of granulomatous uveitis, which is the presence of large gray keratic precipitates. These large keratic precipitates are comprised of collections of macrophages and epithelioid cells. Inflammatory iris nodules are also frequent in granulomatous uveitis, and aqueous humor cells and flare are typically present.

Intermediate Uveitis (Pars Planitis)

Patients with inflammation of the middle portion of the globe, the ciliary body, present with a gradual decrease of vision and often complain of visual floaters. Floaters result from inflammatory debris in the vitreous cavity, which cast a shadow on the retina. Visual changes are usually from accumulation of fluid in the retina (macular edema) secondary to the intraocular inflammation.

Frequently, there are few, if any, external signs of inflammation in patients with intermediate uveitis, and the anterior chamber is normally devoid of inflammatory reaction. Therefore, the diagnosis is based on finding inflammatory exudates in the pars plana, the posterior portion of the ciliary body. These exudates are impossible to visualize without a dilated pupil and indirect ophthalmoscopy. Patients suspected of having intermediate uveitis should be referred to an ophthalmologist for a complete examination.

Posterior Uveitis

The inflammation of posterior uveitis may be focused in the retina or in the choroid; however, the associated symptoms are very similar. The primary complaint of patients with posterior uveitis is decreased vision. As with intermediate uveitis, floaters may also occur secondary to inflammatory debris in the vitreous. Symptoms may be acute or insidious in presentation. Specific symptoms of metamorphopsia (distortion of straight lines) or scotomas (gray or blank spots within the field of vision) may also be present. Metamorphopsia indicates involvement of the macula, the region of the retina responsible for central reading vision.

Clinical findings of posterior uveitis include inflammatory "sheathing" or "cuffing" of the retinal vessels, exudative deposits within and under the retina, focal narrowing of the vessels, and clumps of pigment deposits. If the inflammation is primarily in the

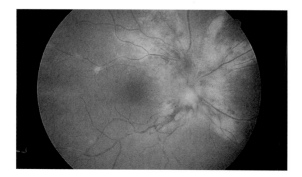

Figure 22.4. Retinitis: inflammation of the retina secondary to cytomegalovirus infection. Note the large areas of white exudate with "feathery" borders and retinal hemorrhages.

retina (retinitis), large areas of the retina may appear white and thickened (Fig. 22.4). The borders between normal and abnormal retina may have a feathery appearance. Retinal ischemia, and even neovascularization may occur. If the inflammation is focused in the choroid (choroiditis), yellowish-white lesions deep to the retina are seen (Fig. 22.5). These lesions are frequently multifocal and distributed throughout the fundus. As choroidal inflammation resolves, the overlying retina may become atrophic and dysfunctional.

Panuveitis

Panuveitis involves the entire eye, therefore signs and symptoms of this disorder are a combination of the clinical findings seen with anterior, intermediate, and posterior uveitis.

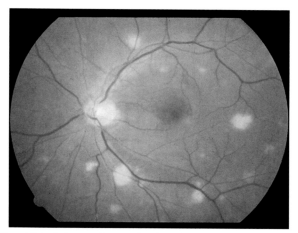

Figure 22.5. Choroiditis. Inflammation confined to the choroid presents with multiple, yellowish-white lesion. The retina may appear normal.

Episcleritis

Episcleritis is generally a benign, self-limited inflammation of the connective tissues overlying the sclera. Episcleritis is usually unilateral. It is usually not associated with systemic disease and does not progress to scleritis. Patients present with mild discomfort and redness that is often limited to one sector of the eye. The involved eye may be very tender. Acute episodes lasting several days to weeks, with frequent recurrences, are common. The etiology of most episcleritis is unknown.

Scleritis

Scleritis is a chronic inflammatory disorder of the sclera that occurs most frequently in women between the ages of 30 and 60 years old. As opposed to episcleritis, scleritis is frequently associated with systemic disease including ankylosing spondylitis, rheumatoid arthritis, Wegner's granulomatosis, and systemic lupus erythematosus (SLE). Most patients with scleritis present with intense ocular pain, redness, and photophobia. The pain may localized to the eye or may involve the periorbita. There is a form of scleritis, necrotizing scleritis without inflammation, which may present with minimal pain. Visual changes are variable and are dependent on whether scleral inflammation is confined to the anterior segment of the eye (anterior scleritis) or to the posterior segment (posterior scleritis). The inflammation of scleritis may extend to adjacent tissue, such as the cornea, episcleral tissues, conjunctiva, or choroid. The inflammation is often severe enough to cause localized areas of scleral thinning.

The most important features of scleritis are its association with a variety of systemic disorders and the possibility of visual complications. Systemic disorders are found in almost all patients with necrotizing scleritis, but are rarely associated with posterior scleritis. Necrotizing scleritis without inflammation may progress to frank scleral perforation (scleromalacia perforans) and is commonly associated with severe rheumatoid arthritis. Severe rheumatoid arthritis may also be associated with thinning of the peripheral cornea (peripheral necrotizing keratitis), which can result in precipitous vision loss (Fig. 22.6).

Differential Diagnosis

Once the diagnosis of uveitis is established, an attempt is made to identify a specific etiology and any associated ocular or systemic disorders. As previously described,

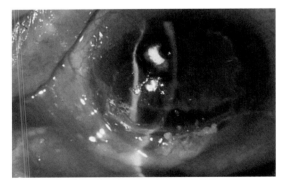

Figure 22.6. Necrotizing keratitis. Note the "gutter-like" thinning of the peripheral inferior cornea in this patient with scleritis and keratitis associated with rheumatoid arthritis.

TABLE 22.3. Common Diagnostic Tests for the Systemic Evaluation of Uveitis

DISORDER	EXAMINATION FINDINGS	DIAGNOSTIC WORKUP MAY INCLUDE
Anterior uveitis	Unilateral Nongranulomatous	Local therapy No further workup
	Bilateral Recurrent Granulomatous	CBC, ESR, PPD, ANA, RPR, FTA-ABS, chest x-ray. Other diagnostic tests based on symptoms (e.g., HLA-B27, sacroiliac x-ray, etc.)
Posterior uveitis	Retinitis	Toxoplasmosis titers, RPR, FTA-ABS, ANA. Other diagnostic tests based on specific retinal findings (e.g., HLA typing, Lyme titers, etc.)
	Choroiditis	PPD, chest x-ray, toxocara titer
	Immunocompromised host	VDRL/FTA-ABS, CMV titers, candida cultures, consider other opportunistic infections
Panuveitis		HLA typing, ACE level, chest x-ray, Lyme titers

many different disease processes can result in inflammation of the uveal tract, including infection, trauma, malignancy, and immune-mediated disorders (Tables 22.1, 22.3, and 22.4). A thorough evaluation of uveitis includes an ocular examination to identify specific clinical characteristics, a systemic history and physical examination, and laboratory evaluation.

Traumatic Uveitis

Blunt, even mild, ocular trauma may result in intraocular inflammation of the uveal tract, usually limited to an anterior uveitis. All patients with uveitis should be questioned about recent ocular trauma. Trauma disrupts the blood-aqueous barrier, allowing serum protein and blood cells to enter the anterior segment of the eye. Symptoms are consistent with other forms of anterior uveitis and include photophobia, mild pain, and redness. Visual acuity is usually unaffected. Traumatic uveitis is typically self-limited, but may require cycloplegic and topical steroid therapy (see "Treatment" in this chapter). As with any ocular trauma, more significant injuries, such as a ruptured globe, should be ruled out with a complete ocular examination (see Chapter 15, "Ocular Trauma").

Anterior Uveitis (Iritis)

The differential diagnosis of acute iritis includes inflammatory autoimmune disorders, infectious diseases, and malignancies. Approximately one-half of patients with acute anterior uveitis are HLA-B27-positive, and half of these will develop an associated autoimmune disorder, including ankylosing spondylitis, Reiter's syndrome, psoriasis, and ulcerative colitis. Other diseases associated with anterior uveitis include Crohn's disease, juvenile rheumatoid arthritis, and sarcoidosis.

Anterior uveitis may also result from an infectious etiology, including syphilis, herpes simplex, herpes zoster, adenovirus, tuberculosis, and human immunodeficiency virus. Finally, a variety of malignancies may masquerade as iritis, including large cell lymphoma, malignant melanoma, leukemia, and retinoblastoma.

duration of action as they provide a drug depot, and they also provide higher levels of the drug to the posterior segment of the eye. These injections are also helpful in the treatment of macular edema which may accompany any form of uveitis. Triamcinolone and dexamethasone are the most frequently injected corticosteroids.

Finally, in cases of severe uveitis, especially if associated with vision loss, systemic corticosteroids may be necessary. Prednisolone (dose 1.0–1.5 mg/kg/day) is preferred and is typically used for several weeks. Oral administration is the most common; however, intravenous therapy may be necessary. Regardless of the route of administration, withdrawal of the corticosteroid therapy should be very slow, as to avoid "rebound" inflammation. Patients who initially require systemic therapy may be tapered and converted to periocular or topical therapy.

Cytotoxic/Cytostatic Immunosuppression

For severe uveitis, systemic cytotoxic therapy may be indicated. Azathioprine, colchicine, methotrexate, cyclosporine, cyclophosphamide, and chlorambucil are the most frequently employed immunosuppressive agents for uveitis. Behçet's syndrome, rheumatoid sclerouveitis, and Vogt-Koyanagi-Harada syndrome are among the absolute indications for cytotoxic therapy. Relative indications for these agents include severe par planitis, retinal vasculitis, and uveitis associated with juvenile rheumatoid arthritis. Cytotoxic/cytostatic therapy requires meticulous monitoring by both a primary care physician and an ophthalmologist. Often, a rheumatologist or oncologist is involved in the administration of cytotoxic immunosuppression.

FREQUENCY OF VISITS

Specific guidelines for the frequency of office visits needed in the treatment of uveitis is difficult because of the diversity of the disease presentations and the highly individualized response to therapy. Generally, after the initial diagnosis, the response to therapy should be assessed weekly and therapy tapered over several weeks to months. For individuals with chronic granulomatous uveitis, ongoing examinations are often required (three to four times per year), because of the high frequency of secondary ocular diseases and lack of symptoms to alert the patient. If the acute episodes are detected early and treated promptly, there is an excellent prognosis for maintaining good vision. Chronic uveitis carries a more guarded prognosis, and retention of vision depends on the underlying etiology.

OCULAR MANIFESTATIONS OF ACQUIRED IMMUNE DEFICIENCY SYNDROME

Patients with human immunodeficiency virus (HIV) infection and acquired immune deficiency syndrome (AIDS) may present with a variety of ocular manifestations. These ocular disorders are usually the result of opportunistic infections or neoplastic diseases. Virtually every part of the eye and its adnexa may be involved, including the eyelids, lacrimal glands, conjunctiva, cornea, anterior segment, and retina. The most common disorders associated with HIV infection are Kaposi's sarcoma, herpes zoster ophthalmicus, infectious keratoconjunctivitis, molluscum contagiosum, and a variety of retinal diseases. Over two-thirds of AIDS patients will have some ocular

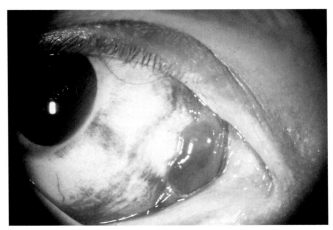

Figure 22.7. Kaposi's sarcoma. Note the typical location in the inferior fornix of the lower eyelid. This lesion appears bright red and may be confused with a subconjunctival hemorrhage.

involvement, with a wide range of possible sequelae from minor cosmetic lesions to total blindness. The potential of severe vision loss is commonly sited as the most feared complication among AIDS patients.

Kaposi's Sarcoma

Kaposi's sarcoma (Fig. 22.7) is the most common external disorder associated with HIV infection and usually presents as a bright red lesion under the conjunctiva. Approximately one-third of AIDS patients will develop this neoplastic disorder. It usually is found in the inferior fornix and may involve the inner eyelid, as well as the globe. It often is confused with a subconjunctival hemorrhage and may rarely extend into the orbit. Kaposi's sarcoma is usually asymptomatic, although foreign body sensation and vision changes may occur. Treatment includes local excision of small lesions and chemotherapy for large, recurrent, multiple, or orbital lesions.

Herpes Zoster Ophthalmicus

Herpes zoster ophthalmicus is very uncommon in patients under the age of 50 years, and HIV infection or other causes of immunosuppression should be suspected in any young patient presenting with this disorder. Herpes zoster ophthalmicus typically presents with a vesicular eruption in the distribution of the trigeminal nerve. A complete discussion of the clinical manifestations, differential diagnosis, and treatment of herpes zoster ophthalmicus are found elsewhere in the text (see Chapter 23, "Ocular Herpetic Infections"). Treatment involves systemic acyclovir (initially intravenous, followed by oral) and control of intraocular inflammation.

Molluscum Contagiosum

Molluscum contagiosum presents as umbilicated, nodular skin lesions on the eyelids and periorbital area. This condition is caused by a DNA-pox virus. Shedding of virus particle into the eye may result in a secondary conjunctivitis, with an accompanying foreign body sensation and ocular irritation. Therapy involves simple surgical excision.

Retinal Disease

Retinal disorders are among the most common ocular abnormalities associated with HIV infection and have the greatest potential for severe vision loss. Because of this, any HIV-positive patient with retinal lesions or visual changes should have a complete ocular examination by an ophthalmologist.

HIV retinopathy is present in many AIDS patients and consists of a retinal vasculitis with cotton wool spots (white infarcts of the retinal nerve fiber layer), retinal hemorrhages, and microaneurysms. The etiology and significance of HIV retinopathy is unknown.

Cytomegalovirus retinitis is the most common ocular opportunistic infection and the most frequent cause of severe vision loss among AIDS patients. The primary symptoms are painless vision loss in one or both eyes. Frequently early in the disease, cytomegalovirus retinitis is asymptomatic as the infection initially involves the peripheral retina and peripheral vision loss is difficult for the patient to detect. A CD4 lymphocyte count of less than 50 cells per mm is highly associated with the development of cytomegalovirus retinitis. The diagnosis of cytomegalovirus retinitis is made by dilated funduscopic examination. The classic findings are multiple, large areas of retinal necrosis (white, atrophic areas) with feathery borders and retinal hemorrhages (Fig. 22.4). This clinical picture has been characterized by the descriptive phrase "pizza pie" retinitis. If the cytomegalovirus infection involves the macular region, severe vision loss is common. An evaluation for systemic cytomegalovirus infection should be performed (urine testing) in any patient suspected of having cytomegalovirus retinitis. Therapy for cytomegalovirus retinitis is evolving, as new antiviral agents become available. The mainstays of therapy presently are ganciclovir and foscarnet. The undesirable side effect of myelosuppression commonly limits the systemic administration of these antiviral agents. Therefore, intravitreal injections and sustained release intraocular implants have been developed.

Other retinal diseases are also associated with HIV infection and include progressive retinal necrosis and infectious retinitis. Progressive retinal necrosis is characterized by acute necrosis of the outer retina, often in HIV-positive individuals without immune compromise. The retina appears white and atrophic. Anterior uveitis may accompany retinal necrosis, and the etiology is believed to be a herpetic virus. Even with treatment, progressive retinal necrosis often results in severe loss of vision. Toxoplasmosis, histoplasmosis, and syphilis are the most common infectious agents that cause retinal infections in immunocompromised patients with HIV.

SUGGESTED READING

Friedberg MA, Rapuano CJ. Uveitis. In: Wills, ed. Eye hospital-office and emergency room diagnosis and treatment of eye disease. Philadelphia: J.B. Lippincott, 1990:331–366.

Hemady R, Tauber J, Foster CS. Immunosuppressive drugs in immune and inflammatory ocular disease. Surv Ophthalmol 1991;35:369–385.

Kanski JJ. Juvenile arthritis and uveitis. Surv Ophthalmol 1990;34:253–267.

Moorthy RS, Rao NA. Uveitis: introduction and classification. In: Wright KW, ed. Textbook of ophthalmology. Baltimore: Williams and Wilkins, 1996:477–479.

Nussenblatt RB, Palestine AG. Uveitis: fundamentals and clinical practice. Chicago: Year Book Medical Publishers, 1989:206–207.

Smith RE, Nozik RA. Uveitis: a clinical approach to diagnosis and management. 2nd ed. Baltimore: Williams and Wilkins, 1989:23–26.

Tamesis RR, Foster CS. Ocular syphilis. Ophthalmology 1990;97:13–22.

Chapter 23 ●❘
Ocular Herpetic Infections

M. A. Terry

INTRODUCTION

Herpetic infections of the eye are common and the primary care physician will often see patients suffering from ocular herpes simplex (HSV or herpes simplex virus) and ocular herpes zoster (HZO or herpes zoster ophthalmicus). The complexity of these two diseases requires early recognition and appropriate therapeutic intervention for the best clinical outcome. Over 95% of the adult United States population has been exposed to herpes simplex type I, and herpes simplex is one of the leading causes of corneal scarring and blindness in industrialized countries. Herpes simplex has been called the "great imitator" and can present as unilateral persistent "conjunctivitis" or nonhealing "corneal abrasion" with a questionable trauma history, making early definitive diagnosis difficult.

The herpes zoster/varicella virus is a common cause of ocular disease in the elderly population. The original virus is usually contracted in childhood as "chicken pox" then resides dormant until adulthood when it reemerges in the zoster form as "shingles." The globe becomes involved when the nasal ciliary branch of cranial nerve V is affected.

The use of topical corticosteroids in the treatment of herpetic eye disease is complex. Corticosteroids are occasionally necessary in the treatment of HSV and frequently in the treatment of HZO. However, the use of steroids for the treatment of herpetic ocular disease requires specialized training to prevent common, and sometimes disastrous, complications of corticosteroid therapy. Chronic topical corticosteroid use frequently causes cataracts and glaucoma. As well, corneal ulceration and globe perforation can quickly occur when steroids are inappropriately used in herpetic eye disease. All patients with herpetic eye disease should be made aware of the special risks involved with topical steroid therapy.

OCULAR HERPES SIMPLEX

CLINICAL MANIFESTATIONS

The primary episode of ocular HSV usually presents as innocuous sores or blisters of the lids or periocular skin (cranial nerve V distribution) in a child or teenager (Fig.

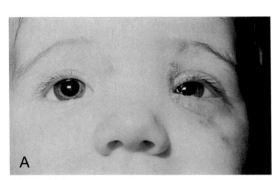
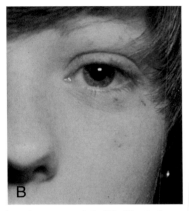

Figure 23.1. Herpes simplex lesions of lids in a child (**A**) and a young adult (**B**). The lesions are typically red blisters that resolve spontaneously.

23.1). Most frequently, there is no involvement of the globe with the primary infection. The lesions resolve without treatment and may go unnoticed by the patient. Subsequent attacks of HSV may involve the conjunctiva or cornea with secondary intraocular inflammation (uveitis). While the primary episode of ocular HSV does not generally require treatment, secondary attacks of HSV may necessitate medical intervention to prevent corneal scarring and visual loss.

Corneal involvement of a secondary HSV infection represents active replicating virus within the corneal epithelium and classically presents as a fluorescein staining "dendrite," indicating a break in the epithelial integrity (Fig. 23.2). The dendritiform pattern of the epithelial defect is common to both ocular HSV and HZO. The epithelial defect has a central linear pattern with multiple branches. These patients may present with a complaint of "irritation" rather than frank pain due to the corneal neuropathy and hypesthesia induced by the virus. Mild tearing, redness, and blurred vision can occur. When multiple dendrites coalesce, a large geographic epithelial defect is seen which may resemble a more typical corneal abrasion. As opposed to the definitive

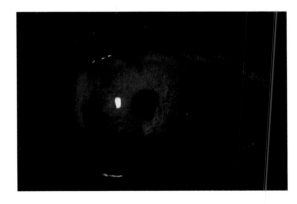

Figure 23.2. Herpes simplex of the cornea. Note the fluorescein staining of the cornea in a "dendritic" pattern. (See also color section.)

history given by most patients with acute traumatic corneal abrasions, when patients with epithelial HSV corneal disease are told that they have an "abrasion," they will often offer a vague history of minor trauma to explain the lesion such as, "I may have rubbed my eye during my sleep." Any patient with an epithelial defect and without an exact history of trauma should be suspected of having ocular HSV.

A simple diagnostic test for a corneal abrasion suspected to be secondary to HSV is the application of a pressure patch for 24 hours. A true corneal abrasion will heal and become smaller, while an HSV lesion will be the same size or larger. When the diagnosis of HSV is suspected, the patient should be referred to an ophthalmologist for evaluation within a few days. The virus is generally not contagious, and it is extremely rare to find bilateral ocular HSV.

Ocular HSV can also involve the corneal stroma and may present as a severely inflamed eye with a necrotizing corneal ulceration or it may present as a relatively white and quiet eye with a central corneal opacity. The active corneal ulceration results from the infectious virus replicating in the depth of the ulcer. The central corneal opacity in a noninflamed eye is known as stromal "disciform disease." These forms of HSV ocular disease usually present in the patient with a past history of epithelial HSV, but can also appear independent of any prior history of dendrite formation.

Necrotizing HSV ulceration of the corneal stroma represents the most serious form of ocular HSV disease. The patient with stromal necrotizing disease will have tearing and redness, but variable pain and vision. Examination reveals an epithelial defect overlying an ulcer with white blood cell infiltrate and vascularization. These ulcerations can often progress to perforation rather quickly if a secondary bacterial infection occurs. Like all corneal ulcers, referral to an ophthalmologist should be immediate (see Chapter 18, "Corneal Abrasions and Corneal Ulcerations"). Patients with HSV stromal disciform disease primarily complain of a sudden decrease in vision, "like looking through a fog." On examination, the epithelium is intact, but the central stroma is swollen and hazy in a "disc" shape obscuring the pupil. A mild uveitis may also be present. This form of HSV represents a purely immune reaction of the eye with no replicating virus. The ophthalmologist will treat this condition with light topical steroids and concurrent antiviral drop coverage. Return of vision usually occurs within a week, but therapy may require weeks or months of tapering dosage.

DIFFERENTIAL DIAGNOSIS

Ocular herpes simplex disease can easily be dismissed as a "chronic conjunctivitis" or "nonhealing epithelial defect" (Table 23.1). Even when the diagnosis of herpes simplex is confirmed, treatment is dictated by the secondary classification of epithelial, stromal disciform, or necrotizing. Finally, each of these forms of ocular HSV may occur independently or concurrently, making the diagnosis and treatment of ocular herpes simplex a challenge to even the most experienced clinician.

TREATMENT

Treatment with trifluridine (Viroptic) is effective in healing the lesion and preventing stromal involvement in most cases of dendritic HSV corneal disease. Stromal involvement occurs when the HSV dendritic form goes untreated, and the virus either gains access to the underlying stromal tissue creating necrosis, or the viral particles incite

◧ TABLE 23.1. Referral Guidelines: Ocular Herpetic Disease

DISEASE	SIGNS AND SYMPTOMS	TREATMENT	WHEN TO REFER
Herpes simplex (054)	"Abrasion" with no clear history of trauma; redness, tearing, mild pain and/or decreased vision	Recognize epithelial form from stromal form; NEVER USE STEROIDS	Refer within 48 hours for dendrites and disciform; refer immediately for necrotizing ulcerative HSV
Herpes zoster (053)	Rash and vesicles in dermatome of CN V; ± redness, photophobia	Begin acyclovir 800 mg p.o. 5× day immediately; pain control	Refer for evaluation of involvement of globe within 72 hours

an inflammatory response with edema and scarring as outlined later. Even with treatment, the patient has a one in three chance of recurrence of the virus in the following 2 years.

Treatment of HSV must be individualized for each patient because the disease has so many unique presentations. A list of the currently used antivirals is presented in Table 23.2. Epithelial HSV usually responds well to a 2-week course of idoxuridine, but toxicity and prolonged use can cause "pseudodendrites" of stromal scarring that can imitate the original disease, further compounding the treatment plan. Stromal disciform HSV is extremely sensitive to topical steroids, but weeks or months of tapering doses may be required to maintain a clear cornea, and the serious threat of active viral replication and subsequent ulceration is always present. Necrotizing HSV ulceration is the most difficult form of HSV to manage. The very delicate balance of antivirals (both topical and systemic) with steroids (topical and occasional systemic) make necrotizing HSV ulceration one of the most challenging clinical problems for the ophthalmologist and corneal subspecialist.

TABLE 23.2. Antiviral Medications

GENERIC NAME	TRADE NAME	MECHANISM OF ACTION	DOSAGE REGIMEN
Trifluridine	Viroptic solution	Abnormal base substitution for mRNA results in faulty viral proteins	Topical 5× daily for 2 weeks
Vidarabine	Vira A ointment	Abnormal sugar results in premature termination of viral DNA synthesis	Topical 5× daily for 2 weeks
Idoxuridine	Herplex solution	Similar to trifluridine but more toxic to host cell metabolism	Topical 5× daily for 2 weeks
Acyclovir	Zovirax tablets	Selectively inhibits HSV and HZ polymerase preventing viral DNA synthesis	Oral 800 mg tablets 5× daily for 10 days
Famciclovir	Famvir tablets	Similar to acyclovir	Oral 500 mg tablets 3× daily for 10 days

Ocular herpes simplex is a chronic and recurrent disease of the eye. With each subsequent attack, sequelae of corneal scarring, vascularization, and corneal thinning may occur. If corneal damage is central, then vision progressively declines. If visual loss causes disability, then corneal transplantation may be necessary to restore vision. Corneal transplantation restores vision, but it does not cure the disease and subsequent attacks of HSV may threaten the future viability of the graft.

Referral Guidelines

Herpes simplex disease of the eye is one of the most complex, chronic, and difficult diseases to manage in the field of ophthalmology and therefore this disease should not be managed by the primary care physician (Table 23.2). Any patient suspected of having HSV should be referred within 48 hours for epithelial or stromal disciform disease. Necrotizing HSV should be referred immediately as an ocular emergency, similar to other ulcerations.

FREQUENCY OF VISITS

Ocular HSV infections are highly varied in their severity of inflammation and damage to the globe. Herpes simplex epithelial disease will usually require an evaluation 3–5 days after the initiation of treatment to verify the response to topical antivirals and then approximately every week for two or three visits. Herpes simplex disciform disease needs to be seen within 48 hours after initiation of steroid therapy and then about every 2–3 weeks for several months as medications are tapered. Herpes simplex stromal necrotizing disease represents a complex ocular emergency and may require daily examinations or emergent surgery until stabilized and then visits every month for 6 months or more. Complicating factors for any of the herpes simplex conditions such as epithelial defects, ulcerations, glaucoma, and secondary infections, can significantly increase the need for more frequent evaluation and increased frequency of visits to the ophthalmologist.

HERPES ZOSTER OPHTHALMICUS

CLINICAL MANIFESTATIONS

Herpes zoster ophthalmicus (HZO) is quite distinctive in its onset and pattern. As in other forms of shingles, the rash and vesicular eruption pattern occurs in a dermatomal pattern and observes the median boundary well. Patients with HZO will show blistering on one side only of the upper face (Fig. 23.3). Vesicular lesions in the scalp on the affected side can also be observed. The distribution is most often confined to the first and second branches of cranial nerve V. As with other herpes zoster infections, dermal involvement often results in permanent scarring after resolution of the initial vesicular eruption. Scrapings of the vesicles will reveal intranuclear inclusions pathognomonic for the disease. While the pain can be severe at the initial presentation, the patient's vision is usually good with a mildly red eye and a watery discharge. Uveitis and epithelial dendrites can occur in over 50% of HZO patients and significant visual loss may occur later in the disease.

The dendritic corneal abrasions associated with HZO are distinctively different

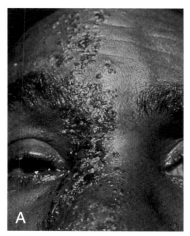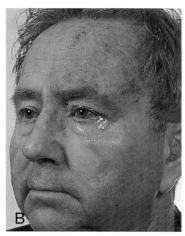

Figure 23.3. Herpes zoster skin lesions. Note the dermatomal pattern of the acute infection (**A**) and the subsequent facial scarring (**B**).

from herpes simplex virus dendrites in that they are generally smaller, plaque-like rather than ulcerative, and do not respond to topical antivirals like trifluridine (Viroptic). Even with treatment, a large proportion of HZO patients develop a chronic uveitis (intraocular inflammation) that can result in extreme damage to intraocular structures. The cornea can also be damaged, resulting in visually debilitating corneal edema. The cornea usually suffers some degree of inflammatory denervation with subsequent loss of sensation (hypesthesia). This hypesthesia, when combined with the variable dry eye of HZO, may result in chronic corneal epithelial drying, epithelial defects, corneal ulcerations, and, occasionally, corneal perforations (Fig. 23.4). The iris can undergo chronic atrophy with sphincter damage leading to chronic pupillary dilation. The lens may become opacified (cataractous) as the result of the chronic inflammation. Chronic intraocular inflammation frequently results in elevated intraocular pressure and glaucoma. Approximately 50% of HZO patients will develop glaucoma. If the inflammation from HZO is concentrated posteriorly in the eye, the retina can become necrotic and

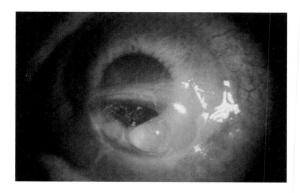

Figure 23.4. Herpes zoster ophthalmicus with corneal ulceration and perforation. Note the thinned, "blistering" inferior cornea and the severe ocular inflammation.

the optic nerve can become severely inflamed, with subsequent dire consequences for vision. External to the globe, HZO may result in lacrimal gland dysfunction and poor tear production. Occasionally, the virus can attack the extraocular muscles causing paralysis and diplopia (double vision) which may become permanent.

DIFFERENTIAL DIAGNOSIS

Most cases of HZO present with a classical onset and distribution of lesions and are not confused with other conditions (Table 23.1). However, in cases where a paucity of skin lesions exists, HZO can resemble ocular herpes simplex, making the appropriate differential diagnosis critical. The worst decision a physician can make is to use the therapy for HZO (topical corticosteroids) for a misdiagnosed case of herpes simplex. Similarly, the conjunctivitis of HZO may appear a few days before the diagnostic skin lesions and may be confused with adenoviral conjunctivitis or allergic conjunctivitis. Therefore, elderly patients with conjunctivitis should be questioned about their associated pain and advised to return for reevaluation sooner if their "conjunctivitis" becomes accompanied by skin blistering on the ipsilateral forehead.

TREATMENT

Treatment of HZO is with Acyclovir 800 mg five times a day for 10 days and should begin at the first sign of a rash or blistering along the dermatomal pattern. Acyclovir has been shown to reduce the duration and severity of the disease, as well as the postherpetic neuralgia, if instituted within the first few days of symptoms. An alternative to Acyclovir is the related compound of famciclovir (Famvir) with a 500-mg three times a day dosing schedule. Topical steroids are a mainstay of therapy and should be instituted at the first sign of globe involvement. Over 60% of patients with cranial nerve V involvement will develop dendrites or uveitis and require topical steroids. Despite the acute treatment of HZO with Acyclovir and topical steroids, long-term complications such as uveitis, dry eye, neurotrophic ulcers, cataracts and glaucoma, can occur. Many patients require chronic tapering doses of topical steroids over months, and even years, to prevent scarring and vision loss.

Referral Guidelines

As soon as the primary care physician suspects HZO, the patient should be placed on Acyclovir. The patient should be referred to an ophthalmologist within 72 hours for a full ocular evaluation and subsequent steroid therapy as indicated. Because of the inherent dangers of topical steroids and the frequent need for prolonged therapy, the management of steroids should only be done by the ophthalmologist.

FREQUENCY OF VISITS

Herpes zoster ophthalmicus will require evaluation and follow-up visits appropriate to the degree of inflammation and extent of ocular damage. Most cases with only superficial skin and conjunctival disease should be seen initially, then subsequently at 1 week, 2 weeks, and 6 weeks after initiation of Acyclovir therapy. In patients with corneal and intraocular involvement, weekly or biweekly visits may be necessary for several months with intermittent exacerbations of inflammation requiring more frequent evaluations. Some patients with intractable intraocular inflammation or extensive corneal involvement will require ongoing ophthalmic specialized management of their chronic disease indefinitely.

SUGGESTED READINGS

Barron B, Gee L, Hauck W, et al. Herpetic eye disease study. A controlled trial of oral acyclovir for herpes simplex stromal keratitis. Ophthalmology 1994;101:1871–1882.

Degreef H, Andrejevic L, Aoki F, et al. Famciclovir, a new oral antiherpes drug. Int J Antimicrobial Agents 1994;4:241–246.

Karbassi M, Raizman M, Schumon J. Herpes zoster ophthalmicus. Surv Ophthalmol 1992;36:395–409.

Liesegang T. Diagnosis and therapy of herpes zoster ophthalmicus. Ophthalmology 1991;98:1216–1229.

Marsh R, Cooper M. Ophthalmic herpes zoster. Eye 1993;7:350–370.

Pepose JS. Herpes simplex keratitis: rose of viral infection versus immune response. Surv Ophthalmol 1991;35:345–352.

Vaughan D. Herpes simplex keratitis. In: Vaughan D, Asbury T, Tabbara K, eds. General ophthalmology. San Mateo, CA: Appleton & Lange, 1989:111–112.

Wilhelmus K, Gee L, Hauck W, et al. Herpetic eye disease study: a controlled trial of topical corticosteroids for herpes simplex stromal keratitis. Ophthalmology 1994;101:1883–1896.

◐❙ TABLE 24.3. Referral Guidelines: Diabetic Retinopathy

DISEASE PROFILE	RECOMMENDED TIME OF FIRST COMPREHENSIVE EYE EXAMINATION	RECOMMENDED MINIMUM FOLLOW-UP (UNLESS RETINOPATHY APPEARS OR INCREASES)
Type I diabetes mellitus (250.01)	5 years after diagnosis and usually not needed before puberty	Annually after first examination
Type II diabetes mellitus (250.02)	Upon diagnosis	Annually after first examination
Pregnancy and type I or type II diabetes mellitus (648.0)	In first trimester	At least in each trimester, more often if retinopathy appears

TABLE 24.4. Management Guidelines: Diabetic Retinopathy by Severity of Disease

SEVERITY OF DIABETIC RETINOPATHY	FOLLOW-UP (MONTHS)	LASER	FLUORESCEIN ANGIOGRAPHY	COLOR FUNDUS PHOTOS
Background diabetic retinopathy (BDR) without cystoid macular edema (362.01)	6–12	No	No	Rarely
Background diabetic retinopathy with edema not yet at threshold for clinical significance (362.83)	4–6	No	Occasionally	Occasionally
Background diabetic retinopathy with cystoid macular edema	2–4	Yes	Yes	Yes
Preproliferative diabetic retinopathy (362.02)	3–4	Usually no	Occasionally	Occasionally
Preproliferative diabetic retinopathy without HRG	2–3*	Usually no	Occasionally	Occasionally
Proliferative diabetic retinopathy without HRG but with background diabetes and cystoid macular edema	2–3*	Yes	Yes	Yes
Proliferative diabetic retinopathy with HRG	3–4	Yes	Occasionally	Occasionally

* Once treated, follow-up every four months
HRG = High risk group characteristics (see Table 24.2)

tive diabetic retinopathy, where fibrous proliferation is extensive, dissection of fibrous membrane is frequently possible, thereby preventing or curing traction retinal detachment.

Unfortunately, not all patients with the most advanced forms of this disease can be successfully treated and blindness still occasionally results. Therefore, it is important for the primary care physician to identify the duration and age of onset of diabetes mellitus in their patients, to determine if their diabetic patients are keeping necessary routine eye appointments, and to question their patients about vision loss.

REFERRAL GUIDELINES

Early treatment of diabetics with clinically significant macular edema in background diabetic retinopathy or high risk characteristics in proliferative diabetic retinopathy is essential. For this reason, Table 24.3 suggests referral guidelines based upon age of onset.

FREQUENCY OF VISITS

Frequency of visits for diabetic retinopathy management based on severity of disease is outlined in Table 24.4. In pregnant diabetic patients, examination in the first trimester is recommended with a minimum follow-up in each succeeding trimester. However, more frequent follow-up may be recommended by an ophthalmologist if retinopathy is increasing. Urgent referral is needed for unexplained vision loss in suspected macular edema or suspected neovascularization on the disc or elsewhere.

SUGGESTED READINGS

Brownlee M, Cerami A, Vlassara H. Advanced glycosylation end products in tissue and the biochemical basis of diabetic complications. N Engl J Med 1988;318(20):1315–1321.

Chase HP, Jackson WE, Hoops SL, Cokerham RS, Archer PG, O'Brien D. Glucose control and the renal and retinal complications of insulin-dependent diabetes. JAMA 1989;261(8):1155–1160.

Engerman RL, Kern TS. Progression of incipient diabetic retinopathy during good glycemic control. Diabetes 1987;36(7):808–812.

Ferris FL. Results of 20 years of research on the treatment of diabetic retinopathy. Prev Med 1994;23:740–742.

Janka HU, Warram JH, Rand LI, Krolewski AS. Risk factors for progression of background diabetic retinopathy in longstanding IDDM. Diabetes 1989;38:460–464.

Klein R, Klein BE, Moss SE, Davis MD, DeMets DL. The Wisconsin epidemiologic survey of diabetic retinopathy, II. Prevalence and risk of diabetic retinopathy when age at diagnosis is less than 30 years. Arch Ophthalmol 1984;102(4):520–526.

Photocoagulation for diabetic macular edema. Early treatment of diabetic retinopathy study, report 1. Arch Ophthalmol 1985;103(12):1796–1806.

Preliminary report on effects of photocoagulation therapy. Am J Ophthalmol 1976;81(4):383–396.

Chapter 25 ◖●❘
Other Retinal Vascular Diseases

C. Ma

INTRODUCTION

There are several noteworthy aspects of the retinal circulation. The eye is the only site where blood vessels can be observed directly. The inner two-thirds of the retina is supplied by the central retinal artery, a small end artery, and has no collateral supply. A cilioretinal artery, arising from the ciliary vessels associated with the optic disc, is present in 25% of eyes. When present it supplies a small area of the retina adjacent to the optic disc. The outer layers of the retina (approximately one-third of the retina's thickness, including the photoreceptors) are supplied by the choroid, which has a higher perfusion than any other tissue in the body. The fovea (the portion of the retina responsible for reading vision) is at the center of an avascular zone 0.5 mm in diameter.

Retinal blood vessels are subject to the conditions and risk factors which exist in the particular patient such as hypertension and cigarette smoking. Arterial and venous occlusions of the retina reflect local and systemic atherosclerotic disease, and tend to occur in the same population as other cardiovascular problems. Abnormalities visualized in retinal blood vessels are also likely to be present in other organs, particularly the central nervous system.

Vascular disease may impair retinal function through ischemia, or because the retina becomes edematous as excess fluid escapes through damaged capillaries. Even small lesions of the retina can be visually significant, because the tissue is so densely organized and proper function is dependent upon the specialized anatomic organization.

The most common retinovascular disease in adults is diabetic retinopathy, and therefore is accorded a separate chapter because of its clinical importance (see Chapter 24, "Diabetic Retinopathy"). In children, congenital vascular malformations of the retina such as Coats disease and angiomatosis retinae in von Hippel-Lindau disease may occur; however, these are rare, and the most important vascular entity to consider in children is retinopathy of prematurity.

DIFFERENTIAL DIAGNOSIS

The most common vascular diseases of the retina, other than diabetic retinopathy, include retinal arterial occlusion, retinal vein occlusion, retinal arterial macroaneurysm,

◼▮ TABLE 25.1. Referral Guidelines: Retinal Vascular Diseases

SYMPTOMS OR SIGNS	DIAGNOSIS	TREATMENT	WHEN TO REFER	LONG-TERM FOLLOW-UP INTERVAL
Floaters, blurred vision; hemoglobinopathy	Sickle cell retinopathy (362.29)	Scatter photocoagulation for neovascularisation	Within 4 weeks	3–6 months
Blurred or distorted vision	Exudative detachment due to ? macroaneurysm (362.17)	FA; laser if threatening fovea; evaluate systemic hypertension	Within 2 weeks	1–3 months
Sudden severe loss of vision in one eye; RAPD, slow blood flow	(Central) Retinal arterial occlusion (362.31)	Within 90 minutes, try to dislodge embolus; investigate for source of emboli	Immediate	Annual
Blurred vision; hemorrhages in sector of retina	Branch retinal vein occlusion (362.36)	FA; grid laser for persistent edema. Investigate for systemic risk factors	Within 4 weeks	Every 3 months if ischæmic
Blurred or dimmed vision; widespread hemorrhages, disc swelling	Central retinal vein occlusion (362.35)	FA; monitor for iris neovascularisation; investigate for systemic risk factors	Within 4 weeks	Every 1–3 months

FA = Fluorescein Angiogram.

and sickle cell retinopathy (Table 25.1). "Cotton wool spots" are small, irregular white patches seen in the inner retina of the posterior pole, which have previously been called "soft exudates," and "cytoid bodies." They represent localized infarcts of the nerve fiber layer caused by obstruction of a terminal retinal arteriole, where opacification is due to interruption of axoplasmic flow and may be seen in many retinal vascular diseases. Observant patients may notice a small scotoma, but cotton wool spots are usually asymptomatic. They usually resolve within 4–12 weeks.

The causes of cotton wool spots are legion, and almost always due to systemic vascular disease, most commonly diabetes mellitus, systemic hypertension, atherosclerotic or septic emboli, background retinopathy associated with HIV infection, and collagen vascular disease. The discovery of a cotton wool spot should prompt an evaluation for these conditions.

RETINAL ARTERIAL OCCLUSION

CLINICAL MANIFESTATIONS

In retinal artery occlusion, the patient typically describes abrupt and painless loss of vision in one eye. If the occlusion occurred in a branch vessel, part of the visual field in one eye is lost, and the patient may notice a horizontal or vertical line of demarcation.

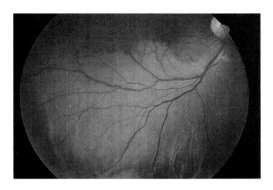

Figure 25.1. Branch retinal artery occlusion with white opacification of inferior retina and attenuation of the retinal arteries. Note embolus in the artery, inferior to the optic nerve.

A small central island of vision may be preserved if part of the retina is supplied by a cilioretinal artery. There may be a prior history of amaurosis fugax, or of cerebral TIAs or stroke.

Visual acuity is usually decreased to a level of counting fingers or worse. An afferent pupillary defect may be the only objective physical sign demonstrable shortly after arterial obstruction. The ocular fundus is initially unremarkable. Careful examination may suggest thinning of the arterioles, and segmentation with slow flow of the blood column ("box-carring") within the venules (Fig. 25.1). An arterial embolus is visible in about 20% of eyes. A "Hollenhorst" plaque glistens, reflecting its cholesterol content, but emboli may also be composed of calcific debris, or clots of fibrin and platelets.

Several hours after the occlusion, the retina develops a white appearance due to edema and to opacification of the ganglion cell layer. Because the foveal region lacks ganglion cells, the normal red color of the central macula is preserved and this area, surrounded by abnormally white retina, gives rise to the appearance of the "cherry red spot."

After several weeks, the white appearance of the retina fades. Recanalization and development of collateral circulation may restore some retinal perfusion, but occurs too late to permit any recovery of vision. Iris neovascularization is a late development in about 15% of eyes.

TREATMENT

Ocular

Several techniques have been described which may dislodge an obstruction and mitigate the ischemic damage to the retina. Ischemic injury of the retina is reversible for up to following 90 minutes under experimental conditions. In practice, arterial occlusion may be subtotal, and the retina may survive for longer. The physician should attempt the noninvasive methods described below if the patient presents with symptoms of less than 2 hours duration, after eliminating other causes of dramatic loss of vision such as retinal detachment or ischemic optic neuropathy. The potential for harming the eye is low, as the vision is already severely reduced.

Short pulses of 1–2 seconds duration may be applied to the globe through the upper lid with a thumb. This may transmit pressure waves to the retinal vessels and dislodge an embolus downstream. Asking the patient to breathe increased CO_2 (5%) and O_2 (95%), or rebreathing into a paper bag, or administering sublingual nitroglycerin have all been attempted in the hope of dislodging the embolus by vasodilation. Systemic administration of antifibrinolytic agents (e.g., streptokinase) has been reported, but not proven to be beneficial. Paracentesis, or aspiration of aqueous humor from the anterior chamber to lower the intraocular pressure, is also of unproven benefit and should only be performed by an ophthalmologist.

Systemic

There is no effective treatment to restore vision in an eye after arterial occlusion, but management should be directed at reducing the risk of further embolic events in the fellow eye, or elsewhere in the central nervous system. A patient with any evidence of arterial embolic disease should be investigated for sources of emboli with carotid and cardiac ultrasound studies, whether they present with complete central retinal arterial occlusion, or an asymptomatic Hollenhorst plaque found on routine examination. About two-thirds of patients with retinal arterial occlusion have systemic hypertension, and one-third of individuals have diabetes. Many also have a history of smoking.

Retinal arterial occlusion may occasionally be due to temporal arteritis, although optic neuropathy is a much more common manifestation of this disease. A sedimentation rate should always be checked in patients over the age of 50.

RETINAL VENOUS OCCLUSION

CLINICAL MANIFESTATIONS

The etiology of retinal vein occlusion is not entirely known, but it is believed that thickening of the wall of an atherosclerotic artery compresses an adjacent vein, causing turbulent blood flow, damage to the endothelium, and thrombosis. In a branch retinal vein occlusion (BRVO), this site of occlusion apparently occurs where an artery crosses over a vein in the retina, whereas in a central retinal vein occlusion (CRVO), the lesion lies within the optic nerve where the central retinal artery and vein have a tortuous and closely related course (Fig. 25.2). Visual recovery after a vein occlusion depends upon the extent of capillary loss and retinal ischemia, which may be principally determined by the sufficiency of arterial perfusion.

Patients usually describe unilateral blurring or dimming of vision. In contrast to arterial occlusions, they are usually not certain when the symptoms began. Indeed, some mild vein occlusions are only discovered incidentally. Occasionally, a patient may present with pain due to neovascular glaucoma, which is a frequent late complication of retinal vein occlusions.

Risk factors may be identified from the history, and include systemic hypertension, diabetes mellitus, cardiovascular disease, and glaucoma. In young patients, there may be a history of collagen vascular disease.

Visual acuity ranges from normal to counting fingers. BRVOs cause sectoral field defects, which are difficult to delineate without formal perimetry. CRVOs produce uniform symptoms and dimming of vision across the entire visual field. A relative afferent pupillary defect is present when a significant area of the retina is ischemic.

The typical fundus appearance after a vein occlusion was historically described as "blood and thunder"–numerous intraretinal hemorrhages, scattered cotton wool

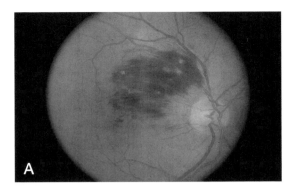

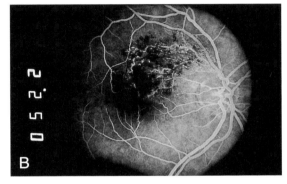

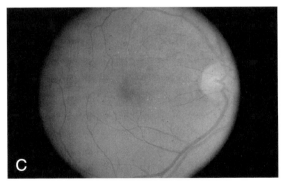

Figure 25.2. **A.** Branch retinal vein occlusion with a large area of retinal hemorrhages and cotton wool spots, reducing acuity to 20/200. The site of occlusion is at arterial-venous crossing above the optic nerve. **B.** Fluorescein angiogram of the same site 3 months later shows microaneurysms and capillary loss in affected sector of the retina, but perifoveal capillaries are intact. **C.** After 7 months and following laser grid photocoagulation, edema has resolved, and the visual acuity has recovered to 20/40.

spots, retinal edema, optic nerve (disc) swelling, and engorgement and tortuosity of the vessels (Fig. 25.3). The clinical appearance is poorly correlated with severity, but the presence of numerous cotton wool spots and thick, dark hemorrhages suggests ischemia and a poor prognosis.

In BRVO, the lesions are limited to a triangular area corresponding to the territory of the occluded vessel, but in CRVO, the findings are visible in all meridians. Hemicentral retinal vein occlusion is a variant of CRVO, in which the fundus changes are seen in either the superior or inferior half of the retina, due to the presence in some

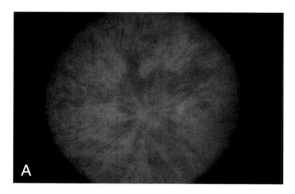

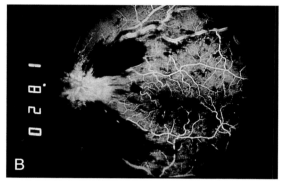

Figure 25.3.   A. Central retinal vein occlusion (CRVO) with diffuse retinal hemorrhages obscuring the view of the optic nerve. **B.** Fluorescein angiogram demonstrates capillary loss even within the macula.

eyes of distinct superior and inferior retinal veins which join more posteriorly in the optic nerve.

The fundus appearance of a vein occlusion may be mistaken for diabetic retinopathy, but the hemorrhages are usually thicker, larger, and almost confluent, and, in the early stages at least, these are unlikely to be hard exudates or visible microaneurysms (Figs. 25.2 and 25.3). BRVO is less likely to be confused with diabetic retinopathy because the changes are only present in one sector of the fundus.

TREATMENT

Ocular

In BRVOs, retinal hemorrhages and cotton wool spots will usually resolve spontaneously after 3–6 months. The visual acuity may also improve, depending on the degree of edema and capillary loss in the central macula. Tortuous collateral vessels often develop in the zone between the normal and affected areas of the fundus. Fluorescein angiography is extremely helpful in determining the extent and severity of vascular damage, and for defining the source of the leakage.

The Branch Vein Occlusion Study showed that laser treatment is likely to improve vision in eyes that have visual acuity less than 20/40 with persistent macular edema for 3 months after the occlusion, provided the perifoveal capillaries are perfused. Laser photocoagulation is applied as a grid of evenly spaced 100–200 μm burns. Denser treatment may be applied if treatment is not effective initially (Fig. 25.2).

About 25% of eyes with extensive (at least one quadrant of the retina) ischemic BRVO develop preretinal neovascularization, sometimes 2–3 years after the original event. These small, abnormal vessels tend to be located peripherally, and are difficult to see with an ophthalmoscope, but leak profusely on fluorescein angiography. They may cause sufficient vitreous hemorrhage to completely obscure vision, and, in rare cases, may lead to preretinal fibrosis and traction retinal detachment. The Branch Vein Occlusion Study found that scatter laser photocoagulation reduced the risk of vitreous hemorrhage in eyes with neovascularization, but concluded that it was not effective to treat ischemic eyes before the abnormal vessels appeared.

In CRVOs, clinical findings such as dense retinal hemorrhages, cotton wool spots, and disc swelling, correlate with a poor outcome. As with branch vein occlusions, the visible signs of CRVO tend to resolve spontaneously over the ensuing months. Collateral vessels, joining the retinal and choroidal venous circulations, frequently appear at the optic disc. They can be distinguished from neovascularization because they are flat on the disc tissue, do not leak on fluorescein angiography, and do not hemorrhage (Fig. 25.3).

The Central Vein Occlusion Study has shown that grid photocoagulation is not helpful for macular edema due to CRVO. There is currently considerable interest in creating retinochoroidal shunt vessels in the peripheral fundus with laser photocoagulation as treatment for CRVO, but this is not yet proven to be of benefit.

The recovery of central and peripheral vision and the probability of complications is dependent upon the severity of macular edema and retinal ischemia. Macular edema and retinal ischemia can only be determined reliably by fluorescein angiography. It is essential to study the midperipheral retina, where the changes are most pronounced, even though this may require the use of a wide-angle fundus camera, or a more skilled photographer to scan these areas during the study. Angiography may not be helpful initially if large areas of the fundus are obscured by dense hemorrhages, but should definitely be performed when the hemorrhages have diminished.

The relative afferent pupillary defect is a simple and helpful clinical assay of retinal ischemia. If greater than 0.9 log units (equivalent to an eightfold disparity with the fellow eye) the prognosis is poor, and there is a high risk of developing neovascular glaucoma.

On the basis of the above findings, CRVOs are usefully divided into two groups: nonischemic and ischemic. In nonischemic CRVO, eyes are likely to have visual acuity better than 20/200, and are at low risk (about 3%) of developing ocular neovascularization. These patients should be reexamined every 3 months, and instructed to report sooner if they experience a drop in vision; there is a probability of about 18% that such eyes will convert to an ischemic CRVO, with the appearance of new hemorrhages and cotton wool spots.

With ischemic CRVO, visual acuity is usually worse than 20/400, with significant loss of peripheral vision. The most important aspect of management is regular monitoring for iris neovascularization, which is a precursor of neovascular glaucoma and develops in two-thirds of these eyes. Neovascular glaucoma is a dramatic elevation of the intraocular pressure due to closure of the trabecular meshwork by abnormal vessels, resulting in pain and blindness. Historically, it was thought to develop after 100 days, but modern research has shown that most cases of neovascular glaucoma manifest between 1 and 30 months after CRVO. These patients should, therefore, have slitlamp examinations and preferably gonioscopy, monthly in the first year. If iris neovascularization appears, panretinal photocoagulation should be applied urgently. The Central Vein Occlusion Study has shown that prophylactic treatment, performed before iris vessels appeared, was not effective. Additional pressure lowering measures such as drainage surgery or ciliary body destruction may be required if the glaucoma is established.

Systemic

The cumulative risk of another retinal vein occlusion occurring in the same eye is 2.5% at 4 years, and 12% for the fellow eye. It is logical to suppose that systemic risk factors are important in the etiology of retinal vein occlusions; however, ocular factors such as the characteristics of the retinal vessels are probably more significant. Several series have shown a statistically significant association between retinal vein occlusions and systemic hypertension, cardiovascular disease, male gender, diabetes mellitus, and open angle glaucoma. The majority of patients are over 60 years of age.

Some specific disease states associated with CRVO are increased blood viscosity due to polycythemia, or Waldenström's macroglobulinemia. Patients with systemic lupus erythematosus may have coagulation abnormalities due to antiphospholipid antibodies, which can lead to ischemic CRVO. Such conditions should be particularly suspected in young patients, especially if there is bilateral or recurrent vein occlusion. Some authors have reported subtle coagulopathies in apparently normal patients with CRVO, but it remains to be seen whether this is of broad clinical significance. It is not known whether lowering the intraocular pressure in a glaucoma patient, or treating systemic hypertension, also reduces the risk of developing a vein occlusion.

Patients with vein occlusions should be examined and evaluated by their primary care physician for the risk factors described earlier. A CBC, ESR, and chemistry profile should be checked, with more unusual tests such as FTA, ANA, PTT, and antiphospholipid antibody titres selected on an individual basis.

RETINAL ARTERIAL MACROANEURYSM

CLINICAL MANIFESTATIONS

Retinal arterial macroaneurysms are small round dilations of retinal arterioles which almost always occur in patients with a history of poorly controlled systemic hypertension, in the fifth to seventh decade of life. Two patterns of presentation are common: exudative retinal detachments and retinal hemorrhages. Exudative retinal detachment (see Chapter 26, "Retinal Detachment") around a macroaneurysm which is sufficiently close to the macula may cause noticeable metamorphopsia or blurring. Such a lesion may involute spontaneously, but most retinal surgeons recommend laser treatment of lesions which threaten central vision (Fig. 25.4).

Loss of vision may occur due to retinal hemorrhages. These hemorrhages may occur under, within, or in front of the retina, or into the vitreous. Management of retinal hemorrhages secondary to arterial macroaneurysms is conservative, as the blood usually clears spontaneously, and is directed at identification of the source. Recovery of vision depends on the quantity of the blood and the proximity to the macula. A macroaneurysm which has bled almost always thromboses, and is therefore unlikely to cause further problems. Patients with retinal arterial macroaneurysms should be

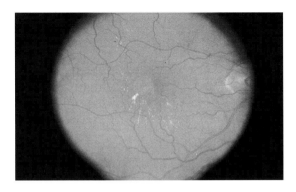

Figure 25.4.   Arterial macroaneurysm causing exudative retinal detachment of the central macula. Hard lipid exudates mark the margin of the detachment.

evaluated for systemic hypertension. The differential diagnosis should include subretinal neovascularization, branch retinal vein occlusion, pigment epithelial detachment, or, in large hemorrhagic lesions, malignant melanoma.

SICKLE CELL RETINOPATHY

Patients with homozygous (SS) sickle cell anemia, although subject to systemic sickling crises, are at low risk of proliferative neovascular retinopathy, probably because they have a low hematocrit. Heterozygotes, with SC or SThal hemoglobinopathies, are paradoxically at high risk of developing blinding complications. However, these heterozygotes may not be recognized until visual complications develop, since their systemic disease and associated anemia are mild with few crises.

Sickle retinopathy is analogous to proliferative diabetic retinopathy, but the ischemic changes develop in the anterior, peripheral retina. Sickling and microvascular occlusions may cause sufficient peripheral retinal ischemia to induce the growth of fronds of preretinal neovascularization which are described as "sea fans." These may lead to vitreous hemorrhage and traction retinal detachment. Nonproliferative lesions include flat intraretinal hemorrhages and arteriovenous shunts.

Patients with sickle cell should be monitored with regular exams of the peripheral retina by an ophthalmologist. Scatter laser treatment of the ischemic periphery appears to be effective in preventing late complications.

SUGGESTED READINGS

Abdel-Khalek MN, Richardson J. Retinal microaneurysm: natural history and guidelines for treatment. Br J Ophthalmol 1986;70:2–11.

Branch Vein Occlusion Study Group. Argon laser scatter photocoagulation for prevention of neovascularization and vitreous hemorrhage in branch vein occlusion. Arch Ophthalmol 1986;104:34–41.

Branch Vein Occlusion Study Group. Argon laser photocoagulation for macular edema in branch vein occlusion. Am J Ophthalmol 1984;98:271–282.

Brown GC. Arterial obstructive disease and the eye. Ophthalmol Clin North Am 1990;3:373–392.

Central Vein Occlusion Study, Group M Report. Evaluation of grid pattern photocoagulation for macular edema in central vein occlusion. Ophthalmology 1995; 102:1425–1433.

Central Vein Occlusion Study, Group N Report. A randomized clinical trial of early panretinal photocoagulation for ischemic central vein occlusion. Ophthalmology 1995;102:1434–1444.

Christensen L. The nature of the cytoid body. Trans Am Ophthalmol Soc 1958;56:451.

Hayreh SS, Rojas, P, Podhajsky P, et al. Ocular neovascularization with retinal vascular occlusion–III. Ophthalmology 1983;90:488–506.

Hayreh SS, Klugman MR, Beri M, et al. Differentiation of ischemic from non-ischemic central retinal vein occlusion during the early acute phase. Graefes Arch Clin Exp Ophthalmol 1990;228:201–217.

Hayreh SS, Zimmerman MB, Podhajsky P. Incidence of various types of retinal vein occlusion and their recurrence and demographic characteristics. Am J Ophthalmol 1994;117:429–441.

The Eye Disease Case-Control Study Group. Risk factors for branch retinal vein occlusion. Am J Ophthalmol 1993;116;286–296.

The Eye Disease Case-Control Study Group. Risk factors for central retinal vein occlusion. Arch Ophthalmol 1996;114:545–554.

Chapter 26 ●◗▮
Retinal Detachment

C. Ma

INTRODUCTION

Retinal detachment is the separation of the retina from its normal position on the interior of the globe. Although retinal detachment is not common, occurring with a frequency of 1 in 10,000 in the general population, this condition deserves special consideration for several reasons. First, the primary symptoms of retinal detachment (floaters and flashes) are a common visual complaint, which may or may not be associated with retinal detachment. Second, retinal detachment is a potentially blinding condition. Finally, it can be repaired surgically, but the visual outcome depends almost entirely upon the speed of delivery of appropriate treatment.

Normal Anatomy

The retina is a thin, delicate sheet of neurosensory tissue, which lines the interior of the globe, extending from the optic disc to the ora serrata (Fig. 26.1). The retina is composed primarily of neurosensory cells (rods and cones) and glial tissue, and is responsible for converting light stimuli into neural signals. These neural signals are transmitted, via the optic nerve, to the brain. The macula is the central region of the retina, composed mainly of cones, which is responsible for the best central "reading" vision. The relative health and function of the retina is dependent on maintenance of its normal anatomy and complex interactions with adjacent tissues. The location of the anterior edge of the retina can be visualized by imagining a line that joins the insertions of the four rectus muscles on the outside of the globe. The retina is closely adherent to the underlying retinal pigment epithelium (RPE), attached by a glue-like layer of mucopolysaccharide and by the constant pumping of fluid by the RPE cells from the vitreous, through the retina, to the choroid. Although the retina and RPE are in close apposition, there are no tight junctions between them. Embryologically, the retina and RPE both arise from the neural ectoderm of the optic vesicle. The two layers face cell apex to cell apex, because the optic cup forms by invagination and obliterates the cavity between the retina and RPE of the optic vesicle. The cavity becomes a potential space, which may fill with fluid if the retina detaches from the RPE.

The vitreous is a gel-like body composed of 99% water, a collagenous meshwork, and hyaluronic acid, which fills the posterior compartment of the eye. It is loosely adherent to the optic disc, macula, and along major retinal vessels. There is a strong adhesion to a narrow band of the anterior retina and pars plana, known as the vitreous base, which is important in the etiology of some retinal detachments.

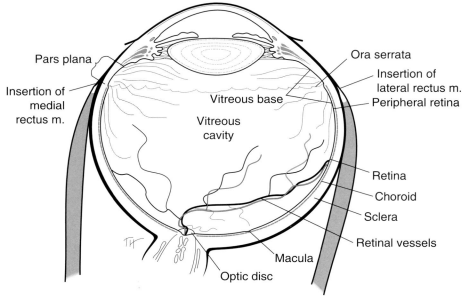

Figure 26.1.   The eye. Note the orientation and anatomy of retina and vitreous body.

Risk Factors

Risk factors for the development of a rhegmatogenous retinal detachment include cataract surgery or any procedure which induces a shift in the vitreous gel. This includes Nd:YAG posterior capsulotomy, which is frequently performed for opacification of the lens capsule after cataract surgery (see Chapter 20, "Adult Cataract"). Blunt trauma, which causes a rapid deformation of the globe, may cause a dialysis of the peripheral retina (an avulsion of the anterior edge of the retina) or the more usual flap tear. High myopia (nearsightedness requiring more than −5 diopters of correction) is an important risk factor for retinal detachment, most likely because the eye is abnormally elongated, with pathological thinning of the tissues (see Chapter 19, "Refractive Errors and Their Correction"). Lattice degeneration is a congenital condition in which patches of the retina are abnormally thin, yet strongly adherent to the overlying vitreous gel. Such areas are prone to tear when the vitreous gel separates.

Pilocarpine and other miotic agents used in the treatment of glaucoma have been implicated in creating retinal tears. These agents induce ciliary body muscular contraction and forward movement of the lens and iris, which may increase vitreous traction, especially when therapy is initiated. With the exception of avoiding direct blows to the eye, such as boxing, there is no evidence that patients can reduce their risk of retinal detachment by limiting activity. Indeed, the rapid eye movements of sleep probably cause as much vitreoretinal traction as any activity that the patient might undertake.

◗❚ TABLE 26.1. Referral Guidelines: Floaters, Flashes, and Retinal Detachment (361.0)

SYMPTOMS OR SIGNS	TREATMENT	WHEN TO REFER
Acute onset of floaters and flashes (379.24)	Dilated exam with depressed exam of peripheral retina	Same day
Progressive peripheral vision loss; extramacular detachment (361.0)	Pneumatic retinopexy or scleral buckle	Same day
Central vision loss; detachment involving macula (361.0)	Pneumatic retinopexy or scleral buckle	Next office day
Chronic detachment (361.05)	Scleral buckle, probably with vitrectomy	Within 1–2 weeks

Differential Diagnosis

Types of Retinal Detachment

It is clinically useful to classify retinal detachments according to the underlying pathogenesis. Three types of retinal detachments, rhegmatogenous, tractional, and exudative, are commonly described.

Rhegmatogenous is derived from the Greek word rhegma, meaning a rent, tear, or fissure. With a rhegmatogenous retinal detachment, the retina is torn by movement of the vitreous gel (Fig. 26.2). Fluid flows rapidly from the vitreous cavity through this tear, into the subretinal space, resulting in detachment and elevation of a steadily enlarging area of the retina. The patient usually notices a corresponding scotoma (blind spot), which enlarges visibly as more fluid collects. This type of detachment is of great clinical importance, because it is the most common, it usually presents in a dramatic fashion, and it often requires urgent surgical treatment to prevent permanent vision loss. The majority of this chapter is devoted to rhegmatogenous retinal detachment.

Tractional retinal detachments result when the retina is pulled away from the retinal pigment epithelium (RPE) secondary to a contraction of the vitreous gel, combined with a pathological adhesion between the vitreous gel and the retina. This occurs commonly in proliferative diabetic retinopathy (see Chapter 24, "Diabetic Retinopathy"), and in chronic or recurrent retinal detachments where fibroblasts proliferate in the vitreous gel and on the surface of the retina. Occasionally, severe traction will cause the retina to tear, producing a combined traction and rhegmatogenous detachment. Traction detachments must be repaired by surgically relieving the traction on the retina.

Exudative retinal detachments occur when a breakdown of the blood-retinal barrier in the vessels of the retinal or choroidal circulation results in collection of fluid under the retina. This may occur in a variety of inflammatory conditions affecting the retina, retinal pigment epithelium, or choroid (e.g., Vogt-Koyanagi-Harada syndrome and posterior scleritis), but increased vascular permeability and exudative retinal detachments may also occur in numerous other diseases (e.g., background diabetic reti-

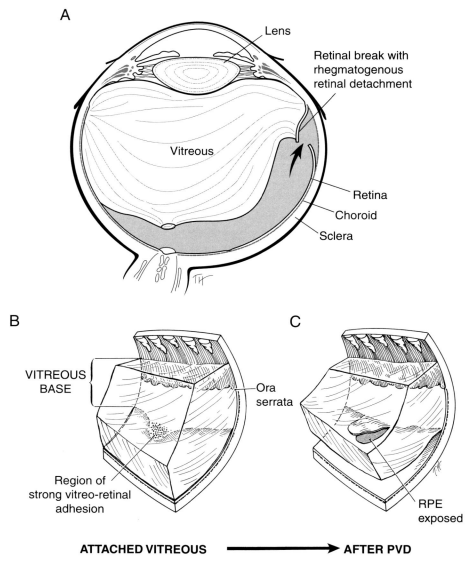

Figure 26.2. Rhegmatogenous retinal detachment. **A.** Note the tear in the retina secondary to pulling from the shifting vitreous. Fluid from the vitreous cavity flows through the tear, under the retina, and causes the detachment. **B.** Enlargement of peripheral retina denoting "vitreous base," an area of strong vitreous attachment to the retina. **C.** With a posterior vitreous detachment (PVD), a horseshoe-shaped retinal tear occurs.

nopathy, subretinal neovascular membrane in age-related macular degeneration, or the abnormal vessels in choroidal melanoma or metastatic ocular tumors).

CLINICAL MANIFESTATIONS

Although the symptoms may seem innocuous, an evolving retinal detachment is one of the few eye diseases where urgent attention is essential, and where the promptness of treatment significantly affects the return or preservation of visual function. If a retinal tear is identified before a detachment develops, it can be treated and sealed with laser therapy, eliminating the need for a surgical procedure. If a retinal detachment is identified and treated before it involves detachment of the macular region, the patient is much more likely to preserve good central vision. Three symptoms are commonly associated with a progressive retinal detachment: floaters and flashes, loss of peripheral vision, and loss of central vision.

The primary event leading to rhegmatogenous retinal detachment is "posterior vitreous detachment" (PVD). PVD is a normal consequence of aging, which results as the hyaluronic acid concentration within the vitreous declines and the collagenous meshwork of the gel collapses. The vitreous separates from the posterior part of the retina and causes traction on the retina at any site where it remains attached. The symptoms which typically accompany this event are floaters and flashes.

There is a 30% risk of developing a retinal detachment within 6 weeks of onset of floaters and flashes. Floaters are due to dispersed blood, pigment, or collagenous condensations in the vitreous gel which cast a visible shadow on the retina. Floaters are more suspicious if they are numerous and small, like spots or "bugs," rather than a veil, or circular ring. The flashes (photopsia) are due to stimulation of the peripheral retina by acute vitreous traction. They are usually unilateral, repetitive, and noticeable when the eyes are either opened or closed. They may be quite bright and distracting to the patient. Although flashes are often reported as occurring in one direction, this symptom has little value in establishing the location of changes within the retina.

Retinal breaks most commonly occur at sites of abnormally strong adhesions between the vitreous and retina. With collapse of the vitreous gel, sufficient stress at these adhesion points tears the retina, instead of the usual vitreous separation (posterior vitreous detachment). Such sites may be present along the posterior border of the vitreous base, or adjacent to retinal vessels, or in areas of abnormal retina (e.g., lattice degeneration). Retinal tears are frequently difficult to identify without a widely dilated pupil and specialized ophthalmoscopy. As there are no unique symptoms that distinguish patients with retinal tears from those with an uncomplicated posterior vitreous detachment, it is necessary to evaluate all patients with flashes or floaters with a full ophthalmic examination.

Later in the course of a progressive retinal detachment, the classic symptom of a "curtain falling across the vision" develops. This occurs as fluid accumulates under the retina in the vicinity of the retinal break. "Curtain" is a misleading term, for many patients use it to describe the myriad of floaters which sometimes seem to form a sheet obscuring vision. When the peripheral retina detaches, there is a corresponding loss in the visual field which enlarges as more fluid accumulates. The loss of peripheral vision is not due to obscuration, but is due to the loss of function of the retina when it is separated from the pigment epithelium. By ophthalmoscopy, the detached retina appears white or gray, compared to the normal pinkish orange color. The interval

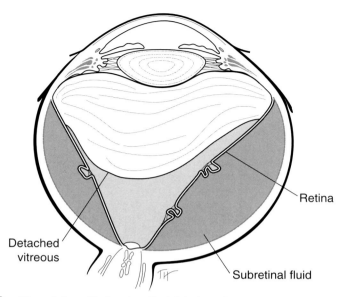

Figure 26.3. "Funnel-shaped" chronic retinal detachment.

between earliest symptoms and development of a scotoma may range from hours to weeks, depending on the location of the retinal tear. The scotoma may fluctuate, because the retina may partially settle under gravity when the patient is upright during the day or asleep overnight.

Patients often dismiss the early symptoms of retinal detachments, but eventually subretinal fluid will track under the macula and cause noticeable loss of central vision. Once the macula detaches, the prognosis for recovery of central vision of 20/50 or better (reading vision) is only 50%.

Long-standing (more than 1 month) retinal detachments may be complicated by the proliferation of fibroglial membranes on the surface of the retina and along the collagen meshwork of the vitreous, known as proliferative vitreoretinopathy. These membranes are produced by glial cells of retinal origin and by fibroblasts derived from the pigment epithelium, which migrate from the subretinal space, through retinal breaks, into the vitreous cavity. As these membranes mature, they contract, drawing the retina into the center of the eye. This results in a so-called funnel detachment, because the retina forms a wide cone anteriorly, leading into a narrow tube connected at the optic disc (Fig. 26.3). Usually the eye will become soft (low intraocular pressure), and may collapse and become irreversibly blind.

TREATMENT
Evaluation of Floaters and Flashes

Patients reporting floaters and flashes symptoms should be evaluated urgently to assess for a retinal tear or frank detachment. These conditions can only be satisfactorily ruled out by examining the peripheral retina through a dilated pupil, with scleral depression to bring the entire anterior retina into view. Seventy percent of patients will not develop retinal disease, but they cannot be distinguished solely on the basis of their symptoms. If examination shows no pathology, patients are told to report back promptly if the symptoms increase, and that a similar event may occur in the fellow eye. Many patients become quite vexed by the increase in floaters which follows posterior vitreous detachment. These patients should be reassured that the symptoms will diminish with time and become less distracting, although they will never entirely disappear.

Prophylactic Treatment of Retinal Breaks

Retinal tears almost always occur in the anterior retina, so far peripherally that the defect in the retina itself is not visually significant (not within the noticeable field of vision). Tears are treated to reduce the risk of progression to retinal detachment and not to close the actual defect in the retina. However, not all retinal tears require prophylactic treatment. The key criterion is the presence of vitreous traction which will tend to elevate the retina and encourage the passage of fluid into the subretinal space. Photopsia is an important clue to continuing traction, because it is caused by mechanical stimulation of the retina.

The purpose of prophylactic treatment is to create a chorioretinal scar, between the retina and pigment epithelium, in attached retina surrounding the retinal break. This does not relieve vitreous traction, but creates a barrier to further accumulation of fluid. The chorioretinal adhesion may be induced by a full thickness freeze through the wall of the eye using a small hand-held cryopexy probe, which is cooled at the tip to $-60°C$ by circulating nitrous oxide. The extent of the freeze is monitored ophthalmoscopically. Alternatively, laser photocoagulation may be employed, which may be more difficult to perform, but possibly induces a more rapid adhesion. Laser treatment is conducted through a contact lens which allows the surgeon to visualize the retinal break with the slitlamp microscope, or through a specially adapted binocular indirect ophthalmoscope. Both laser and cryopexy may usually be performed with topical anesthetic alone.

Patients must be reexamined regularly after treatment to check that subretinal fluid has not broken through the treatment barrier and to evaluate for the possibility of further tears. An increase in floaters or flashes may signal such an event (increased tears or accumulation of subretinal fluid). The treatment scars become visibly pigmented about 1 week after treatment, but will already have developed chorioretinal adhesion within 24–48 hours.

Pneumatic Retinopexy

Pneumatic retinopexy is an office procedure and is effective for retinal detachments which are due to tears in the superior retina (Fig. 26.4). A bubble of sulphur hexafluoride (SF_6), usually about 0.3–0.5 cc in volume, is injected into the vitreous cavity, and the patient positioned so that the tear will be located over the gas bubble and consequently closed by the surface tension effect. Once the flow of fluid through the hole is prevented, existing subretinal fluid is usually pumped away quite quickly by the pigment epithelium, and the retina will reattach within a day or two. Laser treatment or cryopexy can then be applied around the break(s) to seal them permanently. The bubble diffuses gradually into the bloodstream and is eliminated by the lungs over a period of about

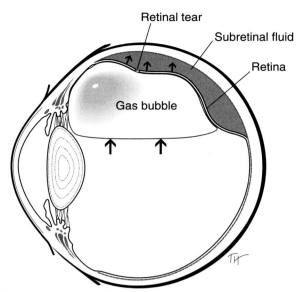

Figure 26.4. Pneumatic retinopexy. The patient's head is positioned so that the intravitreal gas bubble closes the break. The subretinal fluid is then absorbed by the pumping action (*small arrow*) of the retinal pigment epithelium.

5 days. This procedure requires a highly compliant patient, as they must maintain the correct position for that time. The success rate for successful reattachment is 70–81%. The benefits of pneumatic retinopexy are in avoiding the cost of hospitalization and surgery, and in avoiding the use of a permanent explant on the eye.

Scleral Buckle

The principle of scleral buckling is to block the retinal tear by indenting the wall of the globe to bring the pigment epithelium back into apposition with the retina (Fig. 26.5). The sclera is exposed by opening the conjunctiva and elevating the extraocular muscles. The flexible silicone explant is secured and indented into the eye with sutures. It is shaped and positioned to lie under all of the retinal tears. Frequently, the buckle encircles the eye at the equator to support the entire vitreous base. Subretinal fluid is drained by making an incision through sclera and choroid into the subretinal space. Local anesthetic is often sufficient for this operation, with the assistance of an anesthesiologist to administer intravenous sedation.

This technique is much more widely applicable than pneumatic retinopexy, and is successful where there are multiple tears, inferiorly located tears, or mild degrees of proliferative vitreoretinopathy. Postsurgical care is much simpler for the patient, but the buckle must remain in place permanently, and will usually cause some induced nearsightedness, increased astigmatism, or occasionally interfere with the normal action of the extraocular muscles. There is an 80–95% success rate for reattachment with sclera buckling surgery.

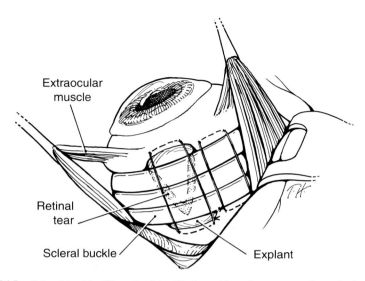

Extraocular
muscle

Retinal
tear

Scleral buckle

Explant

Figure 26.5. Scleral buckle. The scleral buckle is positioned to support the retinal tears (*dotted lines*). The extraocular muscles are elevated with sutures so that the encircling band can be passed around the globe.

Pars Plana Vitrectomy

Detachments which are complicated by very large retinal tears, dense vitreous hemorrhage, or significant preretinal membranes are usually approached internally. An operating microscope is employed to view the retina through the pupil, with a fiber optic probe for endo-ocular illumination. The vitreous gel is removed with suction through a high speed reciprocating cutter. A variety of 20-gauge instruments (scissors, forceps, diathermy, aspirators, laser probes) are introduced to peel membranes, and reposition the retina. The eye is inflated throughout the procedure by an infusion of balanced saline solution.

Intraocular Tamponade

At the close of pars plana vitrectomy, the eye will often be filled with air, frequently mixed with sulphur hexafluoride (SF_6) or octofluoropropane (C_3F_8) gases. The resulting bubble will persist for 1–6 weeks, and is used to maintain the position of the retina by surface tension. The patient will be asked to maintain a certain position (face down, left side down, etc.) to keep the bubble apposed to the area of pathology until a permanent chorioretinal adhesion develops at areas of laser treatment.

When there are very extensive retinal breaks, it may be necessary to maintain tamponade for long periods of several months. This can be accomplished with "silicone oil" (a polymer, dimethylsiloxane), which is highly viscous and remains inert within the eye until it is surgically removed. It is transparent and permits useful vision. One of the more common applications of silicone oil is in the repair of retinal detachments due to cytomegalovirus retinitis.

SUGGESTED READINGS

Davis MD. The natural history of retinal breaks without detachment. Trans Am Ophthalmol Soc 1973;71:343–372.

Fitzgerald CR, Birch DG, Enoch JM. Functional analysis of vision in patients after retinal detachment repair. Arch Ophthalmol 1980;98:1237–1244.

Meredith TA. Sensory experiences with posterior vitreous detachment [Editorial]. Am J Ophthalmol 1996;121:687–689.

Sigelman J. Vitreous base classification of retinal tears: clinical application. Surv Ophthalmol 1980;25:59–74.

Tornambe PE, Hilton GF, Retinal Detachment Study Group. Pneumatic retinopexy: a multicenter randomized, controlled trial comparing pneumatic retinopexy with scleral buckling. Ophthalmology 1989;96:772–783.

Chapter 27 ◖●◗
Age-Related Macular Degeneration

R. F. Dreyer

INTRODUCTION

Age-related macular degeneration (AMD) is a progressive dysfunction of the macula secondary to involutional changes of the subretinal tissues. Age-related macular degeneration is the leading cause of irreversible vision loss after the age of 50 in western developed countries, but it also less commonly occurs in younger individuals. It is believed that there is a genetic predisposition to AMD, although specific genetic markers have not been identified. Certain factors are associated with an increased risk of developing AMD, including a family history of the disease and lightly pigmented irides. Other potential risk factors for AMD include a lifetime of extensive sun exposure, cigarette smoking, cardiovascular disease, and diet. Although there is no proven benefit to altering the dietary patterns of individuals with macular degeneration, there remains a great deal of interest regarding the prevalence of macular degeneration in relation to nutrition, particularly since many elderly patients have inadequate diets. In recent years, interest has centered on dietary supplements of large amounts of zinc and antioxidants including vitamin C, vitamin E, and beta carotene.

The Age-Related Eye Disease Study (AREDS), a prospective, randomized clinical trial supported by the National Institutes of Health, is currently evaluating the effectiveness of antioxidants and zinc in treating early macular degeneration. In addition, this study is evaluating the natural history and risk factors for the development of macular degeneration and cataracts. A recent report identified a lower incidence of macular degeneration in subjects whose dietary intake of dark green leafy vegetables was high. This study does not confirm that individuals should increase intake of these food stuffs, but it may indicate that some benefit occurs from antioxidant vitamins.

Normal Anatomy

The retina is the neurosensory tissue of the eye and is responsible for sensing light stimuli. As previously detailed, the retina lines the posterior segment of the eye, extending just posterior to the iris and ciliary body to the optic nerve (Fig. 27.1). The retina is composed of various neural tissues, vascular elements, and glial support cells. The neurosensory cells (rods and cones) compose the deepest layer of the retina and lie adjacent to the choroid, the posterior vascular coat of the eye. Between the retina and the choroid are the retinal pigment epithelium (RPE) and Bruch's membrane. The retina is normally closely adherent to the underlying retinal pigment epithelium, attached by a glue-like layer of mucopolysaccharide and by the constant pumping of fluid by the retinal pigment epithelium cells from the vitreous, through the retina, to

219

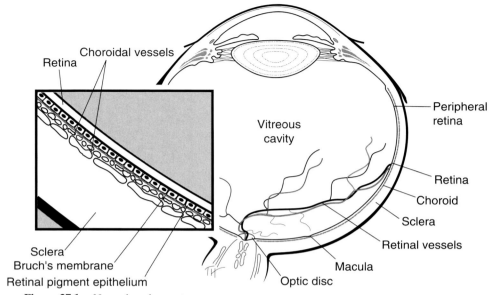

Figure 27.1.   Normal ocular anatomy.

the choroid. Bruch's membrane lies beneath the retinal pigment epithelium and is a relatively impermeable membrane which comprises part of the blood/retinal barrier. The choroid is the vascular coat which lies deep to the Bruch's membrane.

The macula is the central region of the retina. The fovea (the center of the macula) is primarily composed of cones and provides the best central visual acuity (i.e., reading vision). The macula is located temporal to the optic nerve, between the retinal vascular arcades (Fig. 27.2). The macula generally has a slightly more pigmented appearance, compared to the surrounding orange retina. If the macular cones are anatomically distorted or dysfunctional, vision may decrease precipitously.

Pathophysiology

Age-related macular degeneration (AMD) results from involutional changes of the subretinal tissues, the retinal pigment epithelium (RPE), and Bruch's membrane. These changes cause loss of central vision secondary to distortion of the normal macular anatomy or disruption of the normal macular function. However, the exact pathogenesis of AMD remains unknown. There may be a degenerative or abnormal genetic process in either the retina or retinal pigment epithelium, which leads to a buildup of protein-aceous deposits between the retinal pigment epithelium and Bruch's membrane. These deposits are called "drusen" and are the hallmark of AMD (Fig. 27.3). Drusen are associated with defects in the normal anatomy and function of the retinal pigment epithelium and Bruch's membrane.

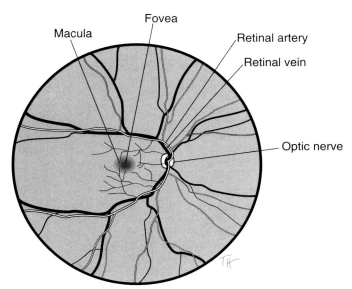

Figure 27.2.   Retina. Note the macula, temporal to the optic nerve and between the retinal vascular arcades. The fovea is at the center of the macula.

CLINICAL MANIFESTATIONS

From a clinical and pathophysiological standpoint, age-related macular degeneration is divided into two categories: the "dry" form and the "wet" form (Table 27.1). The wet form of the disease usually occurs after the dry form has been present for many years.

The symptoms of dry macular degeneration include mild blurring of vision that usually develops slowly. Patients may note parts of words are missing, and they require

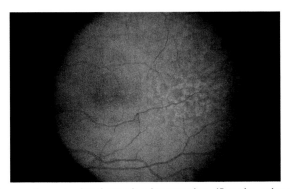

Figure 27.3.   Drusen: dry age-related macular degeneration. (See also color section.)

TABLE 27.1. Ocular Changes With AMD

TYPE OF RETINOPATHY	OCULAR FINDINGS
Dry AMD (362.51)	Drusen (proteinaceous deposits on Bruch's membrane, mimicking yellowish cobblestones clinically)
	Retinal pigment epithelial atrophy
	Retinal pigment epithelial hypertrophy
Wet AMD (362.52)	Choroidal neovascularization (sometimes visible as a flat gray-green network under retina)
	Hemorrhage
	Exudate
	Subretinal fluid

more light or magnification to read. The clinical signs of dry macular degeneration include drusen, hypertrophy of the retinal pigment epithelium, and atrophy of the retinal pigment epithelium (RPE). Drusen may be seen with a direct ophthalmoscope and appear as yellowish deposits in the macula region. Drusen typically have well-defined borders and are almost always present bilaterally (Fig. 27.3). Since the drusen are located under the retina, the overlying macula may appear normal. Retinal pigment epithelium hypertrophy presents as darkly pigmented clumps under the retina. Retinal pigment epithelium atrophy occurs in areas where multiple drusen join together and with advanced retinal pigment epithelium atrophy, a localized deficiency of pigmentation is seen.

As dry AMD progresses, significant central vision loss may occur (typically in the range of 20/40 to 20/100). Clinically, the macular region may have large areas of drusen and retinal pigment epithelium changes. Severe vision loss (20/200 vision or worse) may occur in patients with dry AMD, but more often is secondary to the wet form of the disease. Severe vision loss in dry AMD is typically caused by extensive atrophy of the retinal pigment epithelium and the overlying retina. This combined retinal pigment epithelium and retinal atrophy reduces the number of functional photoreceptors, causing symptoms of progressive central blurring, and when most severe, results in the development of central scotomas, which can restrict the patient's ability to drive and read.

The wet form of AMD occurs when neovascular tissue extends from the choroid through defects in Bruch's membrane under the macular region. These neovascular growths invade the potential space between the retina and pigment epithelium and are termed "choroidal neovascular membranes" or CNVM (Fig. 27.4). Vision loss occurs when these new vessels leak blood or proteinaceous fluid, causing hemorrhagic and serous detachments of the retina, respectively. Patients may experience sudden vision loss in one eye, metamorphopsia (distortion of straight lines), or scotomas (gray or blank spots within the field of vision). Central vision loss may be profound with a large central scotoma and inability to read, but peripheral vision is rarely affected in AMD. Continued growth of a CNVM with subsequent subretinal bleeding and localized retinal detachments results in subretinal and retinal scar tissue formation (Fig. 27.5). This scar tissue results in irreversible vision loss. The incidence of the opposite eye involvement in neovascular or wet AMD is approximately 12% per year.

The clinical signs of the wet AMD include hemorrhages under or in the retina, white exudates in the macular region, and subretinal fluid. Choroidal neovascular

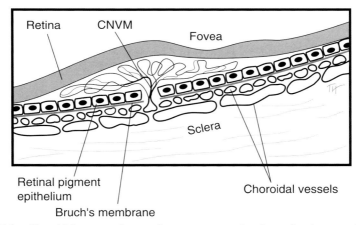

Figure 27.4.   Choroidal neovascular membrane: wet age-related macular degeneration. Note the neovascular tissue extending from the choroid through the Bruch's membrane under the retina.

membranes may sometimes be visible as flat grayish-green spots under the macula. Although the blood vessels of the retina are easy to observe through the transparent ocular media, choroidal neovascular membranes are often hard to identify on clinical examination. Fundus fluorescein angiography employs an intravenous contrast agent to enhance a photographic image, revealing structures which may be too small to resolve with an ophthalmoscope, and highlighting areas of abnormal vascular permeability (see Chapter 32, "Fundus Fluorescein Angiography"). Fundus fluorescein angiography is used diagnostically to identify CNVM, prognostically to aide in patient counseling, and therapeutically to guide laser therapy (Table 27.2). In severe AMD, large white scars may be seen involving the entire macular region (Fig. 27.5).

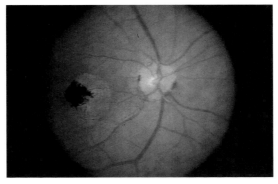

Figure 27.5.   Age-related macular degeneration: large macular scar with overlying hemorrhage (to left of optic nerve).

TABLE 27.2. Management Guidelines for AMD: When to Obtain Fluorescein Angiogram

SYMPTOMS OR SIGNS	OBTAIN FLUORESCEIN ANGIOGRAM	FOLLOW-UP
Minimal or questionable symptoms—no signs or choroidal neovascularization (CNV) (no hemorrhage, exudate, or subretinal fluid)		Give amsler grid and follow-up in 1 month with eye care specialist (ophthalmologist)
Minimal or questionable symptoms with signs of CNV	Obtain fluorescein angiogram	
Definite symptoms (distortion, scotomas) even if no signs of CNV	Obtain fluorescein angiogram	
Definite symptoms or definite signs of CNV	Obtain fluorescein angiogram	
Definite symptoms and signs of CNV but clinical examination shows clearly untreatable CNV		Follow-up in 1–3 months

DIFFERENTIAL DIAGNOSIS

Very few diseases clinically resemble dry AMD (Table 27.3). The classic finding of drusen in the macula and the predilection for elderly patients prevents confusion or misdiagnosis in most patients. Certain individuals have been identified with a familial retinopathy that presents with retinal drusen; however, these drusen typically are seen at an earlier age and are distributed throughout the retina.

However, a variety of ocular disorders may mimic wet AMD. Choroidal neovascular membranes may result from any disease or injury that affects the integrity of the retinal pigment epithelium and Bruch's membrane. These include inflammatory diseases (e.g., ocular histoplasmosis syndrome), high myopia (extreme nearsightedness), or blunt ocular trauma. Most often, these various disorders can be ruled out by history and age of onset.

TABLE 27.3. Management Guidelines for AMD: When to Consider Laser

PATTERN OF CHOROIDAL NEOVASCULARIZATION (CNV)	ARGON LASER	KRYPTON LASER
CNV that is clearly defined on fluorescein angiogram, is symptomatic, is closer than 2500 μm to fovea and is not under the foveal avascular zone	Consider argon photocoagulation	
CNV with above features except that it extends under the foveal avascular zone but not past the center of the foveal avascular zone		Consider krypton photocoagulation
CNV extends past center of foveal avascular zone		Consider photocoagulation in special circumstances

AMSLER RECORDING CHART
A replica of Chart No. 1, printed in black
on white for convenience of recording.

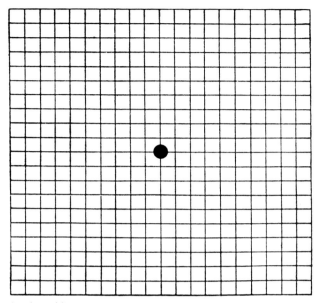

Figure 27.6.   Amsler grid.

TREATMENT

There is no proven therapy for the dry form of macular degeneration. As mentioned, the ongoing Age-Related Eye Disease Study may provide useful guidelines for the treatment of elderly patients with zinc and antioxidants. Fortunately, only 10% of all patients with macular degeneration will experience severe vision loss either from the growth of neovascular tissue (wet AMD), or from severe atrophy of the central retinal pigment epithelium and retina (dry AMD). Most patients who have advanced vision loss from macular degeneration retain peripheral vision, allowing them to ambulate on their own and to perform routine activities of daily living. Therefore, most individuals with AMD lead independent lives even with advanced vision loss. Additionally, low vision aids may be of benefit in assisting some patients with severe central vision loss to see enough to read large print materials and to write checks. State agencies are usually very helpful in providing books and periodicals on tape to patients with advanced vision loss. It is, therefore, a good idea to ask your patients with severe macular degeneration if they have registered with their state agency if they are legally blind.

In patients over the age of 55 or 60 years old, it is important to routinely question if they have vision loss or distortion (one must test the eyes separately to identify this). Because many patients with AMD will take large doses of zinc, copper deficiency anemia may occur if supplemental copper is not being used, and one should question patients about large doses of supplemental zinc. Finally, because macular degeneration

◉❚ TABLE 27.4. Referral Guidelines: AMD (362.5)

SYMPTOMS AND SIGNS	ROUTINE REFERRAL (1–4 WEEKS)	URGENT REFERRAL (WITHIN 3 DAYS)	EMERGENT REFERRAL (SAME DAY)
Asymptomatic, but drusen noted on clinical examination (362.57)	Routine referral if not under care of an ophthalmologist		
Questionable or mild symptoms of blurred vision or missed letters when reading	Routine referral recommended		
Sudden onset of symptoms of blurring, distortion (metamorphopsia) or blank areas in vision (scotomas) but without severe vision loss		Urgent referral recommended	
Sudden, severe vision loss			Emergent referral recommended

is inherited with a multifactorial pattern, it would be helpful to know if there is a positive family history of macular degeneration.

The wet form of AMD may be responsive to laser photocoagulation therapy, depending on the location and extent of the choroidal neovascular membrane. It is, therefore, important to identify potentially treatable patients as early as possible. A useful home screening test for the wet form of the disease employs a grid of straight lines which resembles graph paper (Fig. 27.6). At the center of the graph, a black dot acts as a fixation point. The patient views the grid with one eye at a time, trying to identify the occurrence of any new metamorphopsia (irregular, distorted lines) or scotomas (blank spots), near the point of central fixation. Certainly, any loss of central vision in a patient with a history of dry AMD should be considered highly suspicious for the development of a choroidal neovascular membrane.

Unfortunately, even when recognized early, fewer than 20% of patients with neovascular membranes from macular degeneration can be treated with laser. Photocoagulation of neovascular tissue has been proven effective in a subset of patients, when guidelines established by the Macular Photocoagulation Study (a multicenter, prospective, randomized clinical trial) are met. These guidelines, summarized in Table 27.4, establish parameters for the location and size of neovascular nets which can be effectively treated. When photocoagulation is performed, confluent laser spots are placed to completely cover the neovascular membrane as identified on a fluorescein angiogram. Because the neovascular process is so damaging to central vision, there is interest in other treatments, including the use of interferon-α_{2a} and thalidomide. Ongoing research will determine whether these therapies are of clinical value.

SUGGESTED READINGS

Bressler SB, Maguire MG, Bressler NM, Fine SL. The Macular Photocoagulation Study Group: relationship of drusen and abnormalities of the retinal pigment epithelium to the prognosis of neovascular macular degeneration. Arch Ophthalmol 1990;108:1444–1447.

Green WR, McDonnell PH, Yeo JH. Pathologic features of senile macular degeneration. Ophthalmol 1985;92:615–627.

Macular Photocoagulation Study Group. Argon laser photocoagulation for neovascular maculopathy after five years. Arch Ophthalmol 1991;109:1109–1114.

◖◗ Chapter 28
Optic Nerve Disorders

W. T. Shults

INTRODUCTION

The optic nerve consists of about 1.2 million nerve fibers which originate in ganglion cells distributed over the surface of the retina. These fibers vary in size with smaller diameter fibers originating in the region of the macula and larger diameter fibers from more peripheral retina. The route by which these fibers make their way across the retina to congregate at the sieve-like opening in the sclera (lamina cribrosa), from which they gain egress from the globe, is stereotyped and accounts for the patterns of arcuate or wedge-shaped visual field loss which characterize lesions of this portion of the visual pathway. This chapter discusses some of the more common disorders of the optic nerve–optic neuritis, ischemic optic neuropathy, papilledema, optic nerve tumors, and optic atrophy.

DIFFERENTIAL DIAGNOSIS

OPTIC NEURITIS

CLINICAL MANIFESTATIONS

Optic neuritis, an acute demyelinating disease of the optic nerve, is one of the commonest of neuro-ophthalmic disorders (Table 28.1). Most affected patients are between the ages of 15 and 45 years, with women more often affected than men. The clinical picture is usually easily recognizable and consists of mild to severe loss of vision often accompanied by retrobulbar pain worsened by eye movement, which evolves over a period of hours to several days. In over one-third of patients, the vision loss will be severe (20/200 or less), while the rest will be less severely involved. In some patients, visual loss is preceded by up to a week or more of periorbital and retrobulbar discomfort. Some report flashes of light induced by eye movement—so-called movement phosphenes. Some patients will note worsening of visual function with exercise or increase in body temperature (such as with a hot shower or bath), a symptom referred to as Uhthoff's phenomenon. Though not exclusively seen in patients with demyelinating disease, its occurrence should definitely prompt consideration of such a possibility.

About a third of patients have optic disc swelling (papillitis) (Fig. 28.1), while the remainder have a normal appearing optic nerve head (retrobulbar optic neuritis). Optic nerve head appearance seems to bear no relationship to the prognosis for visual recovery. Optic nerve head swelling, if present, may or may not have accompanying peripapillary hemorrhages and vascular sheathing (a segmental whitened appearance

● TABLE 28.1. Referral Guidelines: Optic Neuritis (377.3)

SYMPTOM OR SIGN	TREATMENT	WHEN TO REFER
Blurred vision, decreased color vision, decreased visual field (368.8)	If typical for optic neuritis, no ancillary testing is necessary beyond that required to confirm the clinical suspicion of optic neuritis i.e., visual acuity, color vision, pupil testing, and visual fields. Treatment with IV methylprednisolone followed by oral prednisone is indicated for bilateral visual loss or reduced vision in an only eye to decrease the period of visual disability	Any patient whose clinical course becomes atypical needs referral, e.g., continued decline in vision over a period of greater than 10 days, persistent pain, recurrent visual loss or bilateral simultaneous visual loss, vision loss outside the typical age range for optic neuritis (15–45 yrs)
Pain on eye movement (379.91)	Aspirin or acetaminophen usually suffices	If pain persists despite treatment with these agents
Progressive decline in vision over/greater than 1 week (369.20)	None	Refer because patient is atypical
Failure to recover vision (369.00)	None	Refer because patient is atypical
Development of additional neurologic symptoms	Depends upon the nature of the symptom. Numbness in one hand may require no treatment while an acute bladder atonicity from a lower cord lesion may require catheterization	If uncomfortable with nature or extent of neurological symptomatology

of the vessel wall appearing as parallel lines on either side of the blood column). The appearance of proteinaceous exudates deposited in a hemi- or complete macular star pattern defines a variant of optic neuritis called "neuroretinitis" (Fig. 28.2). Should such a fundus picture evolve, the risk for the subsequent development of multiple sclerosis (MS) diminishes considerably, as this fundus picture usually arises in children and young adults and suggests optic nerve inflammation on a nondemyelinating basis such as cat scratch disease.

Many patients will develop optic atrophy following resolution of the acute inflammatory process (Fig. 28.3). The appearance of optic atrophy correlates with the presence of fixed deficits of visual function and is more prone to develop in patients whose initial degree of visual loss was severe. Even in those without florid atrophy, subtle slit-like defects in the superior and inferior retinal nerve fiber layer may be detected ophthalmoscopically by viewing with the green light of the ophthalmoscope.

The pupil on the affected side reacts less briskly and less fully than that on the uninvolved side, a feature which is best appreciated through the use of a "swinging

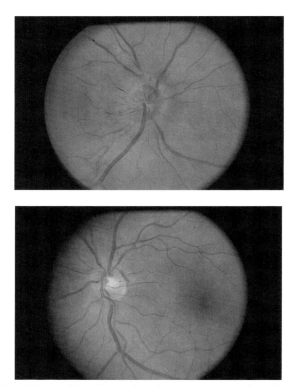

Figure 28.1.   Right (Top) and left (Bottom) optic nerve from a patient with acute optic neuritis in the right eye. The right disc is mildly swollen and hyperemic. The margin of the optic disc is made indistinct by nerve fiber edema. Note the splinter hemorrhages along the superior disc margin. Optic neuritis with this disc picture is termed papillitis. (See also color section.)

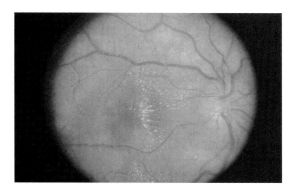

Figure 28.2. Optic disc edema accompanied by a "macular star" pattern of exudate defines the fundus picture of neuroretinitis, an optic nerve inflammation which often results from cat scratch disease. This pattern is not seen in the more common optic neuritis associated with multiple sclerosis. (See also color section.)

flashlight" testing paradigm. In this pupil testing technique, room lighting is reduced and the patient is asked to fix his or her gaze on a distant target. A bright penlight is shined into the "good" eye from a position slightly below the visual axis (so as not to disrupt the patient's ability to maintain steady fixation on the target), and the speed and extent of the pupillary constriction noted. The penlight is then quickly moved across the bridge of the nose and shined into the "bad" eye. When tested in this fashion, the initial response of the pupil in the affected eye will be to dilate rather than constrict, reflecting the relative reduction in light stimulus reaching the pupil centers in the midbrain through the inflamed nerve on that side compared to the uninvolved nerve. This pupillary dilation, when tested with the "swinging flashlight" paradigm, is termed the relative afferent pupillary defect or, less descriptively, the Marcus Gunn pupil, and is an extremely helpful sign of optic nerve disease which is almost always present in patients with optic neuritis.

Color vision is often impaired in patients with optic neuritis and the extent of the reduction is commonly greater than one might expect from the degree of decrease in the patient's visual acuity. Though visual evoked potentials are routinely delayed in optic neuritis, the diagnosis is usually apparent without resorting to the use of such technology (though it may have some utility in defining a "second lesion" in a person with suspected multiple sclerosis).

Central visual field loss is more common, but literally any type of visual field

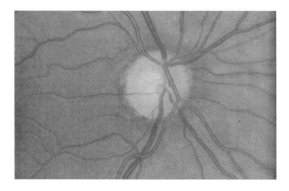

Figure 28.3. Severe optic neuritis can result in axonal death. As the axons in the optic nerve die, the color of the optic nerve head changes from a salmon pink color to a paler shade. If the axonal loss is extensive, the atrophy of nerve fibers results in a chalky white optic disc shown here.

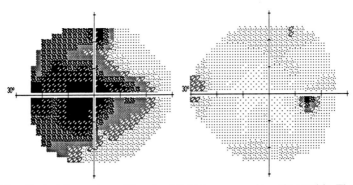

Figure 28.4.   Central depression of the visual field is common in optic neuritis. The young woman whose field is shown had marked loss of central vision, yet a normal fundus appearance.

defect may occur (Fig. 28.4). Recent work has shown that altitudinal field defects occur commonly in patients with optic neuritis making that pattern of field loss less helpful in differentiating optic neuritis from ischemic optic neuropathy than was once believed (Fig. 28.5). Though substantial spontaneous recovery occurs over weeks to months in most patients, subtle residual visual deficits (such as decreases in visual field, color vision, and contrast sensitivity) are common. Thus, lingering complaints of washed out color perception and deceased contrast appreciation are common.

Optic neuritis occurs frequently in patients with known multiple sclerosis and is often the initial manifestation of that disease prompting some to propose that it is a forme fruste of MS . While incidence rates vary in reported series, over 50% of patients presenting with optic neuritis will develop multiple sclerosis within 15 years. About 15% of patients will experience recurrent episodes of optic neuritis in either the same or opposite eye. While usually unilateral, bilateral simultaneous involvement can occur.

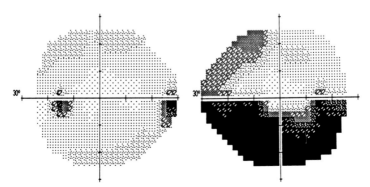

Figure 28.5.   Once thought relatively uncommon in optic neuritis, the altitudinal loss shown here is now recognized to occur relatively frequently in patients with optic neuritis.

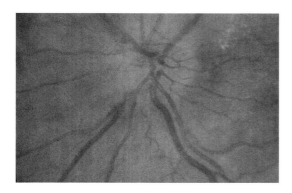

Figure 28.6. Optic disc edema in non-arteritic (idiopathic) anterior ischemic optic neuropathy is more apt to be hyperemic, as shown here, than pallid.

Other causes of acute vision loss must be considered in any patient with optic neuritis. **Ischemic optic neuropathy** produces sudden loss of vision accompanied by optic disc edema and either central or altitudinal visual field loss; however, ischemic optic neuropathy generally affects an older population and pain is not a major feature of ischemic optic neuropathy as it is in optic neuritis. The optic disc swelling in ischemic optic neuropathy is more often focal than is the disc edema of optic neuritis and peripapillary hemorrhages are more common in ischemic disease (Fig. 28.6). Cotton wool spots on the disc surface and pallid swelling are both more often a feature of ischemic optic neuropathy than optic neuritis. However, it must be stated that there are no features of the optic disc appearance that are so distinctive as to allow one to define a cause for disc edema solely on the basis of the disc appearance alone. On the other hand, optic nerve ischemia is rarely retrobulbar and, as such, optic disc swelling is a necessary finding if one is considering that diagnosis. Vision loss in optic neuritis is much more prone to recover than is that associated with ischemic optic neuropathy.

Vascular occlusive events involving the intraocular circulation will rarely prove difficult to distinguish from optic neuritis as the accompanying funduscopic picture is so definitive. **Central or branch retinal artery occlusion** produces cloudy swelling of the retina and a "cherry-red" spot in the fovea if the parafoveal area was supplied by the occluded vessel. **Central or branch retinal vein occlusion** produces a distinctive hemorrhagic retinopathy which cannot be confused with the normal fundus of retrobulbar optic neuritis or the acute disc swelling of papillitis.

Papilledema can produce optic disc swelling which is indistinguishable from that of optic neuritis (Figs. 28.7 and 28.8); however, central vision loss is not an early feature of papilledema and the patient doesn't usually complain of pain on eye movement.

Compressive optic neuropathy from a primary **optic nerve sheath tumor** may be accompanied by optic disc edema and vision loss, but the loss is slowly progressive rather than acute. Such funduscopic changes may be seen with **spheno-optic meningiomas** as well, but the time signature of slow evolution distinguishes such patients from those with optic neuritis. Rarely, intracranial compressive lesions may precisely mimic retrobulbar optic neuritis emphasizing the need to follow patients with presumed optic neuritis to ensure that their clinical course follows the expected pattern. Should it not, then neuroimaging studies would be necessary.

A relatively uncommon disorder, **Leber's hereditary neuroretinopathy**, produces sudden and sequential visual loss in both eyes separated by an interval of days to

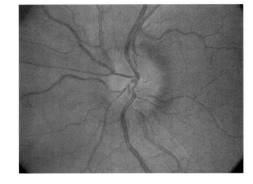

Figure 28.7. Early papilledema. The peripapillary nerve fiber layer striations become smudged and indistinct. Mild venous distention develops and peripapillary hemorrhages may appear. The degree of mounding up of disc tissue is relatively minimal at this stage.

months. This condition, which is inherited via defects in maternal mitochondrial DNA, produces devastating visual loss in otherwise healthy young adults (more rarely in children and older adults) with much less likelihood for recovery than is seen in the typical variety of presumably demyelinative optic neuritis. The lack of recovery, bilateral sequential involvement, and history of other affected family members should suggest this type of optic neuropathy and the presence of one of the known mitochondrial point mutations confirmed with appropriate genetic testing.

Nutritional deficiency (most probably B complex vitamins), **or toxic optic neuropathy** from exposure to such agents as ethambutol or chloromycetin, generally present with slowly progressive loss of central vision and dyschromatopsia (color vision deficits) occurring in both eyes simultaneously (though not necessarily symmetrically) unaccompanied by significant disc edema. If treated promptly with thiamine, folate, and B_{12}, the visual loss is reversible.

TREATMENT

Though corticosteroids have often been used to treat optic neuritis, their efficacy in this condition has been debated since their introduction over 40 years ago. Despite a lack of proof of effectiveness, most ophthalmologists and neurologists used corticosteroids in the management of optic neuritis. Beck et. al. cited a 1986 unpublished report

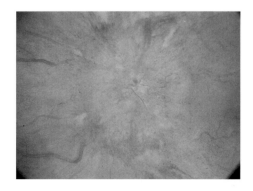

Figure 28.8. Fully developed papilledema. The degree of axonal swelling is such that all normal disc architecture is obscured. Optic nerve vessels are lost in the swollen fibers of the nerve head and cotton wool spots are usually a prominent feature as in this picture.

of an informal mail survey in Florida and Michigan that 65% of ophthalmologists and 90% of neurologists treated optic neuritis patients with corticosteroids, most often in oral form. Despite a lack of long-term benefit demonstrable in previous randomized trials, many physicians continued to use steroids citing a demonstrated hastening of improvement and presumed enhanced degree of ultimate recovery in the absence of significant risks. Those who chose not to treat pointed out that most untreated patients regained excellent visual function without steroids masking the possibility of an alternative diagnosis.

To settle this therapeutic controversy, the National Eye Institute funded the Optic Neuritis Treatment Trial (ONTT) in 1987. The study was designed to define whether either oral prednisone or intravenous methylprednisolone improved the visual outcome in optic neuritis, and whether there was any acceleration of the recovery process. In addition, the contribution of ancillary testing such as MRI scanning and laboratory testing (CBC, VDRL, ANA, chest x-ray, sedimentation rate) to the diagnosis and management of patients with optic neuritis was evaluated in a controlled fashion.

The patient presenting with historical and physical findings typical for optic neuritis does not need an elaborate battery of laboratory tests and neuroimaging studies to confirm the presumptive diagnosis (Optic Neuritis Study Group, 1991). Determinations of blood glucose, antinuclear antibody (ANA), and fluorescent treponemal antibody absorption (FTA-ABS) are of little benefit and are not cost-effective in a patient whose presentation is typical. No patients in the ONTT had an abnormal chest x-ray. In no case was a nondemyelinating cause for optic neuritis suggested from the spinal fluid examination, which was either normal or supported a diagnosis of MS. These results imply that the clinical diagnosis of optic neuritis in a typical case is not benefitted by the use of ancillary testing. Such tests should be reserved for use in those patients with unusual features such as progressive visual loss beyond 1 week, absence of pain or persistence of pain, or age greater than 45 years. Typical optic neuritis is characterized by visual loss progressing over a few days accompanied by retrobulbar pain (often exacerbated by eye movement) with either a normal or swollen optic nerve. The extent of visual acuity and field loss and the pattern of field loss are more variable than had been previously appreciated.

MRI scanning was not helpful in identifying causes of visual impairment other than optic neuritis in the ONTT patients (only 1 of 457 patients had an unsuspected intracranial lesion identified on the initial scan). Its use for purposes of diagnosis seems unreasonable. However, the MRI scan did prove to be the most valuable of all of the prognostic indicators with respect to the subsequent development of MS.

Neither intravenous (1000 mg methylprednisolone daily for 3 days followed by 1 mg/kg per day prednisone for 11 days with 3-day taper) nor oral corticosteroids (1 mg/kg/day prednisone for 14 days followed by a 3-day taper) conferred any long-term visual benefit to patients with acute optic neuritis, though those patients treated with intravenous methylprednisolone followed by oral prednisone did improve quicker during the first several weeks following treatment. Those patients treated with oral prednisone alone, the most commonly used treatment prior to the ONTT, fared no better than those treated with placebo and had a doubling of the incident of subsequent episodes of optic neuritis.

The results of the ONTT require a change in treatment practices for acute optic neuritis. It is no longer acceptable to treat patients with oral prednisone alone. This would be so even if no adverse effects on the incidence of subsequent episodes of optic neuritis had been demonstrated in the prednisone-treated group. Prednisone simply is no better than placebo and therefore should not be used. That it carries an additional burden of increasing the incidence of subsequent episodes of optic neuritis is interesting but unessential information in arriving at a conclusion that prednisone usage (as the sole treatment, not preceded by I.V. methylprednisolone) should be abandoned for treatment of optic neuritis.

While I.V. methylprednisolone followed by oral prednisone improved the speed of recovery by about 10–14 days, it provided no improvement in the extent of visual recovery at 1 year. For patients who have a compelling need to recover visual function quickly, intravenous methylprednisolone followed by oral prednisone should be considered.

Intravenous methylprednisolone followed by oral prednisone treatment seemed to reduce the incidence of nonoptic neuritis neurological events for a period of 2 years following treatment especially in those patients whose initial MRI scan showed greater white matter disease (two or more areas of bright signal of at least 3 mm in size), but this effect waned thereafter.

Many neurologists use 1000 mg of intravenous methylprednisolone as a single daily dose to permit outpatient administration and reduce cost. The data from the ONTT do not permit any assessment of the relative efficacy of this regimen.

The prognosis for recovery of vision in optic neuritis is quite good. In the ONTT, 71% of placebo-treated patients had a visual acuity of 20/20 at 1 year and 95% had a visual acuity of 20/40 or better. In those patients with two or more periventricular bright signal abnormalities (3 mm or greater in size) at the time of presentation with optic neuritis, there was a 36% chance of developing MS within a 2-year period. Though the rate of developing MS was lessened in this group by treatment with I.V. methylprednisolone (from 36% to 16%), the effect waned after 2 years and the rate of conversion to MS was comparable in both the treated and placebo groups thereafter.

FREQUENCY OF VISITS

After the initial visit which establishes the diagnosis of optic neuritis, the patient should return in about 1 week to check on the progress of their disease. Many patients will have begun to recover by this point, while a few others may still be evolving their loss (though vision loss which progresses beyond 10 days should prompt concern for the correctness of the diagnosis). By 3–4 weeks after the onset of vision loss most patients will have begun to experience some measure of visual recovery and it is a good idea to confirm that fact with a brief examination. Thereafter, visual recovery proceeds at a variable pace with most patients regaining maximum visual function by 6 months after the onset of their illness. Any departure from this course should prompt a reexamination.

ISCHEMIC OPTIC NEUROPATHY

Infarction of the optic nerve head is most often idiopathic in origin though it is an important cause of vision loss in systemic vasculitides such as giant cell arteritis as well (Table 28.2). Abrupt, painless visual loss in a middle-aged to elderly person with optic disc swelling is more apt to be related to one of these forms of ischemic optic neuropathy than to any other cause.

●▮ TABLE 28.2. Referral Guidelines: Ischemic Optic Neuropathy (377.41)

SYMPTOM OR SIGN	TREATMENT	WHEN TO REFER
Sudden painless vision loss in otherwise asymptomatic middle-age patient with optic disc edema, peripapillary splinter hemorrhages and visual field loss (likely altitudinal) (369.9)	Get sedimentation rate to rule out temporal arteritis, TA biopsy if patient has suggestive systemic symptoms otherwise unnecessary. No treatment necessary unless suspicion high for temporal arteritis then should cover with systemic prednisone while awaiting biopsy results	Any patient in whom the diagnosis is in doubt. A consultation in this circumstance is far less expensive than an unnecessary neuroimaging study performed for assessment of "papilledema"
Sudden painless vision loss in an elderly patient with pallid optic disc edema and systemic symptoms suggestive of giant cell arteritis (369.9)	Begin systemic steroids immediately (either high dose oral prednisone or I.V. methylprednisolone). Get sedimentation rate and temporal artery biopsy to confirm diagnosis. Monitor disease response with sedimentation rate and patient's symptomatic improvement	It is appropriate to document the extent of visual impairment in all such patients even though treatment will likely not alter the visual outcome. The patient will have numerous questions about their changed visual capacity which may pose problems for the primary care physician.

CLINICAL MANIFESTATIONS
Arteritic Ischemic Optic Neuropathy

Giant cell (temporal) arteritis is a polysymptomatic disorder of the elderly (over age 60 years) characterized by weight loss, low-grade fever, anemia, polymyalgia rheumatica, claudication in the jaw on chewing, temporal artery and scalp tenderness, and generalized malaise in which there is marked tendency for the occurrence of anterior ischemic optic neuropathy. The systemic symptoms are often poorly described making the diagnosis obscure until ischemic optic neuropathy affects the vision in one eye. Rarely, arteritic ischemic optic neuropathy may arise in patients who profess none of the systemic symptomatology–so-called occult giant cell arteritis.

Over one-third of patients will develop ischemic optic neuropathy if the origin of their symptoms is not recognized and treated promptly. In many such patients, total blindness in the affected eye ensues. Laboratory findings suggestive of giant cell arteritis include elevation of the sedimentation rate and alkaline phosphatase, a positive ANA, and a positive temporal artery biopsy. Though the sedimentation rate is usually markedly elevated, there are occasional patients in whom the sedimentation rate is well within the normal range. While ischemic optic neuropathy is the principal ocular consequence of giant cell arteritis, occlusion of cerebral, extremity and coronary arteries may produce stroke, claudication, or myocardial infarction, making early diagnosis and prompt therapy important in order to preserve life and limb as well as vision. Visual loss in arteritic ischemic optic neuropathy may be presaged by amaurosis fugax, a fact which should prompt consideration of giant cell arteritis in any elderly patient with complaints of transient monocular visual loss.

Of the variety of ocular manifestations of giant cell arteritis, ischemic optic neuropathy is the most important. The characteristic disc infarction results from occlusion of the short posterior ciliary arteries at the optic nerve head typically producing sudden severe loss of visual acuity and visual field. The degree of visual loss and disc pallor are both more prominent in arteritic than in idiopathic optic neuropathy. Rarely, the infarct may affect the retrobulbar optic nerve producing retrobulbar ischemic optic neuropathy unaccompanied by optic disc edema. Acutely, the optic disc exhibits pallid or hyperemic edema with or without peripapillary splinter hemorrhages. As this picture clears over several weeks, optic atrophy develops, often with marked cupping of the optic disc, a feature distinguishing arteritic from idiopathic ischemic optic neuropathy, which tends to have no cupping either acutely or once disc swelling has defervesced. Once lost, vision is unlikely to recover to any significant degree. If the patient remains undiagnosed and untreated after infarction of the first optic nerve, over 50% of patients will lose vision from ischemic optic neuropathy occurring sequentially in the opposite eye, a tragedy which occurs all too frequently.

Other, less common, ocular manifestations of giant cell arteritis include ischemic ocular pain, central retinal and ophthalmic artery occlusion, and diplopia from ocular muscle ischemia or ocular motor nerve palsies.

Idiopathic Ischemic Optic Neuropathy

As in giant cell arteritis, visual loss in idiopathic anterior ischemic optic neuropathy (AION) is typically abrupt and painless. While there are exceptions, the extent of visual loss in idiopathic AION is less severe than in the arteritic variety, and there is a greater tendency for at least partial recovery, with 40% of patients improving four or more lines of visual acuity on the standard Snellen chart. Broad arcuate or altitudinal field loss is classical, though almost any pattern of field impairment can be seen. Inferior field loss is more common than superior loss by a three to one margin. Optic disc edema may be diffuse or sectoral, pallid or hyperemic, mild to severe, and be devoid of or accompanied by peripapillary splinter hemorrhages (Fig. 28.6). As in the arteritic variety, optic atrophy follows as acute disc swelling abates, although there is minimal cupping of the disc in contradistinction to the arteritic variety. Patients with idiopathic AION tend to be younger (45–65 years) than their arteritic cohorts and do not have the systemic symptoms which are such a regular accompaniment of giant cell arteritis (although there is a higher incidence of diabetes and systemic hypertension in patients with idiopathic AION than in the general population). Migraineurs and juvenile diabetics may be affected at an even younger age.

Vision loss usually develops over a matter of hours to days with patients often noting their visual impairment upon awakening in the morning. Less commonly, vision decreases over a period of several weeks. While central vision is usually affected, this is not always the case. Altitudinal involvement may spare the macular region or the field loss may affect only a temporal wedge without any central depression. Occasional patients will demonstrate a "presymptomatic" phase of optic disc swelling for days or weeks before acquiring any evidence of impaired function.

There is a substantial tendency (25–40%) for bilateral involvement in this disease with the second eye at risk for an ischemic event occurring days, weeks, months, or years in the future.

Ischemic optic neuropathy shares certain features with other causes of sudden visual loss and is not always easy to distinguish from such entities as **papillitis**. Acute papillitis can mimic AION in the suddenness of loss, disc appearance and type of visual field impairment. Generally, acute papillitis affects a younger age group though there is substantial overlap with the age range of patients with idiopathic ischemic optic neuropathy. AION, especially of the idiopathic variety, is generally unaccompanied by pain while retrobulbar discomfort is a regular feature of optic neuritis. The patient with optic neuritis is much more apt to recover fully or nearly so than the patient with AION, though this fact is not of help in distinguishing these two entities in the acute phase. Neither AION nor optic neuritis is accompanied by the prominent systemic symptoms of arteritic AION, although a history of previous episodes of neurologic symptomatology should be sought as such a history may be helpful in assigning the patient's visual loss to a demyelinating event rather than a vaso-occlusive one.

Because the time course of the patient's visual loss is sometimes unclear, **compressive optic neuropathy**, if it is accompanied by optic disc edema, may occasionally be confused with AION; however, in such patients, the disc edema persists rather than defervesces over a relatively short time as in AION. Optic nerve infarction may rarely be a feature of **primary optic nerve or sheath tumors** initially masking the true origin of the vision loss. Other causes of optic disc edema, such as **papilledema** (optic disc edema secondary to an increase in intracranial pressure), or the infiltrative papillopathy of **sarcoidosis**, or **optic nerve head metastases**, may rarely cause confusion with AION, although the clinical setting and associated symptomatology are usually sufficiently distinct to suggest the correct diagnosis of these other entities.

TREATMENT

Once other causes have been ruled out, the first order of business when faced with a patient with ischemic optic neuropathy is to decide whether the event is idiopathic or arteritic in origin. This is not an academic exercise as the decision to immediately treat the arteritic patient with systemic steroids may prove sight- and even life-saving. A sedimentation rate (preferably Westergren rather than Wintrobe or Zeta) and temporal artery biopsy should be obtained immediately in any patient for whom the diagnosis of giant cell arteritis is being considered and systemic steroids begun in high dosage (80–100 mg oral prednisone or 1000 mg of I.V. methylprednisolone daily infused over about 1 hour) while one waits for the results. It is far wiser to treat a patient with idiopathic AION with a day or two of systemic corticosteroid therapy than to risk visual loss in the remaining eye of an untreated giant cell arteritis patient. The response of the patient's systemic symptoms is quite dramatic with improvement usually evident within 24 hours of beginning therapy. Unfortunately, the prognosis for recovery of vision is poor once the optic nerve is infarcted, but occasional successes have been reported.

It is well-recognized that the sedimentation rate in the elderly patient, even in the absence of temporal arteritis, is higher than the traditionally published "normal" ranges. It is appropriate to use a "normal" rate for males equal to one-half the patient's age and for females the age plus 10 divided by 2. While temporal artery biopsy should be obtained with reasonable promptness, its positivity will not be adversely affected by a week or two of systemic steroid therapy. It cannot be overemphasized that therapy with systemic steroids should not be delayed while waiting for a biopsy. If you are concerned enough about the possibility of giant cell arteritis to obtain a biopsy, then the patient should be covered with steroids while awaiting the scheduling of the procedure and the results—to do otherwise jeopardizes the patient's vision. Unfortunate examples of the consequences of such delayed treatment are legion. If the biopsy is negative on one side, and your clinical suspicion of the disease is strong enough, then the other side should be biopsied. The segment of temporal artery harvested should be several centimeters in length to avoid biopsying a "skip" area (a zone of unaffected artery between affected areas). Rarely, the biopsy will be negative in patients with an otherwise typical presentation for giant cell arteritis. Such patients may well have the disease and should probably be treated using the sedimentation rate to monitor clinical response.

Therapy for idiopathic anterior ischemic optic neuropathy is disappointing. No treatment has been demonstrated to be of value. Though optic nerve sheath decompression was proposed as being of potential benefit (at least in those patients with the more slowly progressive form of the disease), this was shown not to be the case in a recent prospective clinical trial. That study found no improvement in the group treated with optic nerve sheath decompression (a procedure which produces a fenestration in the optic nerve's perineural sheath allowing spinal fluid to percolate into the orbit with resultant decompression of the perineural sheath space), and even suggested that such a procedure increased the risk of visual impairment. Though oral corticosteroids have been used by some practitioners for many years, no conclusive evidence exists supporting their benefit and there are numerous examples of second eyes becoming involved while the patient was being treated for an ischemic event in the first eye. The ultimate visual outcome in idiopathic anterior ischemic optic neuropathy is more variable and less uniformly pessimistic than that in arteritic ischemic optic neuropathy, and in large measure is dependent upon the extent of the initial ischemic insult. The recently completed clinical trial performed to define the efficacy of optic nerve sheath decompression in idiopathic AION found that 40% of untreated patients will recover at least four lines of visual acuity. Even so the final level of visual function may leave the patient with a substantial level of visual impairment in one or both eyes. Even if visual acuity is preserved, altitudinal or temporal wedge visual field defects may impair the patient's ability to perform such important activities of daily living as operating a motor vehicle. Inferior visual field loss often makes the patient hesitant in going down stairs and may contribute to an increased tendency for falling in the elderly patient so afflicted. Because of the suddenness of the change in visual capacity and the tendency for actual or potential bilateral involvement, patients with AION of either idiopathic or arteritic type may develop substantial depression and anger at the sudden loss of independence imposed by their visual deficits. Tact and empathy go a long way toward helping these patients adjust to the limitations their vision loss imposes.

FREQUENCY OF VISITS

Idiopathic Ischemic Optic Neuropathy

Following the initial visit at which the diagnosis is established, it is appropriate to see the patient within 2 weeks to define the clinical course and answer the patient's questions, which will be many if their acuity and visual field have continued to decline since the first visit. Another visit several weeks thereafter is reasonable to define the

■■ TABLE 28.3. Referral Guidelines: Papilledema		
SYMPTOM OR SIGN	**TREATMENT**	**WHEN TO REFER**
Presence of papilledema (377.00)	Depends on the underlying cause. Tumors will require neurosurgical removal while disorders such as pseudotumor cerebri will require initial treatment with weight loss acetazolamide, digoxin, and possible optic nerve sheath decompression	All patients who have papilledema should be seen by an ophthalmologist for determination of their baseline visual function. The need for and frequency of follow-up visits are defined by the patient's response to initial therapeutic measures.

level of visual function, as it will likely be close to its final level by that time and a visit at this point provides a forum for the discussion of practical limitations (such as inability to drive) which the patient's reduced visual function may impose. Low vision aids may be considered and prescribed at this visit as well.

Arteritic Ischemic Optic Neuropathy

Initial follow-up of the patient's visual complaints parallels that described earlier for idiopathic ischemic optic neuropathy. As the patient's steroid dosage is reduced, it is important to follow the sedimentation rate to insure that the vasculitis is remaining quiescent. Any recurrence of visual symptomatology such as transient visual obscurations, should prompt concern that the patient is being tapered too quickly and merits ophthalmologic follow-up to look for evidence of ischemic changes of the disc or retina suggestive of reactivation warranting increasing the steroid dosage. Prolonged treatment (a year or more) with systemic steroids is commonly necessary. The systemic disease should be treated even if the patient has suffered bilateral blindness as substantial morbidity from systemic vascular involvement may ensue.

PAPILLEDEMA

The term papilledema should be reserved exclusively for optic disc swelling resulting from increased intracranial pressure (Table 28.3). While the causes of increased intracranial pressure are numerous, the ways in which the optic nerve head responds to such a pressure increase are relatively few and do not vary with the cause. Papilledema arises from impediment of anterograde axoplasmic transport from the ganglion cell bodies in the retina to the periphery of the nerve fiber (which terminates in the lateral geniculate body of the thalamus). Axoplasmic constipation arises anterior to the lamina cribrosa (the sieve-like opening in the sclera through which the 1.2 million nerve fibers comprising the optic nerve must pass as they leave the globe) with the consequence of a damming of axoplasm in that region. The bulging axons produce a mounding up of tissue at the nerve head so typical of papilledema.

As mentioned earlier, the term papilledema should be reserved for optic disc swelling secondary to increased intracranial pressure. While the most feared cause of

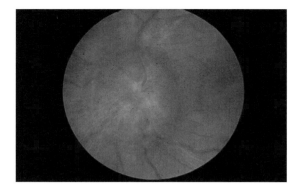

Figure 28.9. Chronic papilledema. As the changes depicted in the fully developed stage evolve, the optic disc develops a mounded swelling, which is often likened to the appearance of a champagne cork.

papilledema is brain tumor, other mass lesions such as aneurysms, cysts, intracranial bleeds, arteriovenous malformations, and brain abscess must be considered. In addition, nonmass lesions such as cerebral venous sinus occlusion, pseudotumor cerebri (benign or idiopathic intracranial hypertension), and increased spinal fluid protein from such conditions as spinal cord tumors or Guillain-Barré syndrome may also cause papilledema.

CLINICAL MANIFESTATIONS

Four stages of papilledema have been described by Hoyt and Beeston: early, fully developed, chronic and atrophic (Figs. 28.7–28.9).

In early papilledema (Fig. 28.7) the normal finely striated pattern of the peripapillary nerve fiber layer becomes smudged and indistinct. Fine capillaries on the disc surface dilate along with the retinal veins and the surface of the optic nerve bulges forward to a variable degree. Venous pulsations, a feature present in about 85–90% of normals, disappear and splinter hemorrhages arise at the disc margin and in the peripapillary retina. Some or all of these findings may be present in any given patient in the early stages of the development of papilledema and no single sign establishes its presence. If uncertain, the most reasonable course to follow is close serial observation if the patient is otherwise asymptomatic.

Fully developed papilledema (Fig. 28.8) demonstrates a greater degree of disc edema, venous distention, vascular tortuosity, peripapillary hemorrhages, and indistinctness of the nerve fiber layer to the point of obscuring retinal arteries and veins on the disc surface, and in the surrounding retina. Cotton wool spots (small grayish-white fluffy areas representing focal zones of infarction of the retinal nerve fiber layer) appear on the disc surface and in the retina near the nerve head. A macular star may form because of leakage from the disc capillaries and retinal hemorrhages secondary to venous obstruction may appear in the posterior pole and even in the retinal periphery.

Chronic papilledema (Fig. 28.9) manifests none of the changes described in the fully developed stage, as these gradually fade leaving a mounded swelling of the optic nerve head whose appearance is often likened to a champagne cork sometimes containing hard exudates. If the intracranial pressure is not alleviated, nerve fiber attrition leads to optic atrophy and the fourth stage of chronic atrophic papilledema. In this phase, the disc often shows a pearly pallor with vascular sheathing. A variable degree of visual field loss accompanies the disc pallor of chronic atrophic papilledema, though it may be extreme.

Papilledema is usually gradual in onset, although under certain circumstances the evolution may occur over a matter of hours (intracranial hemorrhage and abscess formation). Resolution is also gradual with swelling diminishing over the course of several months.

Papilledema is almost always bilateral, although there are exceptions to that general rule. All age groups can display this manifestation of increased intracranial pressure. Though the patient may experience either spontaneous or posturally induced transient episodes of visual whiteouts or blackouts (so-called transient visual obscurations), permanently decreased visual acuity is not an early manifestation of papilledema and is a helpful feature differentiating the disc swelling of papilledema from that of papillitis or AION. Persistent papilledema eventually results in permanent visual field loss. Acute disc infarction may arise if papilledema is severe, and retinal edema in the region of the macula, as well as lipid exudates collecting in the same region, may also impair vision in the patient with chronic disc swelling.

Both papillitis and AION are accompanied by acute visual loss, whereas the patient's central visual function in papilledema is preserved until late in the course (except for the transient visual obscurations mentioned earlier). Infiltrative papillopathy from conditions such as sarcoidosis or metastatic carcinoma to the optic nerve head also produces vision loss from the outset and are rarely the sole manifestation of these underlying conditions. Headache is a prominent symptom in most patients with papilledema, whereas it is not so prominent in papillitis (usually retrobulbar pain on eye movement) or AION (usually painless).

Patients with increased intracranial pressure not uncommonly have diplopia secondary to unilateral or bilateral abducens nerve palsy. Pulsatile tinnitus may also be a complaint, presumably stemming from compression of the venous sinuses. In addition to headache, many patients with increased intracranial pressure will report pain in the neck shoulders, back, and arms. None of these symptoms are features of papillitis or AION.

TREATMENT

Management of papilledema in large measure revolves around treatment of the underlying cause of the patient's increased intracranial pressure. However, relief of increased intracranial pressure is not always possible and steps may be required to relieve the disc swelling before measures directed at the underlying cause have had a chance to be effective, or when such measures fail to achieve the desired result. The range of treatments applied to reduce elevated intracranial pressure is almost as broad as the list of things which cause it, and complete discussion of the treatment options for each of these conditions is not possible because of space limitations.

If medical measures such as the use of corticosteroids, acetazolamide, or digoxin, amongst other measures, do not relieve the increased intracranial pressure, and tests of visual function such as visual acuity, color vision, contrast sensitivity, pupil testing, and visual fields demonstrate loss of optic nerve function, then operative intervention is indicated to preserve function of the remaining axons. In years past, this would have consisted of subtemporal decompression or repeat lumbar punctures. Currently, the two most widely applied therapies are shunting (either lumboperitoneal or ventriculoperitoneal) and optic nerve sheath decompression. Each procedure has its advocates though most authorities now lean toward the use of optic nerve sheath decompression for the management of threatened vision loss. In this procedure, a window or multiple linear slits are made in the retrobulbar optic nerve sheath to provide a route of egress for the perineural spinal fluid thus decompressing the optic nerve behind the lamina cribrosa. Such a procedure, if effective in creating a fistula, reduces optic disc edema and protects the nerve from further axonal attrition and permanent visual impairment. About 40% of patients will also experience improvement of headache implying that the intracranial space may also be decompressed on an ongoing basis in at least some patients. It is clear that not all patients require such invasive measures, but there is no easy way to discern the optimal time for sheath decompression—operate too soon and you may be performing unnecessary surgery; too late and the patient will have lost vision. It is much the same dilemma physicians have faced for years in deciding the approach to possible appendicitis. The key piece of information for the clinician to know in making the decision regarding the timing of optic nerve sheath decompression is the patient's visual status, which requires careful monitoring.

Development of progressive loss despite maximal medical therapy, the presence of severe visual loss (bilateral or unilateral) at the time of presentation, or persistent headache despite treatment, are all indications for operative intervention. It has been estimated that 10–25% of patients with papilledema will develop some degree of permanent visual loss, so the risk is moderately high and the need for careful follow-up must be stressed to the patient to avert preventable visual impairment.

FREQUENCY OF VISITS

From the standpoint of vision, the goal in the patient with papilledema is to prevent permanent impairment. After establishing the patient's baseline visual function, the need for and frequency of follow-up visits are determined by the patient's response to initial therapeutic measures. Thus, a child with acute papilledema due to a posterior fossa brain tumor whose optic disc swelling rapidly defervesces after surgical removal of the tumor is at little risk of ongoing visual loss and would require only one or two follow-up examinations to define the final level of visual function. However, the patient with pseudotumor cerebri being managed with a structured weight-loss program and acetazolamide should be monitored at monthly or shorter intervals for signs of visual failure until such time as clear-cut improvement in the funduscopic picture provides evidence that such measures are working. This judgment requires more than just a fundus exam. Visual function studies, and especially visual fields, are necessary to decide the question of improvement, as a dying optic nerve will also exhibit reduced swelling and may mislead the physician into thinking that improvement is occurring when in fact the opposite is true.

OPTIC ATROPHY

Optic atrophy is the end result of ganglion cell death (Table 28.4). It can be the product of retinal or optic nerve disease and occasionally results from retrogeniculate lesions. In each case, the disorders must be of sufficient severity to not only impair ganglion cell function, but result in destruction of the cell itself. With the consequential dying back of the retinal axons, slits and grooves become visible in the retinal nerve fiber

◗▮ TABLE 28.4. Referral Guidelines: Optic Atrophy

SYMPTOM OR SIGN	TREATMENT	WHEN TO REFER
Optic atrophy (377.1)	Depends on the cause; see discussion of treatment of optic neuritis, ischemic optic neuropathy and papilledema. History of gradual onset mandates investigation of possible compressive, toxic or nutritional and infiltrative causes	Whenever physician's comfort level as to the cause has been exceeded

layer and the optic disc assumes a different color, changing from a healthy salmon-pink to a chalky-white (if the loss of fibers is complete or nearly so). Optic atrophy may be diffuse or focal, and mild or severe. It is not a diagnosis unto itself, but rather a description of a clinical appearance of the optic nerve head, and as such always requires further investigation to establish a cause for the disc pallor. This is so even if the pallor has been present for many years. Long-standing optic atrophy may be the presenting manifestation of a slow growing skull-base tumor such as a meningioma. The fact that atrophy has been documented to have been present for many years does not negate the possibility that it was produced by a brain tumor.

CLINICAL MANIFESTATIONS

Any patient with optic atrophy has impaired visual function, though the degree of lost function may be so minimal and its evolution so gradual that the patient is unaware of the deficit. Decreased visual acuity, color vision, contrast sensitivity, pupillary reactivity, and visual fields, to a greater or lesser degree, are abnormal in patients with atrophy of the optic nerve head. The loss of nerve fiber layer may be diffuse as in a disorder such as postpapilledema optic atrophy (Fig. 28.10), or focal as in segmental disc infarction of

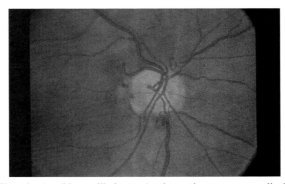

Figure 28.10. Chronic atrophic papilledema. As the optic nerve axons die from unrelieved increased intracranial pressure, the optic nerve head becomes pale. Optociliary shunts may be present as shown here. These vessels connect the retina to the choroidal circulation and arise when there is obstruction of the primary route of egress of venous blood from the eye. Visual field loss invariably accompanies postpapilledema optic atrophy.

AION. There is usually nothing specific about the appearance of most atrophic optic discs which will provide clues to the origin of the atrophy. Such clues come from the patient's history and prior exam findings–whether the loss was slow or rapid; whether there was accompanying pain; whether the atrophy was preceded by a stage of optic disc or retinal edema; and so forth. However, optic disc and retinal appearance can sometimes offer helpful clues. Accompanying narrowing in the caliber of the retinal vessels or the presence of bright plaques in their branching points may suggest prior central retinal artery occlusion. Optociliary shunt vessels (Fig. 28.10) on the disc surface of an atrophic nerve head in a patient with a history of slowly progressive visual loss are strongly suggestive of the diagnosis of optic nerve sheath meningioma.

The atrophic nerve head of AION generally has little or no cupping while that which follows arteritic AION is more apt to be cupped, although such distinctions may be fallible in any individual case. The optic atrophy which develops in tobacco-alcohol or nutritional amblyopia tends to affect the papillomacular bundle, preferentially producing an optic nerve which has greater pallor in the temporal entry zone for those fibers. This is the same area which is most affected in a type of hereditary optic neuropathy known as dominantly inherited optic atrophy.

Band atrophy is the descriptive term applied to the pattern of axonal loss which is produced by compression of the optic chiasm. Retrograde atrophy of the crossing optic nerve fibers in the chiasm produces relatively greater attrition of nasal retinal nerve fibers arising from ganglion cells subserving temporal visual field. These fibers degenerate leaving fibers from temporal retinal ganglion cells intact. These fibers from temporal retinal ganglion cells enter the superior and inferior poles of the optic nerve head, while the nasal retinal fibers degenerate in a "bow tie" pattern in the mid disc producing the characteristic band of relative atrophy horizontally bisecting the disc.

While a cupped, atrophic disc generally connotes end-stage glaucoma, compressive optic neuropathy can occasionally produce similar findings.

As implied earlier, there is a spectrum of optic atrophy ranging from barely detectable to severe. Early on the functional impairment accompanying minimal disc atrophy is itself subtle and may be unassociated with any symptomatic complaints from the patient. Nonetheless, in the face of subtle atrophy, if acuity, color, contrast, pupil function, or visual field testing yield suboptimal results, further investigation is warranted. The differential diagnosis of optic atrophy lies not so much in what can be confused with the clinical picture of a pale disc as it does with the various causes of optic disc pallor. The following list is incomplete, but provides an overview of the differential possibilities which must considered when faced with a patient with optic nerve atrophy:

Compressive lesions
Tumors (Meningiomas, pituitary adenomas, gliomas, etc.)
Aneurysms (Carotid, ophthalmic, anterior cerebral)
Fractures of optic canal
Paranasal sinus mucoceles
Vascular insults
   Central retinal artery occlusion
   Idiopathic and arteritic ischemic optic neuropathy
Optic nerve trauma
   Direct or indirect
Retinal diseases
   Retinitis pigmentosa
   Panretinal photocoagulation

Optic nerve inflammatory diseases
   Optic neuritis
Optic nerve infiltrative disorders
   Sarcoidosis
   Carcinomatous optic neuropathy
Secondary to untreated papilledema
Toxic or nutritional amblyopia
Hereditary optic neuropathy (Leber) or dominantly inherited optic neuropathy

As noted earlier, to a large degree the distinction amongst these varied causes of optic atrophy is defined by the associated history and physical findings rather than the disc appearance itself which may be of little help in distinguishing one cause from another. The time signature of the loss is of great benefit in sorting through the various possibilities. Compressive, toxic/nutritional, and infiltrative etiologies typically produce gradual impairment, while inflammatory, ischemic, and traumatic causes result in a more abrupt loss, often with optic disc edema in the acute phase. In these latter circumstances, the clinician has the opportunity to watch the acutely swollen disc become atrophic, while in the former, the patient presents with a pale optic nerve head likely necessitating neuroimaging to elucidate the cause.

TREATMENT

Given the myriad causes of optic atrophy, no global statement can be made regarding its treatment, as that is totally dependent upon the underlying condition which rendered the optic nerve atrophic in the first place. Treatment of optic neuritis, ischemic optic neuropathy, and papilledema were discussed in greater detail earlier. Compressive optic neuropathy from an intracranial lesion such as a parasellar tumor or aneurysm requires neurosurgical input to determine the optimum management. The proper approach to direct and indirect optic nerve trauma is a controversial topic for which no universally accepted guidelines presently exist. Toxic and nutritional amblyopia should be treated with appropriate replacement vitamins. Sarcoid optic neuropathy frequently responds favorably to high dose oral corticosteroids though the benefits may not prove permanent.

By definition, the presence of optic atrophy connotes some measure of permanent loss of axons in the optic nerve, and as such is accompanied by a lasting deficit of function, though the degree of functional loss may be small and unassociated with any visual symptoms. While the degree of lost function usually roughly parallels the extent of optic atrophy, the linkage is not so tight that one can make reliable predictions regarding the level of ultimate visual recovery in an atrophic nerve. For the most part, the amount of vision recovered in the first 6 months after treatment of the underlying cause of the patient's atrophy represents essentially all the clinically significant improvement one can expect, though, rarely, younger patients may continue to improve over periods of a year or more.

FREQUENCY OF VISITS

No general guidelines are applicable here given the heterogeneous nature of the disorders capable of producing optic atrophy. Frequency-of-visit guidelines for such causes of optic atrophy as optic neuritis, ischemic optic neuropathy, and papilledema are provided in the sections dealing with those disorders.

SUGGESTED READINGS

Albert D, Ruchman M, Keltner J. Skip areas in temporal arteritis. Arch Ophthalmol 1976;94:2072–2077.

Beck R, Cleary P, Trobe J, et al. The effect of corticosteroids for acute optic neuritis on the subsequent development of multiple sclerosis. N Engl J Med 1993;329:1764–1769.

Beck RW, Arrington J, Murtagh FR, et al. Brain magnetic resonance imaging in acute optic neuritis. Arch Neurol 1993;50:841–846.

Beck RW, Cleary PA, Anderson MM Jr, et al. A randomized, controlled trial of corticosteroids in the treatment of acute optic neuritis. N Engl J Med 1992;326:581–588.

Beck RW, Cleary PA, Optic Neuritis Study Group. Optic Neuritis Treatment Trial: one-year follow-up results. Arch Ophthalmol 1993;111:773–775.

Beck RW, Kupersmith MJ, Cleary PA, Katz B, Optic Neuritis Study Group. Fellow eye abnormalities in acute unilateral optic neuritis: experience of the Optic Neuritis Treatment Trial. Ophthalmology 1993;100:691–698.

Bengtsson B, Malmvall B. Prognosis of giant-cell arteritis, including temporal arteritis and polymyalgia rheumatica. Acta Med Scand 1981;209:337–345.

Beri M, Klugman M, Kohler J, Hayreh S. Anterior ischemic optic neuropathy. VII. Incidence of bilaterality and various influencing factors. Ophthalmology 1987;94:1020–1028.

Boghen D, Glaser J. Ischaemic optic neuropathy–the clinical profile and natural history. Brain 1975;98;689–708.

Bowden AN, Bowden PMA, Friedmann AI, Perkin GD, Rose FC. A trial of corticotrophin gelatin injection in acute optic neuritis. J Neurol Neurosurg Psychiatry 1974;37:869–873.

Chrousos GA, Kattah JC, Beck RW, Cleary PA, Optic Neuritis Study Group. Side effects of glucocorticoid treatment: experience of the Optic Neuritis Treatment Trial. JAMA 1993;269:2110–2112.

Davis F, Bergen D, Schauf C, McDonald I, Deutsch W. Movement phosphenes in optic neuritis: a new clinical sign. Neurology 1976;26:1100–1104.

Ebers GC. Optic neuritis and multiple sclerosis. Arch Neurol 1985;42:702–704.

Fleischman JA, Beck RW, Linares OA, Klein JW. Deficits of visual function after resolution of optic neuritis. Ophthalmology 1987;94:1029–1035.

Frisen L, Hoyt W. Insidious atrophy of retinal nerve fibers in multiple sclerosis. Funduscopic identification in patients with and without vision complaints. Arch Ophthalmol 1974;92:91–97.

Galvin R, Sanders M. Peripheral retinal hemorrhages with papilloedema. Br J Ophthalmol 1980;64:262–266.

Gould ES, Bird AC, Leaver PK, McDonald WI. Treatment of optic neuritis by retrobulbar injection of triamcinolone. Br Med J 1977;1:1495–1497.

Griffin J, Wray S. Acquired color vision defects in retrobulbar optic neuritis. Am J Ophthalmol 1978;86:193–201.

Halliday A, McDonald W, Mushin J. Delayed visual evoked response in optic neuritis. Lancet 1972;1:982–985.

Hayreh S. Anterior ischemic optic neuropathy. Arch Neurol 1981;38:675–678.

Hayreh S. Anterior ischemic optic neuropathy. V. Optic disc edema as early sign. Arch Ophthalmol 1981;99:1030–1040.

Hayreh S, Zahoruk R. Anterior ischemic optic neuropathy. VI. In juvenile diabetics. Ophthalmology 1981;182:13–28.

Hoyt W, Beeston D. Papilledema–sign of increased intracranial pressure. In: Hoyt W, Beeston D, eds. The ocular fundus in neurologic disease: a diagnostic manual and stereo atlas. St. Louis: C.V. Mosby, 1966:1–23.

Hoyt W, Rios-Montenegro E, Behrens M, Eckelhoff R. Homonymous hemioptic hypoplasia: funduscopic features in standard and red-free illumination in three patients with congenital hemiplegia. Br J Ophthalmol 1972;56:537–545.

Ischemic Optic Neuropathy Decompression Treatment Research Group. Optic nerve decompression surgery for nonarteritic anterior ischemic optic neuropathy (NAIO) is not effective and may be harmful. JAMA 1995;273:625–632.

Kansu T, Corbett J, Savino P, Schatz N. Giant-cell arteritis with normal sedimentation rate. Arch Neurol 1977;34:624–625.

Katz B. Bilateral sequential migrainous ischemic optic neuropathy. Am J Ophthalmol 1985;99:489.

Keltner J. Giant-cell arteritis. Signs and symptoms. Ophthalmology 1982;89:1101–1110.

Keltner JL, Johnson CA, Spurr JO, Beck RW, Optic Neuritis Study Group. Baseline visual field profile of optic neuritis: the experience of the Optic Neuritis Treatment Trial. Arch Ophthamol 1993;111:231–324.

Kirkham T, Sanders M, Sapp G. Unilateral papilledema in benign intracranial hypertension. Can J Ophthalmol 1973;8:533–538.

Kupersmith M, Krohn D. Cavernous optic atrophy with compressive lesions of the anterior visual pathway [Abstract]. Ann Neurol 1982;12:117.

Miller N, Savino P, Schneider T. Rapid growth of an intracranial aneurysm causing apparent retrobulbar optic neuritis. J Neuroophthalmol 1995;15:212–218.

Monteiro M, Coppetto J, Greco P. Giant-cell arteritis of the posterior circulation presenting with ataxia and ophthalmoplegia. Arch Ophthalmol 1984;102:407–409.

Optic Neuritis Study Group. The clinical profile of optic neuritis. Arch Ophthalmol 1991;109:1673–1678.

Pagani L. The rapid appearance of papilledema. J Neurosurg 1969;30:247–249.

Rawson MD, Liversdege LA. Treatment of retrobulbar neuritis with corticotrophin. Lancet 1969;2:222.

Rawson MD, Liversedge LA, Goldfarb G. Treatment of acute retrobulbar optic neuritis with corticotrophin. Lancet 1966;2:1044–1046.

Repka M, Savino P, Schatz N, Sergott R. Clinical profile and long-term implications of anterior ischemic optic neuropathy. Am J Ophthalmol 1983;96:478–483.

Rizzo J, Lessell S. Risk of developing multiple sclerosis after uncomplicated optic neuritis: a long-term prospective study. Neurology 1988;38:185–190.

Rose AS, Kuzma JW, Kurtzke JF, et al. Cooperative study in the evaluation of therapy in multiple sclerosis. ACTH vs. placebo–final report. Neurology 1970;20:1–59.

Rosenfield S, Kosmorsky G, Lingele T, et al. Treatment of temporal arteritis with ocular involvement. Am J Med 1986;80:143–145.

Sanders EACM, Volkers ACW, van der Poel JC, van Lith GHM. Estimation of visual function after optic neuritis: a comparison of clinical tests. Br J Ophthalmol 1986;70:918–924.

Selhorst J, Saul R, Waybright E. Optic nerve conduction: opposing effects of exercise and hyperventilation. Trans Am Neuro Assoc 1981;106:1–4.

Chapter 29 ◖◗❙
Glaucoma

E. M. Van Buskirk and G. A. Cioffi

INTRODUCTION

Visual loss from glaucoma results from characteristic progressive deterioration of the optic nerve and associated loss of retinal ganglion cells leading to progressive loss of visual field. At least 3 million Americans suffer from glaucoma. Glaucoma is one of the leading causes of adult blindness, and it is also the leading cause of preventable blindness. Most blind subjects are blind in at least one eye at the time of original detection, pointing to the need for better early diagnosis. Because glaucoma usually does not manifest any symptoms until extensive peripheral visual loss becomes apparent in the final stages of the disease, it is often likened to the "sneak thief of sight." Unlike most eye diseases, most varieties of glaucoma are chronic, virtually "lifelong" disorders that can be controlled but not cured. Like diabetes mellitus, systemic hypertension, reactive airway disease, or arthritis, glaucoma requires some modification in lifestyle such as compliance with medical regimens, regular physician visits, and acknowledgment of the disease to achieve successful treatment.

Three areas of ocular anatomy are key to understanding the group of disorders known as glaucoma. These include the anterior optic nerve (referred to as the optic nerve head, the optic disk, or the optic papilla), the ciliary body, and the angle of the anterior chamber. The anatomy of the anterior optic nerve is described in detail later. The ciliary body is the midportion of the uveal tract lying just behind the iris and is the site of production of aqueous humor (Fig. 29.1). The angle of the anterior chamber refers to the region between the cornea and the iris which contains the trabecular meshwork, the principal site of outflow of aqueous humor from the eye. Aqueous humor bathes the anterior segment of the eye, providing oxygen and nutrition to the region. The aqueous humor is produced at a relatively constant rate by the ciliary body. The trabecular meshwork acts as a sieve of tissue that connects, via Schlemm's canal, to the venous system, where the aqueous humor is resorbed into the bloodstream. Intraocular pressure (eye pressure) is dependent on the production of aqueous humor and the resistance of aqueous humor outflow through the trabecular meshwork.

The majority of glaucoma cases in North America and Europe are associated with elevation of the intraocular pressure. Elevated intraocular pressure could result from either an excessive production of aqueous humor from the ciliary body or an obstruction of aqueous humor outflow through the chamber angle (trabecular meshwork). In fact, virtually all elevation of intraocular pressure arises from some form of blockade of aqueous humor outflow through the trabecular meshwork. This blockage occurs either at the trabecular cellular level or from gross blockade of the tissue by fibrosis or circulating material. Some patients exhibit the progressive optic neuropathy

251

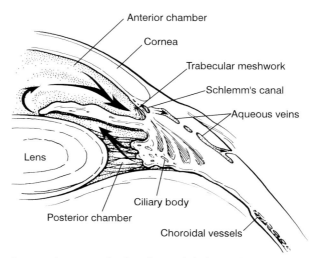

Figure 29.1.   Aqueous humor production, flow and drainage. Aqueous humor is produced by the ciliary body in the posterior chamber, flows between the lens and iris, through the pupil, into the anterior chamber, and out of the eye through the anterior chamber angle (trabecular meshwork). (Reprinted with permission from Cioffi GA. Pathogenesis of glaucoma. In: Wright KW, ed. Textbook of ophthalmology. Ch. 42, Fig. 42.2. Baltimore: Williams and Wilkins, 1996:571.)

of glaucoma, but seldom or never manifest increased intraocular pressure. Controversy exists about whether these individuals have exquisitely pressure-sensitive optic nerves, or whether other damaging factors such as compromised microcirculation cause the optic neuropathy. Evidence suggests that other, nonpressure factors do contribute to glaucomatous optic neuropathy, regardless of intraocular pressure. Glaucomatous optic nerve damage without elevated intraocular pressure is sometimes referred to as "low tension glaucoma" or "normal pressure glaucoma."

The clinical varieties of glaucoma are classified according to three parameters: (a) primary (i.e., idiopathic) or secondary (i.e., associated with some other ocular or systemic conditions); (b) the state of the anterior chamber angle–open angle (i.e., open access of the outflowing aqueous humor to trabecular meshwork) or closed angle (i.e., the trabecular meshwork is blocked by apposition of the peripheral iris); and (c) chronicity–acute or chronic. The vast majority of glaucomas are chronic.

Although most glaucoma patients have the primary open angle type, some 50 different varieties of secondary glaucoma have been described, the most common of which are listed in Table 29.1. In general, these are not specifically attributable to endogenous dysfunction of the trabecular meshwork, but rather to some other ocular or systemic disorders such as inflammation, intraocular neovascularization, congenital anomalies, ocular trauma, or tumors. Although appropriate diagnosis of an unusual secondary glaucoma can make the difference between sight preservation and blindness, most secondary glaucomas are sufficiently uncommon to fall exclusively within the ken of the glaucoma subspecialist. A few are relatively common or afflict a specific group of patients to mandate some familiarity by the primary care physician.

TABLE 29.1. Most Common Secondary Glaucomas

TYPE OF GLAUCOMA	COMMON ASSOCIATED FINDINGS
Traumatic glaucoma	Distant history of ocular trauma, hyphema
Pigmentary glaucoma	Young (30–50 years old); myopia; male
Neovascular glaucoma	Diabetes mellitus; retinal vein occlusion; peripheral vascular disease
Glaucoma associated with elevated episcleral venous pressure	Arteriovenous fistula; Sturge-Weber syndrome; orbital bruit; chronic "red eye" secondary to venous engorgement
Inflammatory glaucoma	Recent ocular trauma or surgery; history of uveitis; ocular inflammatory disease (herpes, rheumatoid arthritis, etc.)
Glaucoma associated with Corticosteroid therapy	Recent use of corticosteroid therapy (topical, nasal, or systemic); family history of glaucoma

Glaucoma refers to a group of diseases of the eye, most of which are chronic and, when unrecognized, produce insidious irreversible visual loss. Blindness from glaucoma can be prevented or greatly reduced by appropriate screening, particularly by eliciting a family history of glaucoma and detecting the presence of glaucomatous optic neuropathy by ophthalmoscopy. Glaucoma, like other chronic diseases, requires establishment of a strong physician-patient relationship, ongoing therapeutic regimen, and regular physician office visits. Patients whose glaucoma is recognized in the early stages usually learn to cope with their disease and retain good functional vision throughout their life. Patients whose diagnosis is delayed until advanced visual field loss develops, who cannot cope with the rigors of chronic disease therapy, or who suffer from nonpressure risk factors have a much worse prognosis for retention of useful vision.

CLINICAL MANIFESTATIONS

Glaucomatous Optic Neuropathy

A characteristic deterioration of the optic nerve associated with cupping and atrophy is the common denominator of all forms of glaucoma (primary or secondary, open or closed angle, chronic or acute). Atrophy of the optic nerve is the primary cause of permanent visual loss in glaucoma. Because of the ready visibility of the anterior optic nerve with any ophthalmoscope, recognition of the early signs of glaucomatous optic neuropathy becomes the single most useful clinical tool for glaucoma screening. With the ophthalmoscope and visualization of the optic nerve head, recognition of the glaucomatous optic neuropathy is not difficult. The circular optic disk border is visualized as the junction between the nerve head and the surrounding retina (Fig. 29.2). The optic nerve is primarily composed of the axons (the retinal nerve fibers) from the retinal ganglion cells and acts as the neural connection between the neurosensory retina and the brain. The optic nerve head represents the perpendicular transition of the retinal nerve fibers from the surface of the retina to the optic nerve as they exit the eye. The normal, healthy optic nerve is composed of approximately 1.2–1.5 million neurons or fibers. With advancing age, there is often some atrophy of the tissue surrounding the optic nerve that gives a pale halo around the disk edge and provides an obvious visual separation of the retina and the optic disk tissue. The neural tissue

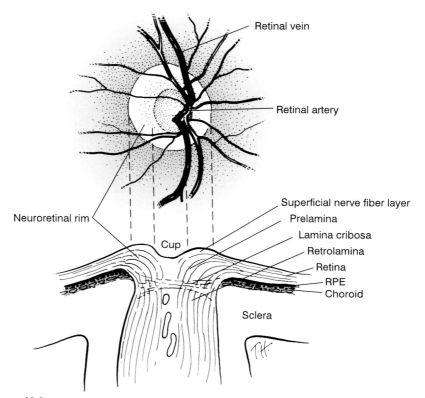

Figure 29.2.   Normal optic nerve (anterior optic nerve head and transverse cross-section, right eye). Note the central cup, neuroretinal rim, and retinal blood vessels. (Reprinted with permission from Cioffi GA. Clinical testing in glaucoma. In: Wright KW, ed. Textbook of ophthalmology. Ch. 43, Fig. 43.4. Baltimore: Williams and Wilkins, 1996:581.)

of the disk has an orange-pinkish hue and has a full, slightly elevated appearance, with a relatively distinct border at the disk edge. Centrally, the orange-pink neural tissue gradually gives way to a yellow-whitish central zone or optic disk cup that is slightly more excavated than the surrounding neural tissue. This renders a bagel-like or doughnut-like appearance to the nerve head, the neural tissue or neural "rim" surrounding the central physiologic cup. The retinal vessels, arteries and veins, enter and exit the globe through the optic nerve in the area of the optic cup. In glaucoma, as the neural tissue atrophies, the central cup appears to enlarge due to the surrounding tissue loss. The ratio of the diameter of the cup to the total diameter of the disk (cup-disk ratio) is usually 0.3 or less; a ratio greater than 0.5 should raise suspicion of glaucoma (Figs. 29.3 and 29.4).

Most individuals will have very similar, symmetric optic disks and cups in each eye. An asymmetry of the cup-disk ratio of 0.2 or greater between the two eyes is easy to recognize and one of the most useful signs of early glaucoma optic nerve

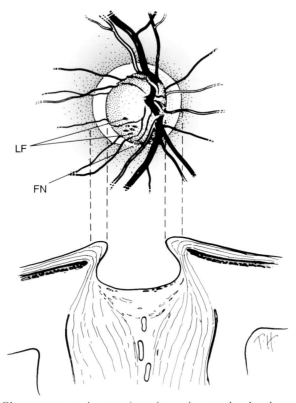

Figure 29.3. Glaucomatous optic nerve (anterior optic nerve head and transverse cross-section, right eye). Note the thinning of the neuroretinal rim, enlargement of the cup, nasal displacement of the retinal blood vessels. The inferior rim is thinned to a focal notch (*FN*) and the fenestrations of the underlying lamina cribrosa (*LF*) can be seen due to neural atrophy. (Reprinted with permission from Cioffi GA. Clinical testing in glaucoma. In: Wright KW, ed. Textbook of ophthalmology. Ch. 43, Fig. 43.5. Baltimore: Williams and Wilkins, 1996:582.)

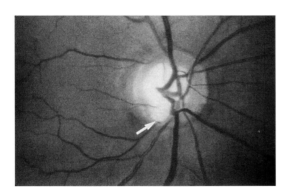

Figure 29.4. Glaucomatous optic nerve (right eye). Note the enlarged cup, thin neuroretinal rim and displaced retinal vessels. The arrow points to a focal notch, area of rim thinning. (See also color section.)

damage (glaucomatous optic neuropathy). This is the most characteristic findings of glaucomatous neural change, and is called cupping. This produces not only side-to-side enlargement of the cup, but also anterior posterior enlargement with retrodisplacement of the support tissue. This posterior displacement causes an obvious backward bowing of the white tissue at the base of the central cup portion of the disk.

In addition to diffuse enlargement of the physiologic cup, focal thinning of the optic nerve rim is also very characteristic of glaucoma. Typically, the lower pole of the nerve head shows a focal defect of the neural rim earlier than the superior pole of the optic nerve. This results in a concomitant defect in the superior visual field. Small, "flame-shaped" hemorrhages at the disk edge are also often harbingers of advancing neural damage and visual field loss, and are quite characteristic of glaucomatous optic neuropathy (Fig. 29.5).

As the central cup enlarges and the neural tissue of the optic nerve recedes, support for the retinal vessels traversing the disk disappears, and the vessels become displaced to the nasal aspect. By the same token, because of the excavation of the nerve tissue, displacement of the vessels may cause the apparent abrupt changes in the course of vessels that suddenly jog in a new direction to accommodate the topographic irregularities of the surrounding neural tissue (Figs. 29.3 and 29.4).

Visual Field Loss

Progressive loss of optic neural fibers leads eventually to progressive loss of visual field, and, finally, to complete loss or blindness. However, in most forms of glaucoma, the individual patient will not experience any symptoms until late in the disease. Early peripheral visual field loss is undetectable to the patient, and its slow progression makes its recognition near impossible without special testing. In its normal physiologic state, greater than 1 million fibers of the optic nerve carry visual information from retinal ganglion cells through the nerve fiber layer of the retina, the optic nerve, and to the lateral geniculate body. Fortunately, there is a certain amount of functional reserve in the optic nerve so that a considerable portion, perhaps even half, of the nerve fibers can be lost before significant visual field loss occurs. This offers the opportunity for early diagnosis of disk changes before significant, impending visual loss transpires. The functional status of the optic nerve can be assessed by specialized testing of the peripheral vision, the "visual field" (see Chapter 34, "Visual Fields").

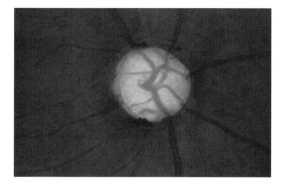

Figure 29.5. Glaucomatous optic nerve with a hemorrhage in the nerve fiber layer at the disc margin (right eye). (See also color section.)

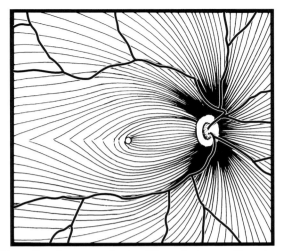

Figure 29.6. Nerve fiber layer organization. The retinal nerve fibers (axons of the ganglion cells) converge on the optic nerve. Arcuate fibers extend from the temporal retina to the optic nerve. Loss of these fibers occurs early in glaucoma, accounting for visual field loss.
(Reprinted with permission from Cioffi GA. Anatomy of the optic nerve. In: Wright KW, ed. Textbook of ophthalmology. Ch. 44, Fig. 44.1. Baltimore: Williams and Wilkins, 1996:592.)

The special anatomy of the nerve fiber layer in the retina produces visual field defects from glaucoma that follow a characteristic pattern. Visual field loss in glaucoma usually arches from the physiologic blind spot of the optic disk, curving around the central region, and ending abruptly along the horizonal axis nasally, corresponding to the nasal raphe of the retinal nerve fiber layer (Fig. 29.6). These arch-shaped defects are known by the eponym of "Bjerrum," or arcuate, scotomas (Fig. 29.7). Loss of the peripheral nasal visual field loss generally occurs first in glaucoma. Following the progressive change and course of these visual field defects becomes the most critical aspect of managing the glaucoma patient.

Intraocular Pressure

In the past, the level of the intraocular pressure was used to define and diagnose glaucoma. However, in recent decades, it has been recognized that many individuals with glaucomatous optic nerve damage lack elevation of the intraocular pressure. Therefore, intraocular pressure is now considered only one of the many risk factors, although possibly the most important, for the development of optic nerve damage. Measurement of intraocular pressure (tonometry) is possible by a variety of techniques, the most accurate of which uses a slitlamp and applanation device. Applanation tonometry indirectly measures the intraocular pressure by assessing the firmness of the globe and the resistance of the round cornea to flattening. Other tonometers, such as a Schiötz tonometer, measure the intraocular pressure by assessing the resistance to indentation. In a firm eye (high intraocular pressure), the resistance to corneal flattening or to indentation will be high, while a soft eye will flatten or indent easily. Measurement

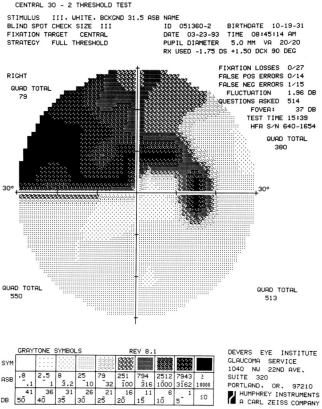

CENTRAL 30 - 2 THRESHOLD TEST

STIMULUS   III, WHITE, BCKGND 31.5 ASB NAME
BLIND SPOT CHECK SIZE III   ID 051360-2   BIRTHDATE 10-19-31
FIXATION TARGET   CENTRAL   DATE 03-23-93 TIME 08:45:14 AM
STRATEGY   FULL THRESHOLD   PUPIL DIAMETER   5.0 MM VA 20/20
                                             RX USED -1.75 DS +1.50 DCX 90 DEG

RIGHT   FIXATION LOSSES 0/27
                                         FALSE POS ERRORS 0/14
QUAD TOTAL   FALSE NEG ERRORS 1/15
    79   FLUCTUATION   1.96 DB
                                        QUESTIONS ASKED   514
                                               FOVEA: 37 DB
                                             TEST TIME 15:39
                                             HFA S/N 640-1654

                                                 QUAD TOTAL
                                                    380

30°   30°

QUAD TOTAL   QUAD TOTAL
   550   513

GRAYTONE SYMBOLS   REV 8.1   DEVERS EYE INSTITUTE
SYM   GLAUCOMA SERVICE
                                           1040 NW 22ND AVE.
ASB .8 2.5 8   25   79 251 794 2512 7943 ≥ SUITE 320
     -.1   1 3.2 10   32 100 316 1000 3162 10000 PORTLAND, OR. 97210
DB   41   36 31   26   21   16   11   6   1   HUMPHREY INSTRUMENTS
     50   40 35   30   25   20   15 10 5   ≤0   A CARL ZEISS COMPANY

Figure 29.7.   Glaucomatous visual field loss, arcuate scotoma (right eye). This printout from an automated Visual Field Test demonstrates a dense superior scotoma extending from the physiologic blind spot (*on the right*). (Reprinted with permission from Cioffi GA. Clinical testing in glaucoma. In: Wright KW, ed. Textbook of ophthalmology. Ch. 43, Fig. 43.10. Baltimore: Williams and Wilkins, 1996:586.)

of the intraocular pressure is used by the ophthalmologist to monitor the adequacy of intraocular pressure-lowering medications. Intraocular pressure in most individuals ranges between 10 and 20 mm Hg, with an average of approximately 16 mm Hg. Intraocular pressure above 20 mm Hg is considered suspicious and may be a precursor to the development of glaucoma.

Ophthalmic Examination for Glaucoma

In addition to the complete medical and ocular history and examination, particular emphasis on examination of the anterior chamber angle (gonioscopy), the optic nerve, and the visual field are essential in the ophthalmic examination for glaucoma. Because the anterior chamber angle structures cannot be seen without special optical prism or mirrored devices, gonioscopy becomes a crucial aspect of the glaucoma examination. Using one of a variety of gonioscopic lenses, the peripheral iris, cornea, and trabecular meshwork can be directly visualized to determine the presence of angle closure, adhesions, inflammatory foci, traumatic injury, masses, or other lesions. Gonioscopy is the most important test for the diagnosis of angle closure glaucoma or the secondary glaucomas discussed earlier.

Since the disorder consists primarily of chronic progressive optic nerve deterioration, once the specific glaucoma diagnosis is confirmed, glaucoma is followed primarily with periodic assessment of optic nerve anatomy (ophthalmoscopy), function (visual field assessment), and assessment of the most common principal causative factor, the intraocular pressure. Glaucomatous optic neuropathy in moderate stages is easily recognized by ophthalmoscopy by the presence of cupping, enlargement of the physiologic cup, or erosion of the neural rim tissue, especially if the erosion is focal within the nerve or asymmetrical between the two eyes. Anatomic changes in the optic nerve head are readily visualized by ophthalmoscopy, but require sophisticated photographic or digital imaging techniques to record for prospective documentation of progressive change. Such change is primarily documented for earlier stages of glaucoma before extensive loss occurs. Ophthalmologists typically examine the optic nerve stereoscopically using the slitlamp biomicroscope and specialized condensing lenses. Modern visual field testing employs automated computer-generated light detection threshold measurements at multiple locations throughout the field of vision.

DIFFERENTIAL DIAGNOSIS (TABLE 29.2)

Primary Open Angle Glaucoma

The vast majority of glaucoma patients have primary open angle glaucoma. These patients manifest a chronic, idiopathic disease associated with progressive degeneration

TABLE 29.2. Referral Guidelines: Adult Glaucoma

SIGNS, SYMPTOMS, OR ASSOCIATED FINDINGS	WHEN TO REFER
Optic nerve abnormality (377.14)	Refer for any of the following: Asymmetry of cup disk ratio between eyes Optic nerve hemorrhage Enlargement of the cup disk ratio (>0.5)
Elevated intraocular pressure (365.04)	Greater than 20 mmHg
Blunt ocular trauma (365.65)	Refer within 24 hours for hyphema
Steroid use (topical, nasal, systemic) (365.03)	Refer for evaluation for chronic use (>4 weeks)
Age	Every individual over 40 years old for complete eye examination
Strong family history of glaucoma (365.01)	Two or more first-degree relatives with glaucoma, refer for routine complete eye examination
Eye pain, redness, and halos around lights (angle closure glaucoma) (365.2)	Refer immediately

TABLE 29.3. Risk Factors for the
Development of Open Angle
Glaucoma

Increased intraocular pressure
Advanced age
African heritage
Family history of glaucoma
Diabetes mellitus
Peripheral vascular disease
Systemic hypertension
Myopia
Corticosteroid therapy

of the anterior optic nerve, known as glaucomatous optic neuropathy (Figs. 29.3 and 29.4). Although elevated intraocular pressure is an important causative risk factor, only about half of the 2–3 million North Americans with glaucoma will manifest elevated intraocular pressure at a single measurement. Therefore, measurement of intraocular pressure alone is a poor screening technique for glaucoma. Like most biologic parameters, eye pressure fluctuates diurnally and with other endogenous and exogenous influences, including hydration, sleep, blood pressure, and body position. With multiple measurements at different testing sessions, most, but not all of these glaucoma subjects, will eventually exhibit elevated intraocular pressure at least part of the time. The rise in intraocular pressure associated with primary open angle glaucoma derives not from a clinically visible obstruction of the trabecular meshwork, but rather from cellular dysfunction of the trabecular meshwork tissue leading to reduced permeability and increased aqueous humor outflow resistance. This outflow obstruction probably is associated with a progressive deterioration and loss of trabecular cells, and a concomitant accumulation and reduced turnover of extracellular matrix within this complex tissue. Risk factors for primary open angle glaucoma include family history, corticosteroid sensitivity, myopia, African-American race, systemic hypertension, ocular hypertension, diabetes mellitus, and age (Table 29.3). In addition to these risk factors, early age of onset of disease and poor compliance with a medical regimen and physician visits are associated with a guarded prognosis. As mentioned earlier, some patients with progressive optic nerve damage characteristic of glaucoma never manifest intraocular pressures above the statistically normal range. These patients are commonly diagnosed with "low pressure glaucoma, low tension glaucoma, or normal pressure glaucoma." While recognizing that nonpressure risk factors may play a stronger role in these than in their high pressure counterparts, these normotensive patients are managed similarly to those with conventional primary open angle glaucoma.

Closed Angle Glaucoma

All physicians need be cognizant of another form of glaucoma, closed angle or angle-closure glaucoma, which may present acutely, or may be silent and chronic. This disorder, quite unrelated to open angle glaucoma, derives entirely from blockade of the trabecular meshwork by the peripheral iris, either by simple and reversible anatomical

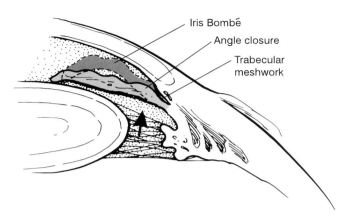

Figure 29.8.   Angle closure glaucoma with pupillary block. The aqueous humor is trapped in the posterior chamber and forces the iris forward (iris bombé), closing of the drainage angle. (Reprinted with permission from Cioffi GA. Clinical manifestations of glaucoma. In: Wright KW, ed. Textbook of ophthalmology. Ch. 45, Fig. 45.2. Baltimore: Williams and Wilkins, 1996:606.)

apposition of the two tissues or by generally irreversible fibrotic adhesion (Fig. 29.8). These irreversible fibrotic adhesions may occur after unrecognized long-standing appositional angle closure (chronic angle closure glaucoma), or from other ocular conditions such as uveitis or neovascularization (secondary angle closure glaucomas).

Classically, angle closure glaucoma is the well-known, less common variety of glaucoma that presents acutely with severe ocular pain, blurring of vision, colored halos around lights (rainbows), nausea, and vomiting. Angle closure usually occurs in the hyperopic (farsighted) eye, which is smaller in diameter than the average eye and thus crowds the iris, cornea, lens, and anterior chamber angle into a smaller than average space. Eventually, usually in the fifth to sixth decade of life, as the lens gradually increases in size with aging, the lens becomes more firmly applied to the posterior pupillary aperture through which aqueous humor from the ciliary body must pass. This relative obstruction of aqueous humor flow at the pupil, known as relative pupillary block, eventually becomes clinically significant, and entraps the aqueous behind the pupil, raising the pressure in the posterior chamber above that in the anterior chamber and driving the iris anteriorly to lie against and block the trabecular meshwork. This trabecular meshwork blockade or angle closure leads to a sudden and dramatic rise of the intraocular pressure from its baseline normal level in the 10–20 mm Hg range to 60 mm Hg or more. This sudden change in pressure leads to edema of the cornea with blurring and visual rainbow halos, and severe ocular pain from iris ischemia and corneal edema. The pupillary margin of the iris becomes most tightly applied to the lens surface when the pupil is in the mid-dilated position; hence, it is often dilation of the pupil by exposure to stress, darkness, or drugs, that precipitates an acute attack.

The immediate treatment of acute angle closure is directed toward reversal of the pupillary block, usually by moving the pupil with constriction. Ultimately, however, the pupillary block can be reversed and prevented by creating a new aqueous channel with peripheral iridectomy (see "Treatment" later in this chapter).

Important Secondary Glaucomas

Glaucoma Associated with Ocular Trauma

Glaucoma may develop after ocular trauma. Penetrating injuries to the globe disrupt, or even destroy, intraocular contents, and may lead to sustained elevation of intraocular pressure and glaucoma (see Chapter 15, "Ocular Trauma"). A more subtle, insidious glaucoma may arise from blunt ocular injury or ocular contusion, as occurs when the globe is struck with a fist, ball, or other object. Blunt injury transiently deforms the globe causing shearing between its internal tissue layers. These shearing forces may tear the insertion of the iris (iridodialysis) or ciliary body (cyclodialysis) from its attachment to the sclera. Most commonly, the fibers of the ciliary muscle that both controls accommodation and modulates aqueous humor outflow become detached, leading to collapse of the trabecular meshwork (known as angle recession) and subsequent secondary glaucoma.

Acutely, the contused eye typically presents with intraocular hemorrhage (hyphema) and the intraocular pressure may be low, normal, or elevated. Angle recession glaucoma may not manifest for months or even years after the original injury. Thus, in any unilateral glaucoma, inquiry about a previous black eye, especially with hyphema, may help identify the underlying diagnosis. Treatment of glaucoma from blunt ocular trauma follows a similar protocol for more common open angle glaucomas, except that these eyes do not respond well to cyclotonic, miotic agents such as pilocarpine because of the damage of the ciliary muscle. In addition, the trabecular meshwork is usually sufficiently damaged so that laser trabeculoplasty is similarly ineffective. Thus, when topical aqueous suppressant agents are ineffective, filtration surgery usually becomes mandated.

Pigmentary Glaucoma

Pigmentary glaucoma is relatively common secondary glaucoma in the young adult and appears to be exclusively an ocular disorder. This disease is significantly relevant because of the potentially severe consequences in young people in the presumed prime of life. Pigmentary glaucoma occurs primarily in young myopic (nearsighted) adults and is more common in males, usually manifesting between ages 20 and 40 years. Melanin pigment granules from the iris circulate freely in the aqueous humor, become deposited or entrapped in the surrounding tissues, the cornea, iris, lens, and particularly within the interstices of the trabecular meshwork. This leads to obstruction of the meshwork, elevation of intraocular pressure, and glaucoma. This condition may manifest with intermittent visual blurring or dull ocular pain, but like other glaucomas may go unnoticed until severe visual loss occurs. Vigorous physical activity or pupillary dilation may induce a shower of pigment granules to be released acutely from the iris in these patients, resulting in a transient, acute rise in eye pressure, corneal edema, blurred vision, and ocular pain. Treatment of pigmentary glaucoma is similar to that for primary open angle glaucoma.

Neovascular Glaucoma

Glaucoma is typically a disease of the middle-aged and the elderly. Thus, its occurrence in children or young adults always raises the question of some associated condition, such as an intraocular tumor. Diabetes mellitus and other vascular disorders are frequently associated with neovascular glaucoma. The devastating consequences of diabetes upon the retinal vasculature and its associated diabetic retinopathy are well known (see Chapter 24, "Diabetic Retinopathy"). In addition to these problems, the diabetic patient may also develop glaucoma as a result of retinal ischemia, known as neovascular glaucoma. Neovascular glaucoma is one of the most devastating varieties of glaucoma. Just as the microangiopathy of the retina results in retinal neovascularization and bleeding, retinal ischemia may also cause proliferation of fibrovascular tissue in the anterior segment of the eye. It is believed that an angiogenic factor is produced by the ischemic retina, leading to new vessel formation inside the eye. Unfortunately, these vessels are aberrant and may cause a variety of vision-threatening sequelae. Neovascular glaucoma derives from fibrovascular proliferation of friable new vessels on the iris (rubeosis irides) and into the chamber angle. The trabecular meshwork provides a fertile template for neovascular growth, that ultimately leads to complete blockade of aqueous humor outflow, marked elevation of intraocular pressure, and severe, often painful, blinding glaucoma. This process can also follow other vascular conditions associated with retinal ischemia including occlusion of the central retinal vein, occlusion of the central retinal artery, and even carotid occlusive disease without manifest retinopathy. Treatment of neovascular glaucoma is multifaceted and involves diligent systemic management of related vascular disease, treatment of retinal ischemia (see Chapter 24, "Diabetic Retinopathy"), and lowering of the intraocular pressure with medical and, often, surgical therapy.

Glaucoma Associated with Increased Episcleral Venous Pressure

Another unusual form of glaucoma is that associated with increased episcleral venous pressure, typically derived from an intracranial arteriovenous shunt. Elevated episcleral venous pressure results in elevated intraocular pressure because the final step in the pathway of aqueous humor drainage is the episcleral venous system. Patients with elevated episcleral venous pressure present with a "red eye," sometimes with proptosis, chemosis, or even a bruit. These findings are associated with an engorged venous system in the eye and orbit. The classic etiology is a carotid artery-cavernous sinus fistula with a high-flow shunt, often following trauma, and is more likely to present with the full spectrum of clinical findings. Those fistulas most commonly referred to the ophthalmologist are the low volume, low-flow shunts spontaneously occurring between dural arterial vessels and the venous system, often in elderly subjects. These present with less severe clinical signs–enlarged, dilated, tortuous episcleral veins that may mimic an inflammatory, red eye from other causes such as conjunctivitis or dysthyroid ophthalmopathy. The absence of other clinical signs of inflammation, the identification of individual dilated, racemose vessels rather than generalized vascular engorgement, and the identification by the clinician or the patient of an orbital bruit help with diagnosis. Because the glaucoma derives from increased episcleral venous pressure, these eyes are usually resistant to medical therapy and require surgical intervention. Successful neuroradiologic intervention with closure of the fistula usually corrects the glaucoma.

Oculofacial hemangioma, associated with the Sturge-Weber syndrome, classically presents with the facial portwine stain and often ipsilateral glaucoma. All patients with Sturge-Weber syndrome should be evaluated for glaucoma. These glaucomas may occur in infancy or early childhood, or milder forms may be delayed until adulthood.

Congenital Glaucoma

Although glaucoma is commonly associated with adult, even elderly, patients, child-hood or infantile glaucomas also exist. The most common, primary congenital open angle glaucoma occurs in children without other identifiable ocular or systemic abnor-malities. Most cases become evident in the first year of life, and often present in the newborn nursery or first few weeks of age. The exact cause of infantile glaucoma is unknown, but appears related to a delay in development of the aqueous humor outflow channels.

Infants with congenital glaucoma present with photophobia (shyness to light), epiphora (tearing), and blepharospasm (see Fig. C.3., Appendix C "Special Pediatric Examination Techniques"). The principal clinical sign is an enlarged cornea, often bilateral. As the disorder advances, the cornea becomes edematous and appears cloudy. The appearance of an enlarged cloudy cornea in an infant is virtually pathognomonic for congenital glaucoma and is obvious to casual penlight examination. Prompt referral to an ophthalmologist for intervention can make the difference between sight and permanent blindness.

Various forms of developmental glaucoma may also be associated with congenital malformations of the anterior chamber angle. Common is the Axenfeld-Rieger syn-drome associated with dental, facial, and other midline developmental abnormalities, adhesions between the cornea and iris, and glaucoma. Aniridia is a bilateral congenital absence of iris that may be inherited by autosomal dominant transmission or may occur spontaneously. These latter, spontaneous cases, may be associated with Wilm's tumor or other anomalies of the genitourinary system. Glaucoma with aniridia usually occurs in early to mid-childhood and is not typically associated with megalocornea.

TREATMENT

Although it is recognized that not all glaucoma patients manifest elevated intraocular pressure and not all glaucomatous optic nerve damage is attributable to pressure damage per se, current standard glaucoma care is devoted almost exclusively to reduc-tion of intraocular pressure. Such pressure reduction, when substantial to the normal or low normal range (17 mm Hg or less), can be expected to arrest progression or dramatically slow its course in the vast majority of cases. At the same time, it must be recognized that some unfortunate individuals, diagnosed late with end-stage neural damage, with an unusually sensitive optic nerve, or who are primarily sensitive to nonpressure factors, will continue to show unabated visual field loss despite maximal pressure lowering. These are the individuals to whom future research regarding other nonpressure causative factors and their treatment must be directed.

Three modalities for glaucoma hypotensive treatment are available–medical (usu-ally topical), laser, and surgical–all of which are designed only to lower intraocular pressure. Since the threshold of pressure damage varies among patients, the only reliable indicator of glaucoma stabilization is stability of the visual field, arresting of visual field loss, and prevention of optic nerve damage. As with systemic hypertension, controversy exists about the appropriate time to institute hypotensive therapy and whether it should be medical or surgical. In the usual glaucoma therapy, intraocular pressure may be lowered by any or all of three methods (medical, laser, and surgery). In a normal, nonglaucomatous population, intraocular pressure averages approximately 16 mm Hg, and most (95%) will fall between 10 and 24 mm Hg, the most frequently

TABLE 29.4. Classifications of Common Glaucoma Medications

CLASSIFICATION	MECHANISM OF ACTION	GENERIC NAMES	COMMON SIDE EFFECTS
Cholinergic agonists	Increased aqueous humor outflow	Carbachol; pilocarpine	Miosis; blurred vision
α-Adrenergic agonists	Decreased aqueous humor production	Apraclonidine; brimonidine	Allergic conjunctivitis
β-Adrenergic antagonists	Decreased aqueous humor production	Timolol; levobunolol; betaxolol; carteolol; metapranolol	Fatigue; bradycardia; bronchospasm (same as systemic β-blockers)
Adrenergic agonists	Increased aqueous humor outflow	Epinephrine; dipivefrin	Tachycardia; palpitations
Prostaglandins	Increased aqueous humor outflow	Latanoprost	Increased iris pigmentation
Carbonic anhydrase inhibitors	Decreased aqueous humor production	Acetazolamide (oral); methazolamide (oral); dorzolamide (topical)	GI upset; fatigue; weight loss; depression; renal calculi; eye irritation

cited normal range. In the glaucomatous population, the mean intraocular pressure is somewhat higher, the range much broader, even as high as 70 mm Hg where arterial circulation to the eye begins to be compromised. Typically, however, the early untreated open angle glaucoma patient will manifest an eye pressure in the mid-20s. Measurement of intraocular pressure at different times of the day establishes the degree of pressure variability before hypotensive therapy is started. The experienced practitioner typically will determine a "target pressure" as a goal to achieve with hypotensive therapy, recognizing that the estimated tension may have to be revised based on further assessment of the visual field.

Topical ocular therapy is an excellent route for systemic drug administration by way of the nasolacrimal passages. Although systemic β-adrenergic blockade from topical therapy is the most common and best known, all ocular drugs demonstrate some systemic absorption and can be associated with systemic effects. At the present time, most subjects are treated first with medical agents, then laser, and finally surgery. However, immediate surgical therapy for early glaucoma is favored in Great Britain and is controversial in the United States. Financial outcome analysis demonstrates surgical therapy to be most cost-effective after 2 years and is associated with the best long-term average pressure control. However, the potential for surgical complications of cataract or intraocular hemorrhage can be visually devastating to individual eyes.

Medical Therapy

Most chronic open angle glaucomas are initially treated with medical hypotensive agents. (Table 29.4). These are most often administered as eye drops from one to four times daily. It is essential to recall that the conjunctival sac is an excellent mode for administration of systemic, as well as ocular, medication. Approximately 50% of an administered eye drop is promptly pumped by the blinking mechanism into the nasolacrimal system–into the nasopharynx where it is immediately absorbed into the nasopharyngeal veins. Thus, this ocular administration is more akin to intravenous than to oral administration of a drug, bypassing the hepatic first pass metabolic effects of oral agents. This accounts for the surprising systemic activity of seemingly low-dose administration of some ocular agents such as β-adrenergic antagonists. Most ocular hypotensive agents stimulate or antagonize receptors of the autonomic nervous system of the anterior segment of the eye; these include cholinergic agonists, cholinesterase inhibitors, adrenergic agonists, and adrenergic antagonists. Inhibitors of the ubiquitous enzyme carbonic anhydrase also reduce aqueous humor formation and reduce intraocular pressure.

The most common agents now used in glaucoma therapy are the β-adrenergic antagonists. These achieve their hypotensive effect by reduction of aqueous humor inflow by blocking β-adrenergic receptors in the ciliary body. Both nonselective and cardioselective β_1-antagonists (such as betaxolol) are effective hypotensive agents. Most agents are administered one or two times daily. A cardioselective agent may be preferable in subjects with concomitant reactive airway disease, but selectivity is relative and β-adrenergic blocking agents should be avoided in such patients. Because of their systemic absorption through the nasolacrimal sac, virtually every reported systemic effect of β blockade has been reported after β-adrenergic antagonist eye drops, including bradycardia, inhibition of exercise-induced tachycardia, bronchospasm, psychotropic effects, fatigue, and many others. β-Adrenergic antagonist ocular therapy is extremely common and the vast majority of glaucoma patients tolerate the treatment well without side effects. However, any patient on a β-blocking adrenergic eye drop should be advised to keep their eyes closed for at least 3 minutes after instillation of the drops to inhibit system absorption. Occlusion of the nasolacrimal duct by compression of the inner canthal region is also helpful but difficult to perform correctly by most patients.

Adrenergic agonists are also used in glaucoma therapy. For many decades, topical epinephrine has been known to lower intraocular pressure. It is administered in a 0.25–2% solution two times daily. System effects such as tachycardia, palpitations, and elevated blood pressure can also be seen from epinephrine ocular therapy. A safer and much more common approach for the past decade, has been with the use of the epinephrine prodrug, dipivefrin, administered as a 0.1% solution. The active epinephrine is then released in the anterior chamber to stimulate aqueous humor outflow, and thereby reduce intraocular pressure. The α-adrenergic agonist clonidine also has some ocular hypotensive effect through inhibition of aqueous humor inflow, but concomitant systemic, primarily central nervous system, effects prevent its use in glaucoma. However, an analog of clonidine, apraclonidine, an α_2-adrenergic agonist, is an effective agent, blocks aqueous inflow, and does not produce the system clonidine effects. Other α_2 agonists, such as brimonidine, are also effective hypotensive agents.

The oldest agent used in glaucoma therapy is the cholinergic agonist pilocarpine, having been prescribed for glaucoma since the latter part of the 19th century. Pilocarpine stimulates contraction of the ciliary muscle, which, in turn, mechanically stretches the trabecular meshwork and reduces its resistance to fluid transduction. Thus, pilocarpine is a stimulant of aqueous humor outflow. Unfortunately, pilocarpine also stimulates contraction of the iris sphincter muscle causing miosis and concomitant dimming of vision, especially in reduced light settings. Its induced contraction and spasm of ciliary muscle may also cause prolonged headache, especially when the drug is first introduced. Pilocarpine is typically administered four times daily placing special demands upon the ability of a patient to comply with a medical regimen. A similar, but somewhat more potent and less tolerated, agent is carbachol. Even less well tolerated are the cholinesterase inhibitors, echothiophate iodide and bremacarium, that also act as indirect cholinergic stimulators.

Most recently, an entirely new medical strategy for reducing intraocular pressure has been introduced in the form of a prostaglandin agent, latanoprost, which enhances aqueous humor outflow. In the normal eye, aqueous humor leaves primarily by way of the trabecular meshwork, but a portion seeps through the ciliary muscle, anterior uvea, and sclera, known as the uveoscleral outflow route. Latanoprost facilitates this pathway and holds great promise for glaucoma therapy.

Another class of ocular hypotensive agents is the carbonic anhydrase inhibitors, which inhibit carbonic anhydrase activity in the ciliary body epithelium and reduce aqueous inflow. Side effects of systemic carbonic anhydrase inhibitor therapy are typically dose-related. Almost all patients develop digital paresthesia. Loss of appetite, fatigue, gastrointestinal upset, and weight loss are all common complaints associated with carbonic anhydrase inhibitor therapy. Severe depression and decreased libido are less common side effects. All carbonic anhydrase inhibitors increase urinary excretion. Carbonic anhydrase inhibitors may exacerbate potassium depletion, especially in individuals on other diuretics. Calcium oxalate and calcium phosphate renal calculi may result from carbonic anhydrase inhibitor use. Rarely, blood dyscrasia, and even aplastic anemia, may result from these medications. Finally, because of the chemical derivation of carbonic anhydrase inhibitors from sulfonamide drugs, there can be allergic cross-reactivity between these classes of drugs. The prototype systemic carbonic anhydrase inhibiter is acetazolamide, but methazolamide is also often prescribed. Until recently, these agents were available only as systemic medications and their chronic use was limited by the induced systemic metabolic acidosis. Recently, a topical carbonic anhydrase inhibitor, dorzolamide, has been introduced as a three times daily agent. This topical agent has rapidly replaced systemic therapy and appears to be free of the common systemic side effects. Allergic, idiosyncratic toxicity, or other nondose-related effects such as bone marrow dyscrasia will not be prevented by topical therapy. Dorzolamide and other topical carbonic anhydrase inhibitors likely will see a major role as antiglaucoma therapy in the near future.

Hyperosmotic agents are systemically administered medications which lower intraocular pressure by increasing the blood osmolality, resulting in vitreous dehydration. Fluid is osmotically drawn from the vitreous cavity into the circulation. These agents rapidly reduce intraocular pressure. Mannitol, glycerine, and isosorbide are the most frequently used hyperosmotic agents. Hyperosmotic agents are only used as a short-term therapy. Glycerine and isosorbide are administered orally, while mannitol is administered intravenously.

Laser Therapy

Argon Laser Trabeculoplasty (Open Angle Glaucoma)

During the early 1970s, attempts were made with a variety of lasers to enhance aqueous humor outflow through the trabecular meshwork in open angle glaucoma by puncturing the trabecular meshwork with the laser energy. Despite the failure of these procedures to create holes in the trabecular meshwork, subsequent decrease in the intraocular

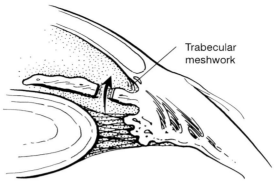

Figure 29.9.   Peripheral iridotomy. The iridotomy allows the aqueous humor flow into the anterior chamber and the iris relaxes posteriorly. This opens the chamber angle allowing outflow through the trabecular meshwork. (Reprinted with permission from Cioffi GA. Clinical manifestations of glaucoma. In: Wright KW, ed. Textbook of ophthalmology. Ch. 45, Fig. 45.3. Baltimore: Williams and Wilkins, 1996:607.)

pressure, several days to weeks following some of the procedures, was observed. In 1979, Wise and Witter published a pilot study describing an argon laser procedure for the control of intraocular pressure. The authors placed evenly spaced argon laser burns for the entire circumference of the trabecular meshwork. Approximately 75% of their patients experienced significant lowering of the intraocular pressure, some lasting for several years. This technique, known as argon laser trabeculoplasty, has changed little since its original description. Many theories attempting to explain the effect of the trabeculoplasty laser burns have emerged. It is now thought that a cascade of biological events that involves renewal of trabecular meshwork cells and accelerated turnover of the extracellular matrix enhances outflow through the trabecular meshwork following laser treatment. Argon laser trabeculoplasty is a relatively uncomplicated office procedure and has gained wide acceptance in the treatment of open angle glaucoma. In approximately 80% of eyes treated with argon laser trabeculoplasty, a significant lowering of the intraocular pressure will be achieved. However, the intraocular pressure lowering effect will diminish over time and approximately 10% of initially successful treatments will fail with each passing year. In patients in whom the initial laser trabeculoplasty was successful, additional laser therapy may be warranted.

Laser Iridotomy (Angle Closure Glaucoma)

Relief of the relative pupillary block (Fig. 29.8) allows the iris to move posteriorly and the anterior chamber drainage angle to open, allowing escape of aqueous humor and lowering of the intraocular pressure. This is now commonly and simply done by fabricating a small hole in the iris with laser (laser iridotomy) which equalizes the pressure between the posterior and anterior chambers and allows the iris to fall back to its normal anatomic position and away from the trabecular surface (Fig. 29.9). With the advancements in lasers during the 1950s and 1960s, the treatment of angle closure glaucoma was greatly altered. Laser iridotomy became the preferred form of treatment for angle closure glaucoma associated with pupillary block. The complications associated with surgical iridectomies are almost entirely eliminated by this therapy. In addition, prophylactic laser iridotomies may be placed in eyes with appositionally closed drainage angles which may be predisposed to either acute episodes of angle closure or chronic angle closure glaucoma. Surgical iridectomies are still rarely performed when extensive corneal edema or corneal opacification prevents adequate visualization of the iris and the placement of laser iridotomy.

Surgical Therapy

Filtering Operations

Trabeculectomy is the most frequently performed incisional operation for the control of elevated intraocular pressure in adult glaucoma. Various filtering procedures have been developed to shunt the aqueous humor from the anterior chamber to a subconjunctival reservoir. These procedures provide an alternative low-resistance pathway for aqueous humor egress from the eye. It is believed that the aqueous humor either filters through the conjunctiva from the reservoir mixing with the tears, or it is absorbed by the vascular tissue of the episclera and conjunctiva. Postoperative management includes topical cycloplegics and antibiotics for the first 1–2 weeks following surgery. Topical corticosteroids are also used to suppress intraocular, conjunctival, and episcleral inflammation. The corticosteroid therapy is thought to reduce scar formation and failure of the filtering bleb. Since trabeculectomy surgery involves creation of an open, guarded fistula, between the anterior chamber and the subconjunctival space, excessive fibroproliferation within the wound leads to scarring, occlusion of the fistula or reservoir (bleb) and failure. Youth, skin pigmentation, previous surgery, and secondary glaucoma greatly increase the risk of failure. Individuals at increased risk, often the majority of surgical patients, receive some form of adjunctive antimetabolite therapy either during surgery by sponge application or postoperatively as subconjunctival injections. 5-Fluorouracil or mitomycin-C are the most commonly used antimetabolite adjuncts to trabeculectomy surgery. In addition, a variety of artificial drainage devices are available that employ a plastic shunt tube to divert the aqueous humor from the anterior chamber into the retrobulbar space where it is resorbed. These glaucoma tube shunts are generally reserved for eyes in which trabeculectomy surgery has failed or in which failure is likely due to extensive scar tissue formation, such as neovascular glaucoma.

Cyclodestructive Surgical Procedures

Just as medical therapy may either increase aqueous outflow from the eye or decrease aqueous production, so may surgical procedures. Filtration operations involve increasing aqueous outflow from the eye, while cyclodestructive procedures reduce the aqueous production. The two most common cyclodestructive procedures are cyclocryotherapy and transscleral cyclophotocoagulation. In cyclocryotherapy, a nitrous oxide or carbon dioxide gas cryotherapy probe is used, cooled to $-60°C$ to $-70°C$, to produce transscleral freezing of the ciliary processes. Transscleral cyclophotocoagulation is also used to suppress aqueous formation by destroying the ciliary epithelium using a variety of lasers including neodymium:YAG lasers, argon lasers, krypton laser, and semiconductor diode lasers. Retrofocusing of the laser energy allows the maximal laser energy to be delivered internally, in the eye, at the level of the ciliary body. These lasers also destroy the ciliary body epithelium by inducing ischemic necrosis and result in marked atrophy of the ciliary processes. Preoperative retrobulbar anesthesia is needed for both

TABLE 29.5. Average Annual Glaucoma Care Visits and Tests Adjusted for Severity of Illness

	ELEVATED IOP & NORMAL VF	EARLY VF LOSS	ADVANCED VF LOSS	VF LOSS WITHIN CENTRAL 5°	MULTIRISK FACTORS	"LOW TENSION GLAUCOMA"
Number of annual visits	1–2	2–3	3–4	4	4–6	6
Visual fields per year	0.5–1	1	2	2	2–3	2–3
Dilated fundus examination per year	1	1	2	2	2	2–3
Optic nerve photography	Initial exam	1/3	1/2	1/2	1/2	1/2

IOP = Intraocular Pressure; VF = Visual Field Testing

cyclocryotherapy and transscleral cyclophotocoagulation. Postoperative complications include both transient and permanent intraocular pressure elevations, intraocular inflammation, and hypotony. Pain, which is the result of intraocular inflammation, is the most frequent postoperative complaint. Suppression of the postoperative inflammation and control of pain with corticosteroid therapy and oral analgesics are almost always necessary. Cycloplegics also help control postoperative pain following these procedures.

FREQUENCY OF VISITS

After the initial examination and diagnosis, glaucoma patients are managed much like patients with other chronic disease, requiring regular visits to assess disease severity and response to therapy. The primary criterion for disease status is the visual field since it is the most accurate measure of visual function in this disorder. Average open angle glaucoma requires management much like other chronic disorders, with periodic medical examinations, diagnostic testing for progression or new findings, and titration of management with drugs or procedures as needed. Once the diagnosis and treatment regimen are established, the average patient needs to be seen 3–4 times yearly with 1–2 visual field tests per year (Table 29.5). Frequency of visits and testing depends upon risks for progressive damage and severity of illness. Because subject performance of visual field testing shows some endogenous and exogenous variability, decisions based upon apparent visual field deterioration for significant changes in management require confirmatory retesting of the visual field.

SUGGESTED READING

Cioffi GA, Van Buskirk EM. What is glaucoma? In: Wright KW, ed. Textbook of ophthalmology. Baltimore: Williams and Wilkins, 1996:563–568.

Cioffi GA, Van Buskirk EM. Glaucoma therapy. In: Wright KW, ed. Textbook of ophthalmology. Baltimore: Williams and Wilkins, 1996:627–648.

Shields MB. Textbook of glaucoma. 3rd ed. Baltimore: Williams and Wilkins, 1992.

Van Buskirk EM, Cioffi GA. Glaucomatous optic neuropathy. Am J Ophthalmol 1992;113(4):447–452.

◖◗❙ Chapter 30
Adult Intraocular Tumors

C. Ma

INTRODUCTION

A wide variety of tumors occur in the eye, including metastatic tumors, malignant melanomas, hemangiomas, osteomas, and lymphomas. The most common intraocular tumors are metastases from extraocular sites. It is estimated that 10% of patients who die from cancer have metastatic foci in the eye. This chapter focuses on the most common of adult tumors, malignant melanoma and metastatic tumors, most of which arise in the uveal tract, the highly vascular and pigmented tissue comprising the iris, ciliary body, and choroid (Fig. 30.1).

The rich vascular supply of the uveal tract, especially the choroid, makes it a likely site for metastatic implantation. The most common metastatic carcinomas found in the eye arise from the lung (male) and the breast (female). By the time metastatic lesions are noted in the eye, the vast majority of patients have already been diagnosed with cancer, but this depends on the primary site. Stephens and Shields found that 91% of women with choroidal metastases from breast carcinoma had already been diagnosed, but in 10 patients with metastases from bronchogenic carcinoma, only 30% had been diagnosed. The prognosis for patients with choroidal metastases is poor, with a median survival of less than 1 year. Therefore, therapy for metastatic intraocular tumors is usually palliative and is provided in conjunction with systemic cancer therapy. The relative frequency of primary site depends upon gender, and reflects the prevalence of those tumors (Table 30.1).

Malignant melanoma of the choroid is the most common primary intraocular tumor in adults, but is relatively rare with an incidence of six cases per million per year. It is associated with a mortality of 50% at 10–15 years. Although recognized for decades, the treatment of choroidal melanoma remains controversial. Choroidal nevi are benign, usually pigmented, tumors of the eye, which are much more common (estimated prevalence of 1–5% of the general population). Choroidal nevi do not cause significant visual problems; therefore, their chief clinical significance lies in distinguishing them from malignant melanoma.

CLINICAL MANIFESTATIONS

Many intraocular tumors are asymptomatic, especially if located under the peripheral retina or iris. Therefore, intraocular tumors are often only detected on routine ophthalmic examination. Tumors of the iris are usually brown (primary) or translucent (metastatic) masses, which are best identified and monitored with the slitlamp biomicroscope. Tumors isolated to the ciliary body, either primary or metastatic, are very rare. Choroi-

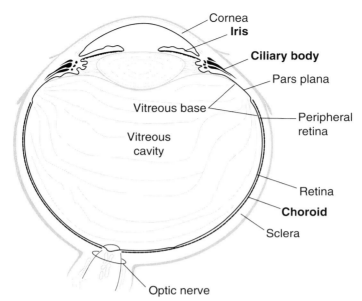

Cornea
Iris
Ciliary body
Pars plana
Vitreous base
Peripheral retina
Vitreous cavity
Retina
Choroid
Sclera
Optic nerve

Figure 30.1. Uveal tract of the eye. The highly vascularized and pigmented layer of the eye is the most frequent site of both metastatic and primary intraocular tumors in adults. The uveal tract is the choroid, the ciliary body and the iris.

dal tumors are usually discrete, elevated lesions under the retina. Choroidal melanomas are typically slate-gray or brown, but metastatic tumors are usually hypopigmented. Metastatic choroidal lesions are frequently found in both eyes at the time of diagnosis and are usually white or yellow in color. These clinical features are often difficult to appreciate with direct ophthalmoscopy and may only be identified with a dilated pupil and binocular indirect ophthalmoscopy, which provides a stereoscopic view across a wide field of the retina.

Visual symptoms vary widely and are not usually helpful in differentiating primary from metastatic lesions. The pattern of visual disturbance primarily depends upon the location, rather than the type of neoplasm. Symptoms of loss of peripheral vision or photopsia (flashes of light) may arise when a lesion impinges on the macula or optic nerve, or produces an exudative retinal detachment. Tumors located in the ciliary body or iris may distort the pupil and/or crystalline lens, thereby hindering the focusing mechanisms of the eye. When visual symptoms occur from intraocular tumors, they

TABLE 30.1. Primary Sites Associated with Ocular Metastases (listed by relative frequency)

FEMALE	%	MALE	%
Breast	78–85	Lung	35–54
Lung	8–12	Unknown primary	24–25
Unknown primary	4–8	Cutaneous melanoma	18
GI (including pancreas)	4	Kidney	6–8
Cutaneous melanoma	<1	Prostate	2

| | TABLE 30.2. Referral Guidelines: Uveal Tumors in Adults |

SYMPTOMS OR SIGNS	TREATMENT	WHEN TO REFER	LONG-TERM FOLLOW-UP INTERVAL
Flat pigmented lesion, no change in appearance or symptoms (224.6)	Observation with ophthalmoscopy and fundus photography	Routine	Every 1–2 years
Elevated lesion <2 mm height, with/without pigmentation (224.6)	Observation with photography, echography	Within 4 weeks	Every 3–6 months, yearly if stable
Tumor 4–10 mm height, or 2–4 mm height with evidence of growth (190.6)	Diagnostic workup, investigate for metastases; radiation or enucleation	Within 2 weeks	Every 3–6 months after treatment
Large tumor, >10 mm height, involvement of posterior pole or ciliary body (190.6)	Diagnostic workup, investigate for metastases; enucleation	Within 2 weeks	Every 6–12 months after treatment

are usually associated with recent growth of the tumor. As a general rule, metastases from nonocular primaries more often present with vision loss, possibly because they are more likely to be associated with exudative retinal detachments and occur more frequently in the posterior pole (the macular region).

Occasionally, a patient will present with a blind, painful eye because a chronic, undetected tumor has resulted in a secondary glaucoma with highly elevated intraocular pressure, intraocular inflammation, or scleral perforation.

DIFFERENTIAL DIAGNOSIS

The identification of a malignant melanoma of the choroid can usually be made on the basis of an ophthalmoscopic examination (Table 30.2). Further diagnostic tests may be necessary to confirm the diagnosis, particularly echographic examination (see Chapter 33, "Ophthalmic Ultrasound").

Choroidal nevi are slate-gray in color, like a melanoma, but nevi usually have a smooth appearance and are flat (less than 2 mm in height as measured by ultrasound) (Fig. 30.2). Nevi may show features which suggest stability such as overlying drusen (yellow deposits), surrounding margins of hypopigmentation, or subretinal choroidal neovascular membranes. Choroidal neovascular membranes are neovascular tissue extending from the choroid, which invade the potential space between the retina and pigment epithelium (see Chapter 27, "Age-Related Macular Degeneration"). If the diagnosis of a choroidal nevi is in doubt, it is helpful to reexamine the lesion after 3 months, as any evidence of enlargement would indicate a slow-growing melanoma.

Melanomas are typically slate-gray, although pigmentation may be uneven (Fig.

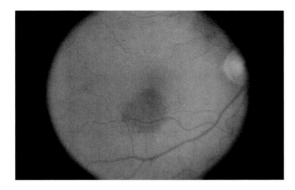

Figure 30.2. Benign choroidal nevus. Note the slate-gray nevus, inferior to the macula. The overlying retinal vessels are not disturbed by this flat choroidal lesion. (See also color section.)

30.3). Orange clumps of lipofuscin are often seen on the surface of melanomas. The tumors may be domed, but the pathognomonic shape is a "collar button," which develops when part of the tumor grows through a defect in Bruch's membrane. An exudative retinal detachment (see Chapter 26, "Retinal Detachment") often overlies a large tumor, but hemorrhage is rare. A number of lesions may simulate a melanoma. A disciform scar is a dark elevated hemorrhage caused by growth of a choroidal neovascular membrane in diseases such as age-related macular degeneration (AMD). There will usually be other evidence of AMD, such as drusen and bilateral macular changes. An arterial macroaneurysm of a retinal vessel may cause both subretinal and preretinal hemorrhage with a dark massive appearance. There are a number of pigmented lesions of the retinal pigment epithelium which may be congenital or develop after trauma or inflammation, but these are usually more darkly pigmented, flat, and often occur in groups.

Diagnostic Testing

Echography is indispensable in the diagnosis and management of choroidal melanoma (see Chapter 33, "Ophthalmic Ultrasound"). On A-scan ultrasonography, the characteristic features of a malignant melanoma are a high initial spike at the tumor anterior surface and low, fairly uniform spikes, representing "low reflectivity" within the tumor

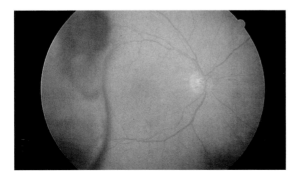

Figure 30.3. Malignant choroidal melanoma. Note the large, pigmented mass (temporal to the macula).

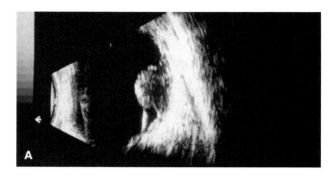

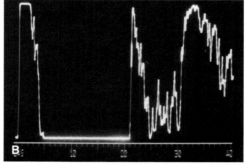

Figure 30.4. Ultrasound of an intraocular malignant melanoma. The melanoma assumes a "mushroom shape" on the B-scan (**A**) and shows an initial high reflectivity spike followed by low internal reflectivity on the A-scan (**B**). (Reprinted with permission from de Juan E, et al. Choroidal and retinal tumors. In: Wright KW, ed. Textbook of ophthalmology. Chap. 62, Fig. 62.2. Baltimore: Williams and Wilkins, 1996:879.)

(Fig. 30.4). This appearance is due to the fairly uniform internal structure of a melanoma. The vascularity of a tumor may cause fluctuation or Doppler shifts of these internal spikes. In contrast, most other lesions which are confused with melanoma have a very mixed histology and are, therefore, highly reflective on ultrasound. Precise measurements (± 0.2 mm) can be made of tumor height with ultrasonography. B-scan ultrasonography can give a clear image of the tumor contour, which may be particularly important in detecting scleral excavation or even extraocular extension through a scleral perforation.

Fluorescein angiography (see Chapter 32, "Fundus Fluorescein Angiography") is not as effective diagnostically as echography, but is useful in identifying disorders such as subretinal hemorrhage, retinal scars, or inflammatory masses. The angiographic appearance of a melanoma is highly variable, depending on the alterations in the retinal pigment epithelium and the vascularity of the tumor.

The ^{32}P uptake test has been largely superceded by ultrasound, but is still occasionally performed. ^{32}P is injected intravenously and is preferentially incorporated into DNA by actively dividing tumor cells. Beta-radiation is detected by a small counter placed directly over the base of the lesion and the activity compared with counts made elsewhere on the same eye. Sensitivity and specificity are greater than 95%.

Fine needle aspiration biopsy is performed with a 25-gauge needle introduced into the tumor through the wall of the eye. The specimen is examined by a cytopathologist, and, in skilled hands, accurate diagnosis can be reached in 90% of cases. The procedure may be complicated by intraocular hemorrhage, but overall the reported morbidity is low. There have been no reports of orbital seeding of tumor, even though tumor cells have been identified along the tract of the needle. This technique is reserved for tumors which pose particular diagnostic difficulties and is not widely performed.

TREATMENT
Systemic Evaluation

About 2.5% of patients with choroidal melanoma have detectable metastases at the time of presentation. The median life expectancy after detection of metastases is 3–8 months, and the results of chemotherapy are generally disappointing. The most common site of extraocular spread is the liver, followed by skin, lung, bone, brain, gastrointestinal tract and lymph nodes.

Before initiating local treatment of an intraocular melanoma, all patients should have a thorough physical examination, with serum liver function tests, blood count, and chest radiographs. An abdominal CT scan is often obtained, but is definitely obtained if there is any clinical or biochemical indication of hepatic involvement. Metastases are most often found in the first 5 years after treatment, and it is presumed that micrometastases are already present but undetectable at presentation.

Small Pigmented Choroidal Tumors

A difficult dilemma arises in the management of small, pigmented choroidal tumors, which may be benign or early small melanomas. The crucial question is whether the tumor has the potential to metastasize. Presently, the metastatic potential of small tumors is unknown, but an ongoing multicenter, prospective study (the Collaborative Ocular Melanoma Study) will contribute to the understanding of the natural history of these lesions. The treatment dilemma is frequently heightened by the absence of any visual impairment, and by the fact that therapy will usually cause significant or total loss of vision.

Several studies suggest that small tumors (defined by volume of less than 200 mm^3, or height less than 2 mm) may be observed for evidence of growth without significantly affecting mortality. Small tumors should be carefully documented clinically, with photographs and echographic measurements, and repeated at 3–6 month intervals to detect any growth.

Large and Medium Pigmented Choroidal Tumors

For many years, the standard treatment for malignant melanoma has been enucleation of the eye. The Collaborative Ocular Melanoma Study is also examining the relative risks and benefits of various treatment options for these tumors. In an enucleation, the extraocular muscles are detached from the globe, the optic nerve is transsected deep within the orbit, and a spherical implant is inserted to fill the void. Usually, the muscles are reattached to the implant to improve long-term retention and to impart some movement to the prosthesis. This implant is completely covered by connective tissue and conjunctiva. A potential space remains between these tissues and the eyelids, into which space the cosmetic prosthesis is fitted. The prosthesis is usually a button-shaped piece of polymethyl-methacrylate onto which an image of the eye is painted to match the fellow eye. When skillfully made and fitted to move in conjunction with the fellow eye, the result is extremely life-like and deceives casual observers and unsuspecting physicians alike.

Radiation therapy was first developed by Stallard at St. Bartholmew's Hospital in London, in the 1930s, using ^{60}Co seeds sutured temporarily to the sclera under the tumor. This method has been refined. Today ^{125}I seeds are most commonly used, supported on a gold plaque to position the radiation source under the tumor and shield the adjacent tissues of the orbit. The plaque is designed to completely cover the base of the tumor, and to deliver a dose of 80–100 Gray. In the operating room, the sclera is exposed and the plaque is secured with sutures after its position has been verified with B-scan ultrasound. It is left in position for 1 week. Often the first visible change in the tumor is hemorrhage or resolution of exudative retinal detachment. During the ensuing weeks, the tumor will usually diminish in size. More importantly, echographic examination will show increasing internal reflectivity, indicating necrosis and fibrosis within the tumor.

External beam radiation therapy has also been applied to choroidal melanomas, using protons and helium ions. Such beams show little scatter, can be accurately aimed, and can deliver radiation more uniformly within the tumor than with an external plaque (which delivers a higher dose to the base of the lesion). A surgical procedure is still necessary as the base of the tumor must be marked with tantalum clips to permit aiming of the beam in subsequent treatment sessions.

SUGGESTED READINGS

Char DH. Metastatic choroidal melanoma. Am J Ophthalmol 1978;86:76–80.

Char DH, Hogan MJ. Management of small elevated pigmented choroidal lesions. Br J Ophthalmol 1977;61:54–58.

Freedman MI, Folk JC. Metastatic tumors to the eye and orbit; patient survival and clinical characteristics. Arch Ophthalmol 1987;105:1215–1219.

Ferry AP, Font RL. Carcinoma metastatic to the eye and orbit. I. A clinico-pathologic study of 227 cases. Arch Ophthalmol 1974;92:276–286.

Gass JDM. Comparison of uveal melanoma growth rates with mitotic index and mortality. Arch Ophthalmol 1985;103:924–931.

Packer S, Stoller S, Lesser ML, Mandel FS, Finger PT. Long-term results of iodine 125 irradiation of uveal melanoma. Ophthalmology 1992;99(5):767–773.

Stephens RF, Shields JA. Diagnosis and management of cancer metastatic to the uvea: a study of 70 cases. Ophthalmology 1979;86:1336–1349.

Thomas JV, Green WR, Maumenee AE. Small choroidal melanomas. A long-term follow-up study. Arch Ophthalmol 1979;97:861–864.

Chapter 31 ◖●◗

Pediatric Intraocular Tumor: Retinoblastoma

A. C. Tongue

INTRODUCTION

Retinoblastoma is a malignant tumor of the retina which affects approximately 11 out of 1 million children under 5 years of age. About 60% of cases are unilateral; of these, 15% are hereditary, and 85% are sporadic isolated single cell mutations. All bilateral cases are hereditary and affect germinal cell mutation.

The retinoblastoma gene (Rb) has been identified on chromosome 13, region q 14. Its function is to suppress growth and if the gene is inhibited growth in retinal cells is unchecked. Since all individuals have two Rb genes and one is sufficient for growth suppression, both Rb genes in an individual have to be nonfunctioning in a retinal cell for retinoblastoma to occur. In hereditary retinoblastoma, the individual has one abnormal, or nonfunctioning, Rb gene in each retinal cell, as well as one normal Rb gene. If an event occurs in any one retinal cell that inhibits the one normal Rb gene from functioning, then retinoblastoma occurs. Since there are millions of retinal cells the odds of this occurring in more than one cell in the individual with hereditary retinoblastoma is high.

Hereditary retinoblastoma, therefore, often has more than one site of tumor origin. In nonhereditary retinoblastoma, both Rb genes are presumably normal and an event has to occur within a retinal cell that will shut both Rb genes off. That this would happen is statistically exceedingly rare, and unilateral retinoblastoma therefore occurs relatively rarely in the population. This also explains why the tumor in nonhereditary retinoblastoma is almost always of single cell origin and is a single tumor. Individuals who have unilateral retinoblastoma with several different tumors sites have hereditary retinoblastoma.

Children with retinoblastoma and a gross deletion in the 13q14 chromosome (3% of retinoblastoma patients) have associated mild facial dysmorphoria, low set ears, and developmental delay. In the overwhelming majority of retinoblastoma patients who do not have a gross deletion in the 13q14 region, identification of the abnormality in the Rb gene sequence (over 200,000 base pairs) is expensive and time-consuming. However, once the specific mutation in a given family has been identified, identification of other family members who have this mutation is more practical. More efficient methods of identifying the mutation are being researched and hopefully will provide a less expensive way of identifying carriers of the gene in the future.

Offspring of retinoblastoma patients have a 50% chance of inheriting the abnormal Rb gene. However, the expressivity is not 100% because of the need for a second

TABLE 31.1. Risk for Retinoblastoma (Rb)

BILATERAL Rb FOUND IN	PATIENT RISK (%) FOR ABNORMAL Rb GENE	PATIENT RISK (%) FOR Rb
Parent	50	45
Sibling	5	2.7
Aunt, uncle	0.5	0.3
First cousin	0.05	0.003
Grandparent (parent normal)	0.5	0.3

UNILATERAL Rb FOUND IN	PATIENT RISK (%) FOR ABNORMAL Rb GENE	PATIENT RISK (%) FOR Rb
Parent	7.5	5.7
Sibling	0.8	0.4
Aunt, uncle	0.08	0.04
First cousin	0.008	0.004
Grandparent (parent normal)	0.08	0.04

mutation to occur to shut off the normal Rb gene in a retinal cell. About 90% of those who have the abnormal inherited gene will develop retinoblastoma. Parents of a child with retinoblastoma are most often normal (90% of cases) and the mutation probably occurs within the sperm or ovum around the time of conception, thereby giving rise to the new hereditary mutation in that particular child. Siblings of offspring with hereditary retinoblastoma, but whose parents are normal, have a 5% risk for inheriting an abnormal retinoblastoma gene (see Table 31.1).

CLINICAL MANIFESTATIONS

The presenting signs of retinoblastoma are leukocoria or an abnormal reflex from the pupil (56%) (Fig. 31.1). Often the parent is the first to notice a "glint" or peculiar reflex. On direct examination or inspection of the eye, nothing abnormal may be noted since the tumor does not have to be in the posterior pole and the parent may have seen light reflected from it at an angle. If the tumor is large and fills most of the eye,

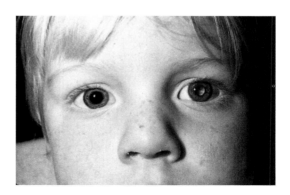

Figure 31.1. Leukocoria left eye, unilateral retinoblastoma. (See also color section.) (Courtesy of A. Tongue, M.D.)

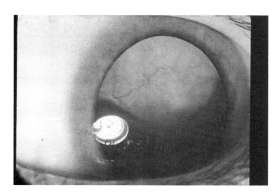

Figure 31.2. Retinoblastoma left eye, causing solid retinal detachment. The retinal vessels are visible on surface of tumor. (Courtesy of A. Tongue, M.D.)

a yellowish pink reflex may be seen in the pupil. If the tumor has grown underneath the retina and caused a solid retinal detachment retinal vessels may be seen on the surface of the tumor (Fig. 31.2). Smaller tumors within the visual axis in the posterior pole may give a yellow or whitish reflex with the red reflex test or show up as a yellow or whitish pupillary reflex in photographs of the child.

The second most common sign is strabismus (20%). This occurs when the tumor interferes with vision. The tumor can be relatively small and not visible to the naked eye on external ophthalmologic examination if it is in the macula (see Chapter 17, "Pediatric and Adult Strabismus", Fig. 17.2).

Other presenting signs which occur less frequently are inflammation and uveitis, glaucoma (Fig. 31.3), hyphema, hypopyon, periorbital cellulitis, poor visual function, and nystagmus. Routine examination rarely detects unsuspected retinoblastoma. Most

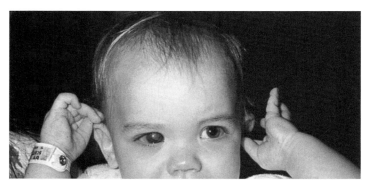

Figure 31.3. Bilateral retinoblastoma presenting as acute angle closure glaucoma with corneal edema, red, painful right eye. The patient died of osteogenic sarcoma. (See also color section.) (Courtesy of A. Tongue, M.D.)

◼ TABLE 31.2. Referral Guidelines: Retinoblastoma (190.5)

SIGNS AND SYMPTOMS	TREATMENT	WHEN TO REFER
Leukocoria, peculiar glint, or light reflex Strabismus Poor vision Red, painful eye Orbital cellulitis Hyphema Hypopyon Uveitis Glaucoma Family history and at-risk 13q14 deletion	Examination of both eyes by ophthalmologist with sedation or anesthesia. CT of orbit and brain. Ultrasound of globe and MRI when indicated. Local ablation, radiation, chemotherapy, and/or enucleation as indicated. Close monitoring for tumor response to treatment, recurrence, and metastases. Fitting of prosthesis, treatment of ocular and systemic complications and metastatic disease. Annual physical examination and prompt attention to signs or symptoms of potential secondary malignancy. Referral to appropriate specialists and agencies. Examination of at-risk family members. Genetic counseling and evaluation.	If any noted signs or symptoms occur. A history of a peculiar light reflex or glint cannot be ignored! All infants and children with unilateral strabismus or poor vision in one or both eyes need a comprehensive ophthalmologic examination. At-risk infants and children need thorough retinal examinations starting at birth. Referral by ophthalmologists may be to centers and individuals specializing in treating retinoblastoma patients, to geneticists, oncologists, radiation therapists, oculoplastic surgeons, glaucoma and corneal specialists, low vision aid centers, and social service agencies.

retinoblastoma discovered by routine examination is in patients at risk for the hereditary form.

DIFFERENTIAL DIAGNOSIS

Any patient presenting with a history of abnormal pupil reflex as noted by a family member or who presents with frank leukocoria (white, gray, yellow pupil reflex) should be considered a retinoblastoma suspect (Table 31.2). Even if a tumor is not seen, immediate referral to an ophthalmologist for a fully dilated examination is in order based on the history alone. Other causes of leukocoria are noted in Table 31.3.

Infants and children with unilateral strabismus also need to have a full ophthalmologic examination to rule out retinoblastoma. The type of strabismus varies and may be esotropic, exotropic, or hypertropic.

TREATMENT

Enucleation of an eye with no evidence of tumor extension has a greater than 90% cure rate. Tumor spread into the optic nerve or out of the eye diminishes the prognosis for life considerably (to 60% if tumor cells are within the optic nerve; 20% if tumor

TABLE 31.3. Leukocoria—
Differential Diagnoses[a]

Cataract
Persistent primary hyperplastic vitreous
Coats' disease
Retrolental fibroplasia
Retinal detachment
Idiopathic
Traumatic
Norrie's disease
Juvenile retinoschisis
Organized vitreous
Toxocara canis
Vitreous inflammation, uveitis
Other intraocular tumors
Coloboma of retina and optic nerve
Myelinated nerve fibers
Endophthalmitis
Hypopyon

[a] Not all inclusive

is at cut end of the optic nerve). Early detection is therefore highly desirable for the patient. Not only does early detection provide a better life prognosis, but also a better vision prognosis. Small tumors can be treated with local ablation and vision may be spared.

For unilateral patients, the treatment of choice is enucleation if the visual prognosis for the eye is poor. Bilateral patients present a more complex dilemma if they have advanced tumor formation in both eyes. Small tumors may be treated with cryotherapy, photocoagulation, locally applied radioactive plaques. Chemotherapy, with VP-16, vincristine, and carboplatin, may be combined with local ablative treatment. External beam radiation is used for tumors which are large, when vitreous seeding is present, and when the tumors are over the optic nerve or in the macula. About 85% of patients who receive external beam radiation have a good response; however, about 40% require further treatment, and one-third eventually undergo enucleation. External beam radiation also has the complication of cranial bone growth retardation often leading to depression of the temporal bone area. Secondary tumors also are seen more frequently in the field of radiation in retinoblastoma patients.

The spread of retinoblastoma is primarily local with invasion of the optic nerve and into the cerebrospinal fluid. Hematogenous spread also occurs, most frequently to the bone marrow and bones. Routine spinal taps and bone marrow aspiration is not performed unless there is suspicion of CNS or hematogenous spread. CT scans using contrast are routinely performed in retinoblastoma patients. Ultrasonography may be employed in some cases as an adjunctive or alternate test. CT scans are very sensitive to calcium deposits, which occur in retinoblastoma but do not occur in other entities causing leukocoria or tumor formation in the eye. CT scans also delineate the extent of tumor involvement of the eye (Fig. 31.4).

Children who have no evidence of recurrence or metastatic disease 3 years after treatment are considered cured. However, hereditary retinoblastoma (which includes

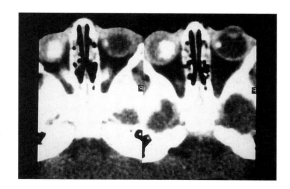

Figure 31.4. CT scan, bilateral retinoblastoma. Note large tumor filling most of the vitreous cavity of right eye and small multiple tumors in the left eye. (Courtesy of A. Tongue, M.D.)

all bilateral cases) has a high risk of developing secondary neoplasms. The most common is osteogenic sarcoma which occurs with greater frequency in the field of radiation, but also occurs outside the field of radiation. Risk and incidence data vary somewhat. In the initial study which emphasized this risk, 89 of 693 bilateral retinoblastoma patients developed secondary neoplasms at a mean of 10 years postretinoblastoma diagnosis. Of the neoplasms, 58 were in the field of radiation, 31 out of the field. Of 18 unilateral retinoblastoma patients, 5 had secondary tumors, 2 in the field of radiation, 3 out of the field. Of the five unilateral, two had a family history of retinoblastoma. Life-time risk data (taken from three different studies) project that 6–20% of hereditary retinoblastoma patients develop secondary malignant neoplasms within 10 years, 14–50% within 20 years, and 19–90% within 30 years. Secondary neoplasms described to date in these patients are primarily sarcomas, particularly osteogenic sarcoma, but can involve any organ and be of any type (including leukemia, Hodgkin's disease, breast cancer, Wilms' tumor, testicular carcinoma, etc.). These patients should be considered likely candidates for developing malignancies and this should be kept in mind if the patient presents with medical complaints. Routine yearly physical examinations are recommended for these patients.

Family members of retinoblastoma patients should have ophthalmologic examinations. Parents should have examinations to rule out any evidence of spontaneously regressed retinoblastoma, which occurs rarely but would indicate that the parent carries the Rb gene. Offspring and siblings of retinoblastoma patients should be examined at least every 4 months for the first 3 years of life with the first examination during the neonatal period. The frequency of examination should be determined by the examining ophthalmologist.

Offspring of retinoblastoma patients have the highest risk, 50%, for inheriting the Rb gene. Most hereditary retinoblastoma presents before age 3, and often before age 1. General anesthesia may be required for examination of the peripheral retina, since early lesions are small, not particularly elevated, avascular, and can be easily ablated with cryotherapy or photocoagulation. Risk data for relatives of retinoblastoma patients are summarized in Table 31.1.

Nieces, nephews, and first cousins of retinoblastoma patients should also have eye examinations, but most likely do not need it at the same intensive intervals as mentioned earlier with general anesthesia examinations. Office examinations interspersed with general anesthesia examinations may be adequate. However, since 10% of abnormal Rb gene carriers do not manifest the disease, there is clearly a risk for a first cousin of a retinoblastoma patient, or a niece, or nephew to have inherited the abnormal Rb gene and develop the tumor. The risk is still over 100- to 200-fold as great as it is for children who have no family members with retinoblastoma.

Retinoblastoma occurs rarely, but is a life-threatening disease. Early detection improves the prognosis for sight and life. A parental history of seeing a peculiar reflex from the pupil cannot be ignored and should be considered retinoblastoma until proven otherwise. Strabismus in infants and toddlers may be the only sign of retinoblastoma.

The treatment varies depending on the size and location of the tumor, and whether it is unilateral or bilateral. Enucleation is the treatment of choice in large sight-robbing unilateral retinoblastoma. The treatment of bilateral retinoblastoma is more complex and may include a number of different modalities. The follow-up of retinoblastoma patients by an ophthalmologist is life-long. Even in initial tumor cures, about 11% develop other retinoblastomas which require further intervention. Hereditary retinoblastoma patients are at significant risk for developing secondary malignancies anywhere in the body, most commonly in bone. Family members of retinoblastoma patients require ophthalmologic evaluation and close scrutiny for at least the first 6 years of life because of the risk developing the tumor.

SUGGESTED READINGS

Abramson DH, Ellsworth RM, Kitchin FD, Tung G. Second non-ocular tumors in retinoblastoma survivors: are they radiation induced? Ophthalmology 1984;91:1351–1355.

Christensen LE, Murphree AL. Retinoblastoma and malignant intraocular tumors. In: Wright KW, ed. Pediatric ophthalmology and strabismus. St. Louis: C.V. Mosby, 1994:495–506.

Moore A. Retinoblastoma. In: Taylor D, ed. Pediatric ophthalmology. Boston: Blackwell Scientific, 1990:348–364.

Musarella MA, Gallie BL. A simplified scheme for genetic counselling in retinoblastoma. J Pediatr Ophthalmol Strabismus 1987;24:124–125.

Nicholson DH, Green WR. Ocular tumors in children. In: Nelson LB, Calhoun JH, Harley RD, eds. Pediatric ophthalmology. 3rd ed. Philadelphia: W.B. Saunders, 1991:382–392.

SPECIALIZED OPHTHALMIC TESTING

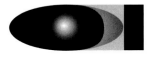

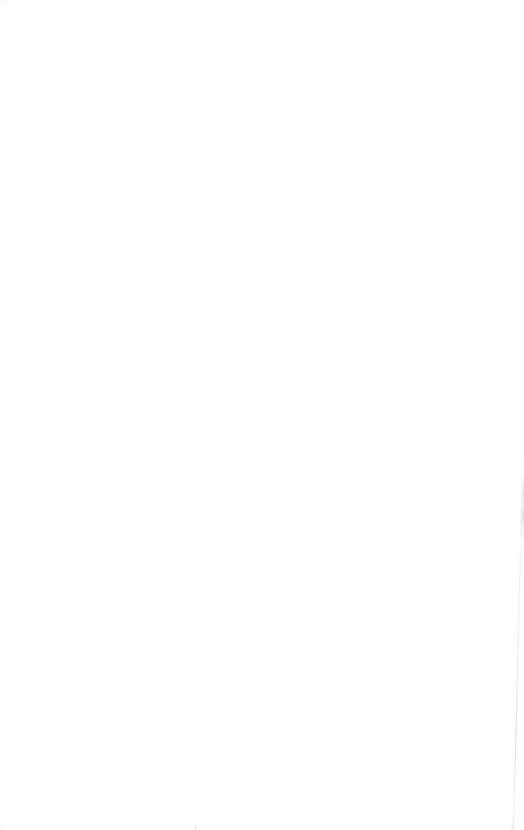

Chapter 32 ●◗▮
Fundus Fluorescein Angiography

C. Ma

INDICATIONS

The blood vessels of the retina are easy to observe through the transparent ocular media, and many diseases can be recognized simply by clinical examination. Fundus fluorescein angiography employs an intravenous contrast agent to enhance a photographic image, revealing structures which may be too small to resolve with an ophthalmoscope, demonstrating the pattern of circulation through an abnormal area of the eye, or highlighting areas of abnormal vascular permeability. Because the retina is not covered by any opaque tissues, this information can be obtained without radiation or the radiopaque dyes used in other types of angiography.

There are several situations in which the technique is indispensable in clinical management:

Diabetic retinopathy—identifying regions of capillary leakage and destruction for treatment of macular edema.
Age-related macular degeneration—identifying subretinal neovascularization and determining the feasibility of treatment.
Identifying patterns of inflammation in the choroid and retinal vessels.

TECHNIQUE

Sodium fluorescein is used as the contrast agent. This substance is excited by blue light (465–490 nm), but emits at a yellow-green wavelength (520–530 nm). For ocular angiography, a 5 cc bolus of dye is injected into the antecubital vein and photographed as it passes through the retinal and choroidal vessels. The fundus is illuminated by a blue flash, and the "barrier" filter incorporated into the camera allows only the light emitted by fluorescein molecules to reach the film. Although simple in principle, fluorescein angiography is subject to many practical pitfalls, not least of which is the difficulty of focusing the retinal image under extremely dim viewing illumination. It is usually performed by a skilled medical photographer.

Contrast usually arrives at the eye 10–20 seconds after injection (Fig. 32.1). It is first manifest within the choroidal vessels, which are highly permeable, and therefore visualized as a homogeneous background "flush." Normally the overlying retinal pigment epithelium is only partially transparent, so that apparent variations in the brightness of the choroidal background may provide information about disease in the pigment epithelium.

Retinal arterioles fill shortly after the choroid, followed by the retinal veins which

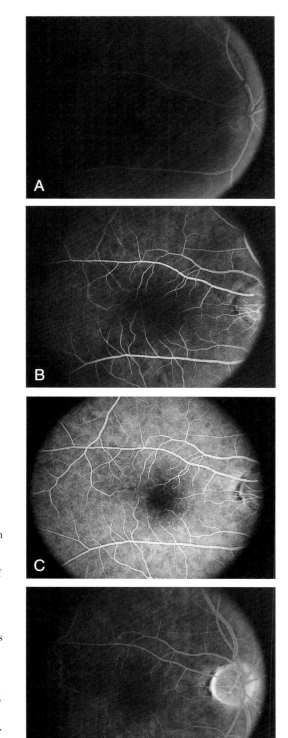

Figure 32.1. Selected frames from a normal fluorescein angiogram. **A.** Contrast (*white*) fills retinal arteries, early in the filling phase of the angiogram. **B.** Venous laminar phase, with "tramline" appearance of retinal vessels. Due to laminar flow, the peripheral blood column fills with the dye first. **C.** Capillaries become visible when sufficient contrast fills them. Note the capillaries surrounding the foveal avascular zone. The lobular pattern of the choriocapillaris (the capillary layer of the choroid) is also demonstrated. **D.** Late in the study, contrast is washed out of most structures, with some late staining of the optic disc.

have a "tramline" appearance due to laminar flow within the vessel. Finally, the capillaries are visible 30–45 seconds after injection. The fine capillaries encircling the foveal avascular zone are an important landmark, and can be seen in any good study, usually between 30 and 100 seconds after injection. In the normal eye, fluorescein is confined within retinal vessels by the blood-retinal barrier, and a normal angiogram will show only those vessels. Extravascular collections of fluorescein mark sites where this barrier has been disrupted by disease.

Photography continues for 10 minutes after injection, by which time fluorescein has usually washed out of normal tissues. Usually a fast, high-resolution monochrome film is employed which can be processed to yield the results of the test in about 1 hour.

ADVERSE REACTIONS

Local extravasation of sodium fluorescein at the injection site can be intensely painful, but usually responds to simple palliative measures.

Systemic reactions to fluorescein include transient nausea or itching (1 in 20), urticaria (1 in 100), and bronchospasm. Pretreatment with antihistamines may effectively block minor reactions, but some patients develop increasingly severe reactions with each subsequent study, and must be monitored carefully during and after the test.

FUTURE DEVELOPMENTS

Several other methods for fundus angiography are presently under active development and may shortly reach wider clinical application. Laser scanning and digital image processing permit significant improvements in both spatial and temporal resolution, making it possible to observe movement of contrast through microvasculature in real time. Images can be obtained despite media opacities, and small pupils.

An important limitation of fluorescein angiography is the obscuration of useful details by blood, turbid subretinal fluid, and the retinal pigment epithelium. There is great interest in the use of indocyanine green for fundus angiography because it emits in the infrared spectrum, and would, in theory, provide valuable information in those disease states. Furthermore, it is hoped that it will be possible to study the choroid and retinal pigment epithelium, regions which are largely invisible to current techniques.

●❙ Chapter 33
Ophthalmic Ultrasound

C. Ma

INDICATIONS

Ultrasonic imaging is useful in ophthalmology for the study of the opaque tissues of the orbit, or when disease causes opacification of the normally transparent ocular media:

Assessment of the posterior segment when the ocular media are opaque, e.g., vitreous hemorrhage or dense cataract.

Quantitative measurement of ultrasound transmission ("reflectivity") within mass lesions, e.g., to differentiate choroidal melanoma from an elevated hemorrhagic scar.

Localization, characterization, and measurement of orbital masses and tumors, enlarged optic nerve, and extraocular muscles.

Axial length measurement for calculation of intraocular lens power prior to cataract surgery.

TECHNIQUE

Topical anaesthetic is applied to the eye and the ultrasound probe is placed on the lids, or directly upon the sclera or cornea. A viscous gel is usually employed as a coupling agent. The operator views the results on a cathode ray screen and records images photographically. The series of images are indexed by the meridian of the globe in the ultrasound beam, posterior or anterior orientation, as well as transverse or axial orientations of the probe.

Two modes are in common use. **A-scan** is performed with a small lightweight probe emitting an unfocused beam at 8 MHz. Echoes are displayed on an oscilloscope screen as spikes along a baseline, such that the height of the spike represents the amplitude of the returning soundwave and the spacing of the spikes represents the distance between the reflecting surfaces (Fig. 33.1). The dimensions of lesions within the orbit can be measured with great accuracy, and the small size of the probe allows examinations to be made with minimal discomfort to the patient. Indeed, in skilled hands, it is possible to safely examine a ruptured globe.

B-scan employs a narrow focused beam at about 10 MHz. The transducer oscillates within the head of the probe producing a two-dimensional acoustic section which is displayed on a screen (Fig. 33.2). The brightness of the spot represents the amplitude at that point, and the pattern of spots corresponds to the reflecting planes of tissue. The probe is significantly larger than for A-scan, and the resolution is not as fine, but the topographic appearance is much easier to visualize with this mode.

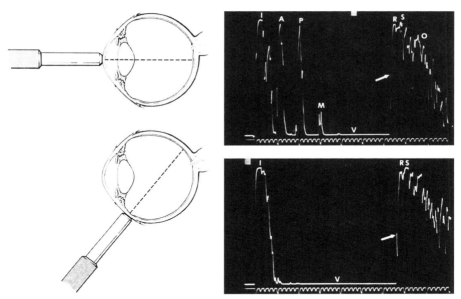

Figure 33.1. Normal standardized A-scan echograms. **Top:** Probe placed on cornea with sound beam directed through lens. **Bottom:** Probe placement to avoid lens. *I*, Initial spike corresponding to probe tip (corneal spike hidden by initial spike); *A*, anterior lens; *P*, posterior lens; *M*, multiple signal; *V*, echo-free vitreous cavity; *R*, retina; *S*, sclera; *O*, orbital soft tissue. (Reprinted with permission from Green RL, Byrne SF. Diagnostic ophthalmic ultrasound. In: Ryan SJ, ed. Retina. 2d ed. Vol. 1, Fig. 17.1. St. Louis: C.V. Mosby, 1989:219.)

Standardized echography refers to a system of examination which combines B-scan, A-scan, and Doppler modes. The instruments are calibrated so that measurements of attenuation within the tissue are reproducible between different laboratories. Accurate and reproducible measurements obtained in this way are particularly helpful in the diagnosis and monitoring of intraocular tumors.

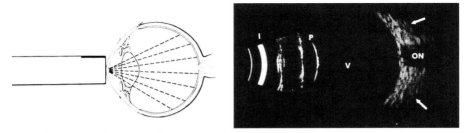

Figure 33.2. Oscillating transducer within B-scan probe creates two-dimensional acoustic section through normal eye. *I*, Initial line corresponding to probe face on cornea; *P*, posterior lens surface; *V*, vitreous cavity; *ON*, optic nerve; *arrows*, orbital soft tissue. (Reprinted with permission from Green RL, Byrne SF. Diagnostic ophthalmic ultrasound. In: Ryan SJ, ed. Retina. 2d ed. Vol. 1, Fig. 17.3. St. Louis: C.V. Mosby, 1989:220.)

FUTURE DEVELOPMENTS

Several enhancements have been described for echography, but are not yet widely available. Real-time Doppler instruments can show a topographic image with a superimposed color-coded display to indicate the direction (relative to the probe) and quantity of blood flow within vessels. Various methods have been developed for combining data from a series of scans and displaying it as a pseudo three-dimensional image. Whereas current ultrasound can demonstrate relatively little detail in the anterior segment, the ultrasound biomicroscope, operating at 50 MHz, can show very detailed images of the anterior segment with a resolution of 50 μ.

Chapter 34 ◖◼
Visual Fields

W. T. Shults

Visual function may be characterized in many different ways including visual acuity, color vision, contrast sensitivity, and pupillary function. Assessment of the field of vision is one of the more helpful and localizing methods of defining visual dysfunction. The visual field defines that zone within which a patient sees a target of a specified size and brightness while maintaining steady fixation on a single point. The normal field of vision for each eye extends horizontally from about 60° nasal to 100° temporal to fixation and vertically from about 60° above to 70° below the point of fixation. The binocular field is about 200° wide and 130° tall.

Lesions at different locations in the visual pathway produce different patterns of visual field loss and a knowledge of those patterns is invaluable in localizing and defining the differential diagnostic possibilities. Thus, arcuate defects result from either retinal or optic nerve disease, while bitemporal and homonymous hemianopsias derive from involvement of the chiasm and retrochiasmal locales, respectively. The location of a lesion within the visual pathway which produces a visual field deficit is defined by the pattern rather than the density of the loss.

Several methods, ranging from simple to more complex, are useful in assessing the field of vision.

CONFRONTATION VISUAL FIELD TESTING

In testing the field of vision with confrontation techniques, the tools are simple but the amount of information obtained may be great (Fig. 34.1). In confrontation testing of the visual field, the fixation target is most often the examiner's nose, while the targets used are the examiner's hands or fingers, or hat pins, or swizzle sticks.

The patient is asked to fixate on a target (the examiner's nose) and to report when he or she first sees a target (the examiner's hand or fingers, the hat pin, etc.) as it is moved into the field of view from various positions in the periphery. This method, though relatively crude, often provides the most information in patients with limited attention span or altered level of consciousness. By asking the patient to compare the qualitative clarity or brightness of color of simultaneously presented targets in each hemifield, the sensitivity of this technique improves. Thus, a patient with a subtle right homonymous hemianopic field depression may report that a hand held in the right hemifield is less clearly seen than one in the left hemifield.

Similarly, "temporal red desaturation testing" in patients with suspected chiasmal compression is a useful screening tool of great reliability in selected patients. In this test, the patient is asked to compare the color of two identically colored red objects

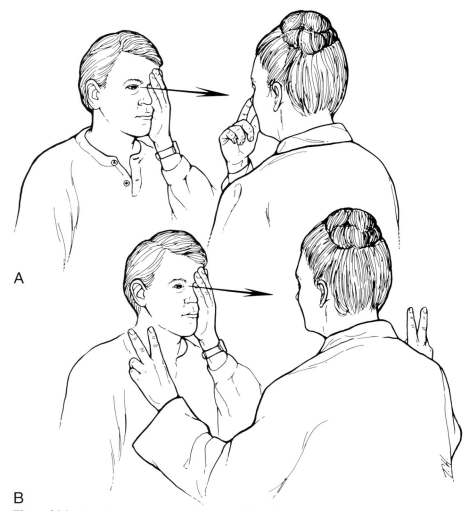

Figure 34.1. Confrontation testing of the visual field. The patient is instructed to look at the examiner's nose (**A**) while the targets are presented in the periphery. The patient is asked to respond when he or she sees the target (**B**). Further refinement of the field and verification of the patient's responses can be obtained by asking the patient to report how many fingers are being displayed in each field.

held simultaneously in each hemifield. The patient with chiasmal compression will report that the red object in the temporal field is less bright or more washed out (desaturated) than is the object held in the nasal visual field.

TANGENT SCREEN EXAMINATION

Confrontation testing of the field of vision, by its very nature, is rather imprecise as the testing distance of the examiner from the patient and the target sizes used are not

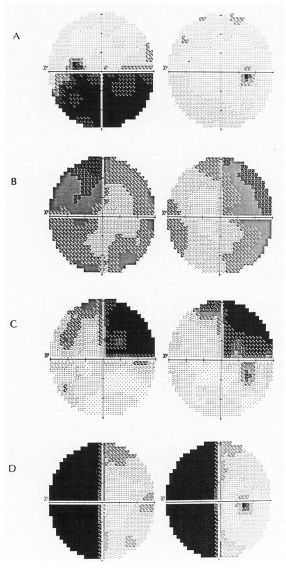

Figure 34.2. Examples of visual field defects as plotted on an automated static threshold perimeter (Humphrey Visual Field Analyzer). By convention, visual fields are always displayed from the patient's view rather than the examiner's, thus the visual field for the left eye will always be on the left of a pair of visual fields. **A.** Inferior altitudinal loss in the left eye from anterior ischemic optic neuropathy. **B.** Relative bitemporal hemianopsia from chiasmal compression due to a pituitary tumor. **C.** Right superior quadrantanopsia resulting from removal of a temporal lobe tumor. **D.** Left homonymous hemianopsia resulting from a right occipital lobe infarction.

standardized or specified in any precise way. Tangent screen examination at least partially corrects these deficiencies. In this method, the patient is seated a specified distance–usually 1 or 2 meters–from the tangent screen (a large square piece of black felt hung on a wall) and is instructed to maintain steady gaze at a central target in the center of the screen. The examiner, who stands to one side of the screen, presents targets of a specified size mounted on a black felt-covered wand from various points in the visual field periphery. The patient reports when these targets are first seen and the location of those points recorded. Connecting those points forms what is termed an isopter. A complete tangent screen examination will consist of several isopters plotted by testing the visual field with targets of several different sizes. The depiction of these isopters provides a pattern of visual impairment which can be assigned to a particular location in the visual pathway.

Virtually all of the early work in defining the important patterns of visual field loss was done on the tangent screen and it is still very useful in quickly assessing the nature of suspected visual field loss though later methods have virtually replaced it for quantifying the extent of visual field loss and following its progression.

One area in which the tangent screen is still very helpful is in the assessment of patients with suspected functional loss of the visual field. Often such patients will report marked constriction of the visual field periphery. Instead of the size of the field expanding in a physiologic fashion as the patient moves further back from the tangent screen, the field in the functional patient with "tubular" fields will remain the same, or actually diminish in size, when the patient is tested at increasing distances. Such testing can only be easily done at the tangent screen.

KINETIC PERIMETRY

As valuable as confrontation and tangent screen field testing may be, they suffer from a lack of standardization of testing conditions and methods for recording and comparing results from consecutively performed tests. This makes it difficult to quantitatively follow changes in the visual field over time. So-called "formal" methods of visual field examination provide a standardized testing and reporting format which permits comparison of results over time. Formal methods are divided into kinetic and static types. In the past, **kinetic** (moving target; Goldmann) perimetry was the standard method for quantitatively assessing the field of vision. It is still the best method for assessing the full extent of visual field loss which involves more than the central 30° of the visual field. However, the frequency of its use has decreased in recent years because quality results are very dependent upon skilled operators who are in increasingly short supply. In addition, kinetic perimetry is less sensitive in detecting early visual field impairment than is static threshold perimetry.

Kinetic perimetry derives its name from the fact that the patient is asked to report when he first sees a moving target (in this regard, tangent screen perimetry is also kinetic). The patient is seated at a machine consisting of a large, vertically oriented bowl positioned 33 cm in front of him or her. Through an ingenious mechanical arm projection system, targets are projected onto the inner surface of the bowl as the patient fixates a central target. The patient presses a button when the target is first seen and an isopter is plotted for that size target. Background lighting conditions are standardized, as are target sizes and brightness, allowing for reproducible testing conditions and permitting comparison of results to detect evidence of progression.

Such information is of critical importance in many ocular disorders, most importantly the glaucomas.

In some elderly patients, kinetic perimetry is the preferred testing method as it is considered to be more "user friendly" than static perimetry and can yield results when the more taxing static methods fail.

STATIC PERIMETRY

Static threshold perimetry with computerized instruments such as the Humphrey Field Analyzer, has largely supplanted kinetic (Goldmann) techniques (Fig. 34.2). This method very accurately assesses the central 30° of field by presenting stationary targets of varying brightness in a grid-like pattern and defining the dimmest target detectable by the patient at each spot in the grid. Though the targets move around as they are presented in different parts of the visual field, the patient is not looking at a moving target, but rather is responding to stationary targets presented in differing locations in the visual field. The information is presented as a printout of numerical "brightness" values in each of the tested points, as well as a grayscale depiction allowing a quick assessment of pathology. Static threshold perimetry is very sensitive in detecting early defects in patients with glaucomatous optic neuropathy, or in detecting subtle residual deficits in patients who have recovered from optic neuritis.

Classical patterns such as arcuate scotomas, altitudinal defects, bitemporal hemianopsias, homonymous hemianopsias, and temporal crescent defects help to define the site of pathology and serve to direct further investigations.

However, visual field data rarely stand alone in defining the patient's problem. Other historical and examination findings such as the time signature of visual loss, the presence or absence of abnormal pupillary reactivity, or optic disc cupping, or atrophy, weigh on the decision for further testing.

FUTURE DEVELOPMENTS

While Goldmann perimetry and static threshold automated perimetry have served us well in the detection and quantification of visual field defects, several other methods which hold promise for the future have been devised for assessing the visual field. Short wave-length automated perimetry using blue targets on a yellow background offers promise in earlier detection of glaucomatous optic nerve damage. Future testing strategies will try to further reduce the testing time for patients, a particularly laudable goal in elderly patients who often have difficulty maintaining concentration for the entire duration of the current testing paradigms.

◗❙ Chapter 35
Neuroimaging

W. T. Shults

INDICATIONS

Scanning of the brain with either computerized tomography (CT) or magnetic resonance imaging (MRI) techniques is an enormously powerful diagnostic tool which has revolutionized the approach to neurodiagnosis. These tools are particularly helpful in assessing patients with proptosis, unexplained visual loss, cryptic optic disc edema, papilledema, ocular motility disturbances, and visual field deficits.

TECHNIQUES
CT Scanning

Computerized tomography utilizes differential x-ray absorption by elements with higher atomic numbers such as calcium, iodine, and iron to create computer-generated two-dimensional images in axial and coronal planes (Table 35.1). Sagittal images are obtainable through reformatting techniques.

 CT scanning is particularly well suited to use in the evaluation of orbital disorders as orbital tissues such as bone, nerve, and fat naturally possess different absorption characteristics making the differentiation of normal from abnormal tissues easier, and often eliminating the need for contrast enhancement. Thin slices will afford the best definition of orbital anatomy. Assessment of orbital tumors (optic nerve gliomas and optic nerve sheath meningiomas) and thyroid ophthalmopathy is well-performed by CT (Fig. 35.1). Contrast enhancement improves the ability to define intracranial extension of sheath meningiomas and optic gliomas.

MRI Scanning

MRI has supplanted CT for most neuro-ophthalmic disorders (Table 35.2). It offers clear benefits in deciding which optic neuritis patients might benefit most from treatment. It is clearly superior to CT in defining disorders of cavernous sinus and parasellar area (Fig. 35.2), skull base, and brainstem, and can define parenchymal mischief with greater precision than CT. The ability to "image" flowing blood is very helpful in diagnosing aneurysms, arteriovenous malformations, and venous sinus occlusions.

USE

Properly used, CT and MRI scanning are clearly cost-effective; used haphazardly without proper indications they increase cost and may delay diagnosis. Despite the

TABLE 35.1. CT Scanning: Advantages and Disadvantages

ADVANTAGES	DISADVANTAGES
1. It is less apt to produce claustrophobia than MRI.	1. Uses ionizing radiation to produce image. This may be a major factor in deciding which imaging modality to use in a child with a suspected optic nerve glioma or an adult with a sheath meningioma who may need repeated scanning over a lifetime. With CT scanning the risk of eventual cataract formation is high due to the repeated exposure of the crystalline lens to ionizing radiation.
2. Not contraindicated in patients with pacemakers.	2. Direct sagittal views not available but must be created from reformatting.
3. Provides better definition of bone and calcium than MRI.	3. Not as sensitive to the differentiation of soft tissues or edema as MRI. MS plaques are much better defined with MRI than CT.
4. Is faster than MRI.	4. Not able to distinguish flowing blood or spinal fluid as with MRI.
5. May be very helpful in localization of intraocular metallic foreign bodies where MRI scanning is contraindicated.	5. Affected more by so-called bone-hardening artifact which impairs views of brainstem because of artifact produced by the petrous pyramids.
	6. Contrast agent allergies (iodine-containing compound) can be a problem with some patients and renal disease may preclude the use of such agents.

advances wrought by CT and MRI technology, certain caveats apply. Indiscriminate ordering of scans on marginal clinical grounds unnecessarily increases the cost of medical care while incomplete imaging of the area of interest or incorrect scan interpretation by a radiologist who has received scant clinical data from the referring physician interferes with timely diagnosis. It is often better not to scan the patient at all than to obtain an incorrect report of a "negative" scan, as all thought stops for a time after such a "reassuring" report.

Proper utilization of modern neuroimaging tools demands effective communication between clinician and radiologist. The primary care physician has an immense advantage over the radiologist in that the primary care physician has seen the patient. If the clinical setting strongly suggests an intracranial lesion but none was found, then the primary care physician should commune with the radiologist and personally review the scan with the radiologist. Such review may disclose that the area of interest was not adequately seen because the slice thickness was too great, or gadolinium was not used when it should have been, or orbital fat suppression was not employed. A repeat scan done properly and at little additional expense to the patient may yield the answer and convert a "negative" scan into one which provides the correct answer. It is not surprising that neuro-ophthalmology has been defined as "the reinterpretation of allegedly negative neuro-imaging studies" (W. F. Hoyt, M.D., personal communication).

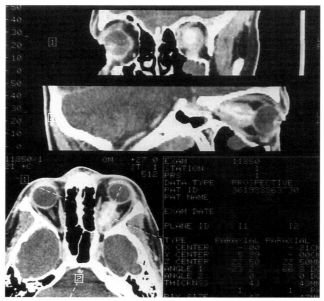

Figure 35.1. CT scan, axial (*below*), off-axis sagittal (*middle*), and coronal reconstruction (*above*) optic nerve sheath meningioma. Thin-section computed tomography is particularly suited to imaging orbital pathology as in this patient with an optic nerve sheath meningioma. The optic nerve is highlighted in the orbit because of calcium within the nerve sheath tumor which produces a bright image on CT (so-called tram-tracking sign). The *upper* and *middle* images are created by a computerized reformatting process in which images acquired in the axial plane are reconstituted in an off-axis sagittal (*center*) and coronal (*top*) plane defined by the *dotted lines* through the optic nerve in the lower image. In this manner, "lateral" and "anteroposterior" views of the orbit are produced from images originally obtained in the axial plane.

FUTURE DEVELOPMENTS

Advances in neuroimaging have irrevocably changed neurodiagnosis. Plain skull films, polytomography, and pneumoencephalography have been supplanted by computed tomography and magnetic resonance imaging. The use of paramagnetic materials such as gadolinium-diethylene penta-acetic acid (Gd-DTPA), and the development of new imaging sequences which permit fat suppression such as short inversion time inversion recovery (STIR), have further refined our abilities to define disease in the orbit and visual pathways. No doubt further developments in imaging sequences (e.g., diffusion-weighted MRI, perfusion imaging, and magnetic resonance spectroscopy) will continue to enhance our abilities. Magnetic resonance angiography permits the identification of flowing blood in vascular structures, a technique which has proven very useful in assessing patients with suspected aneurysms, arteriovenous malformations, and venous sinus occlusions. New methods based upon the use of radionuclides such as single

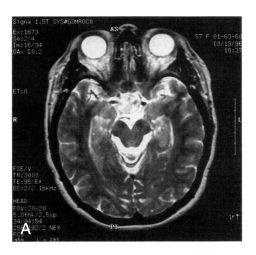
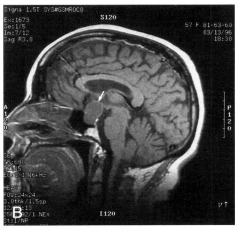
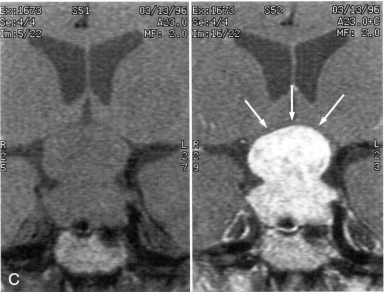

Figure 35.2. MRI scan in axial, sagittal, and coronal planes, pituitary adenoma. MRI is superior to CT in imaging most intracranial pathology, and particularly in imaging disease at the skull base such as the pituitary adenoma shown here. The relationship of the chiasm (*arrow*) to the tumor is elegantly defined in three planes (**A**) axial, (**B**) sagittal, and (**C**) coronal. The coronal images were obtained without (*left*) and with (*right*) paramagnetic "contrast" agent (gadolinium).

TABLE 35.2. MRI: Advantages and Disadvantages

ADVANTAGES	DISADVANTAGES
1. Superior to CT in differentiating gray from white matter and in detecting subtle white or gray matter changes.	1. Not universally available.
2. Produces superior images of posterior fossa structures.	2. Relatively more expensive than CT.
3. Able to define flowing blood and cerebrospinal fluid so useful in the assessment of patients with possible aneurysms, AVM's, venous sinus occlusions, and aqueductal stenosis.	3. Not as good at imaging bone as CT.
4. Much more sensitive in defining demyelinating disease than CT.	4. Claustrophobia is a significant problem requiring sedation in about 20% of patients, and occasionally requiring general anesthesia.
5. Better at defining intracavernous sinus disease than CT.	5. Exam time is longer than CT making it difficult to scan uncooperative patients who are unable to hold still for the longer exam time required by MRI scanning.
6. Superior at defining extension of optic nerve gliomas into the optic chiasm and tracts than CT.	6. Unable to scan patients with pacemakers or with suspected intraocular foreign bodies.
7. Parasellar lesions are better displayed because of the capacity to define anatomical relationships in three planes (coronal, sagittal, and axial) (Fig. 35.2)	

photon emission computed tomography (SPECT) and positron emission tomography (PET) permit functional assessment of normal and abnormal tissues. Recently, so-called functional magnetic resonance imaging has been able to demonstrate changes in neuronal activity of cortical areas, suggesting that in the future we may well be able to more closely correlate structure with function.

SECTION IV

APPENDICES

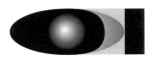

Basic Orbital and Ocular Anatomy

W. T. Shults and G. A. Cioffi

ORBITAL ANATOMY

The orbit is a pyramidal shaped space with the base of the pyramid directed anteriorly. The apex of the pyramid is connected with the intracranial space via the optic canal (Fig. A.1) Other passageways permitting communication of neural and vascular structures to and from the orbit include the superior and inferior orbital fissures, which extend along the corresponding posterior temporal margins of the pyramidal space. The walls of the orbital space are comprised of seven bones (frontal, maxillary, zygomatic, ethmoid, sphenoid, palatine, and temporal) which vary in size and thickness. Through the optic canal pass the optic nerve, ophthalmic artery, and sympathetic nerves, while through the superior orbital fissure, the oculomotor (III), trochlear (IV), and abducens (VI) nerves pass. As well, the first division of the trigeminal nerve (V) and some sympathetic fibers enter through this opening. Venous blood leaves the orbit through the superior ophthalmic and inferior orbital veins which exit through the superior and inferior orbital fissures, respectively. The superior ophthalmic vein drains to the cavernous sinus, while the inferior orbital vein drains to the pterygoid plexus. Lacking valves, the orbital venous system permits the accumulation of profound edema and prominent venous engorgement in response to conditions such as carotid cavernous fistulas, which reverse flow and increase intraluminal pressure in these veins.

Five of the six ocular muscles originate from the annulus of Zinn (Fig. A.2), an ovoid fibrous structure through which the optic nerve passes. The six ocular motor muscles are the four rectus muscles (superior, inferior, lateral, and medial) and the two oblique muscles (superior and inferior). These muscles control the direction of gaze of the globes. In disorders such as thyroid optic neuropathy, the optic nerve may be compressed by enlargement of the ocular muscle bellies in the apex of the orbit, as the bony confines preclude outward expansion of the enlarged muscles with potential disastrous consequences for the optic nerve. From the globe to the orbital apex, the optic nerve travels within a space defined by the ocular muscles and their interconnecting intermuscular membrane–the intraconal space.

The orbit is surrounded by the paranasal sinuses–the ethmoid (medially), sphenoid (posteromedially), maxillary (inferiorly), and frontal (superiorly). Infection in these thin-walled spaces can easily spread to the orbit producing orbital cellulitis or abscess, while mucoceles which originate in the ethmoid or frontal sinuses commonly produce proptosis (protrusion of the globe). Orbital fat fills all potential space within the orbit. Atrophy of this adipose tissue can result from trauma, infection, or inflammation with resultant enophthalmos (a sinking back of the globe into the orbital space), a helpful clinical sign of previous orbital disease.

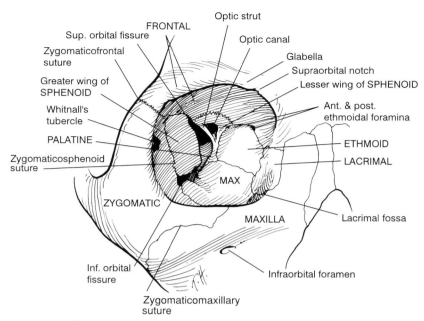

Figure A.1. Orbital anatomy. (Reprinted with permission from Lemke B. Orbital and ocular anatomy. In: Wright K, ed. Textbook of ophthalmology. Fig. 1.1. Baltimore: Williams and Wilkins, 1997:3.)

EYELIDS AND NASOLACRIMAL SYSTEM

The eyelids are specialized structures designed to protect the eye and lubricate the cornea, while maintaining an aperture for vision. The eyelids measure approximately 30 mm in length horizontally. The palpebral fissure is the opening between the upper and lower eyelid, and it measures 10–12 mm in height. The eyelids are most simply thought of as opposing anterior and posterior lamella (Fig. A.3).

The anterior lamella of the eyelid is a myocutaneous layer, composed of skin and the orbicularis oculi. The eyelid skin is keratinized epidermis overlying a modified dermis with associated skin appendages. The orbicularis oculi consists of pretarsal, preseptal, and orbital portions. Each portion of this muscle contributes to proper eyelid closure. The pretarsal and preseptal portions help to form the medial and lateral canthal tendons which stabilize the eyelids.

The orbital septum divides the anterior and posterior lamella. The septum arises from the periorbita (the periosteal lining of the orbit) and acts as a barrier against the spread of infection and the herniation of orbital fat.

The posterior lamella includes the eyelid retractors, the tarsus, and the conjunctiva. The upper eyelid retractors are the levator palpebrae superioris and Müller's muscle. The levator palpebrae superioris arises at the orbital apex from the lesser wing of the sphenoid. It overlies the superior rectus muscle. Anteriorly, the levator becomes an aponeurotic sheet that attaches to the medial and lateral orbital walls and to the anterior tarsal surface. Müller's muscle arises from the posterior surface of the levator

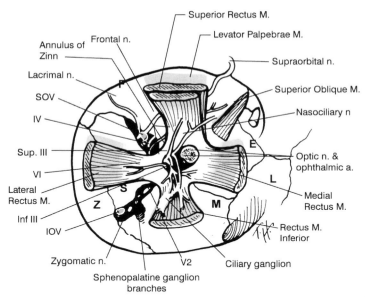

Superior Rectus M.

Levator Palpebrae M.

Annulus of Zinn

Frontal n.

Lacrimal n.

SOV

IV

Sup. III

VI

Lateral Rectus M.

Inf III

IOV

Supraorbital n.

Superior Oblique M.

Nasociliary n

Optic n. & ophthalmic a.

Medial Rectus M.

Rectus M. Inferior

Zygomatic n.

V2

Ciliary ganglion

Sphenopalatine ganglion branches

Figure A.2. Orbital apex. The four rectus muscles and the superior oblique muscle originate in the apex. *SOV*, superior ophthalmic vein. (Reprinted with permission from Lemke B. Orbital and ocular anatomy. In: Wright K, ed. Textbook of ophthalmology. Fig. 1.3. Baltimore: Williams and Wilkins, 1997:6.)

aponeurosis and attaches to the superior tarsal border, within the upper eyelid. The lower lid retractors are analogous to their upper lid counterparts; however, they do not arise from the orbital apex, but rather from an anterior extension of the inferior rectus muscle. The eyelid retractors are innervated by the third cranial nerve and sympathetics that travel with the internal carotid artery through the cavernous sinus. The levator palpebrae superioris is innervated by the superior division of the third cranial nerve. Müller's muscle and the inferior tarsal muscle receive sympathetic innervation.

The tarsi (tarsal plates) are dense connective tissue plates which give form to each eyelid. The tarsal plates border the eyelid margin. The superior tarsus measures 10 mm in height, while the inferior tarsus measures 4 mm in height. Each of the tarsi contains meibomian glands that drain onto the eyelid margin. The conjunctiva is a mucosal surface tightly adherent to posterior tarsal surface. It joins with the skin on the lid margin and is reflected onto the ocular surface at both superior and inferior fornices. The accessory lacrimal glands of Krause and Wolfring are located within the conjunctival fornices.

Tears are produced both by the major lacrimal gland, located in the superior temporal quadrant of the orbit, and by accessory lacrimal glands (Krause and Wolfring), which are found along the internal surface of both the upper and lower eyelids (Fig. A.4). The accessory lacrimal glands are responsible for basic tear secretion, while the major lacrimal gland provides much of the aqueous portion of reflex tearing. Tears serve the useful purposes of maintaining a smooth optical surface on the anterior

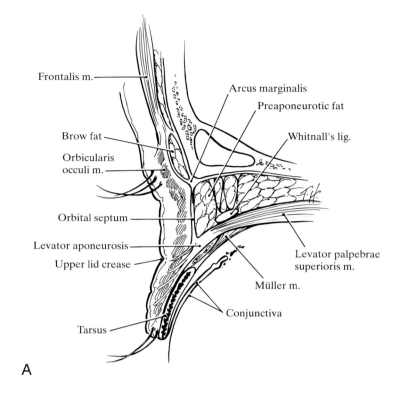

Frontalis m.

Arcus marginalis

Preaponeurotic fat

Brow fat

Whitnall's lig.

Orbicularis
occuli m.

Orbital septum

Levator aponeurosis

Upper lid crease

Levator palpebrae
superioris m.

Müller m.

Conjunctiva

Tarsus

A

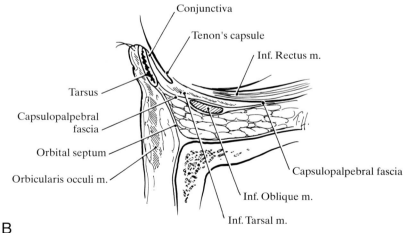

Conjunctiva

Tenon's capsule

Inf. Rectus m.

Tarsus

Capsulopalpebral
fascia

Orbital septum

Orbicularis occuli m.

Capsulopalpebral fascia

Inf. Oblique m.

Inf. Tarsal m.

B

Figure A.3. Upper and lower eyelid diagrams illustrating the anterior of myocutaneous lamella, the orbital septum, and the posterior lamella consisting of the eyelid retractors, the tarsus, and the conjunctiva.

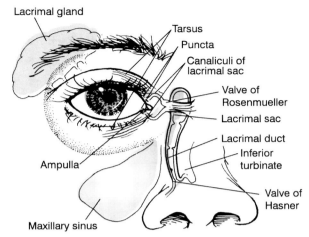

Figure A.4. Nasolacrimal system. (Reprinted with permission from Lemke B. Orbital and ocular anatomy. In: Wright K, ed. Textbook of ophthalmology. Fig. 1.5A. Baltimore: Williams and Wilkins, 1997:7.)

portion of the eye, as well as providing anti-infective agents and removing foreign particulate from the anterior surface of the eye.

Tears are drained from the ocular surface through two puncta at the medial aspect of each of the upper and lower eyelids (Fig. A.5). These puncta, or drainage holes, lead to a single canaliculus which drains into the lacrimal sac. The lacrimal sac is situated along the lateral nasal bridge and drains into the nasal cavity via the nasolacrimal duct.

EYEBALL

The normal adult globe is spherical and has a diameter of 24 mm (Fig. A.6) The eyeball is fluid-filled and can be divided into an anterior segment and a posterior segment separated by the lens. The anterior segment is filled with a clear fluid, aqueous humor. The posterior segment is filled with a gel-like body, vitreous humor.

The ciliary body is the midportion of the uveal tract lying just behind the iris and is the site of production of aqueous humor. Aqueous humor bathes the anterior segment of the eye, providing oxygen and nutrition to the region. The vitreous humor is composed of 99% water, a collagenous meshwork, and hyaluronic acid. The vitreous humor is loosely adherent to the optic disc, macula, and along major retinal vessels.

The cornea is the primary refractive element of the eye. It is the clear dome of tissue which makes up the anterior surface of the globe, and is vulnerable to injury from external disease or trauma. The adult cornea is approximately 12 mm in diameter and approximately 0.5 mm thick. The cornea is composed of three anatomically separate layers: the superficial epithelium, the central stroma, and the endothelium which faces the anterior chamber. The epithelium is nonkeratinized, stratified squamous cells. The stroma accounts for 90% of the corneal thickness and is predominantly composed of collagen. The endothelium is a monolayer of cells, which pumps fluid from the

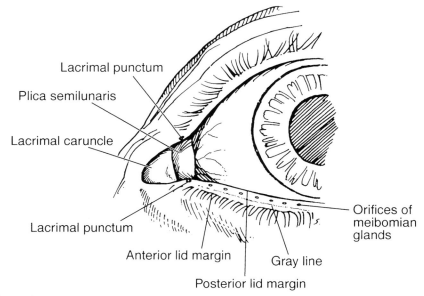

Figure A.5. Tear drainage punctum (medial, left eye). (Reprinted with permission from Lemke B. Orbital and ocular anatomy. In: Wright K, ed. Textbook of ophthalmology. Fig. 1.5B. Baltimore: Williams and Wilkins, 1997:7.)

stroma into the anterior chamber. This pumping action keeps the cornea in a relatively dehydrated state, which is necessary for corneal clarity.

The sclera is the dense connective tissue which composes 80% of the wall of the globe. Like the cornea, the sclera is primarily composed of collagen; but unlike the cornea, the scleral collagen is irregularly arranged and therefore has an opaque appearance. The anterior sclera, the *white of the eye*, is cover by conjunctiva. The conjunctiva is a mucous membrane which lines the internal surface of the eyelids and the anterior sclera. The sclera has a posterior opening which allows the optic nerve to exit the globe.

The crystalline lens is a biconvex structure and is made up of three principal parts: an external capsule, the cortex, and the central nucleus (Fig. A.7). A thin capsule comprises the outer coat of the lens and is composed primarily of basement membrane material. Between the external capsule and the central nucleus is a soft cortical material. The central nucleus is much harder and more dense than the cortical material. The lens consists of approximately 65% water and 35% crystalline and albuminoid proteins. The lens is supported, just posterior to the iris and pupil, and anterior to the vitreous space, by hundreds of fibers known as zonules, which attach to the equator of the lens and the muscular ciliary body within the wall of the eye. The lens, in conjunction with the cornea, focuses light onto the retina. In youth, the crystalline lens is pliable and its shape can be changed by altering the tension on the zonules. Muscular tension exerted on the zonules alters the curvature of the anterior and posterior surface of the lens. This change of shape allows for a variable focus and the clear viewing of objects both close to the eye and in the distance. With age, the composition of the lens changes, and the lens becomes less pliable.

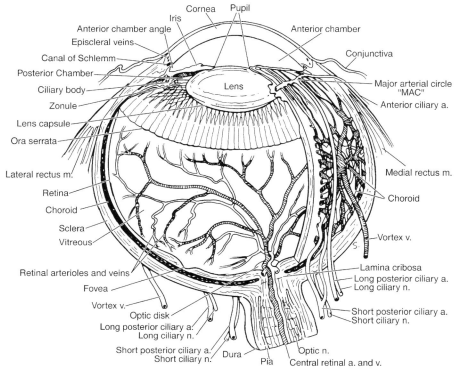

Figure A.6. Anatomy of the eye. (Reprinted with permission from Lemke B. Orbital and ocular anatomy. In: Wright K, ed. Textbook of ophthalmology. Fig. 1.12. Baltimore: Williams and Wilkins, 1997:19.)

The uveal tract refers to the middle layer or "coat" of the eye and is composed of the iris (anteriorly), the ciliary body (middle), and the choroid (posteriorly). This layer anatomically comprises the center tract of the eye and is predominantly composed of muscular and vascular tissues. The iris is the muscular sphincter that regulates the pupillary aperture, while the ciliary body is a muscular structure, posterior to the iris, which controls accommodation and the focusing ability of the crystalline lens. The anterior ciliary body also produces the aqueous humor. The choroid, the vascular layer between the retina and sclera, is the primary blood supply to the outer retina.

RETINA AND OPTIC NERVE

The retina is a thin, delicate sheet of tissue, which lines the interior of the globe, extending from the ora serrata (just behind the ciliary body) to the optic nerve. The retina is the neurosensory tissue of the eye, responsible for converting light stimuli into neural signals and transmitting visual information via the optic nerve to the brain. The retina is composed of various neural tissues, vascular elements, and glial support cells. The retina may be separated into several anatomically distinct layers. The neuro-

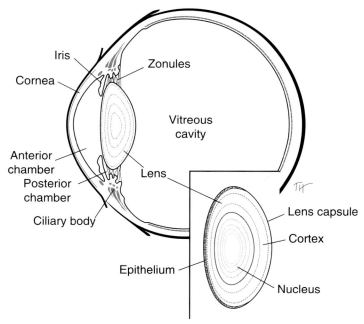

Figure A.7. The location and components of the lens of the eye.

sensory cells (rods and cones) compose the deepest layer of the retina. Rods predominantly detect black and white stimuli, while cones provide color vision.

The neurosensory cells lie adjacent to the choroid, the posterior vascular coat of the eye. Between the retina and the choroid are the retinal pigment epithelium (RPE) and Bruch's membrane. The retina is normally closely adherent to the underlying RPE, attached by a glue-like layer of mucopolysaccharide and by the constant pumping of fluid by the RPE cells from the vitreous, through the retina, to the choroid. Bruch's membrane lies beneath the RPE and is a relatively impermeable membrane which comprises part of the blood-retinal barrier. The choroid is the vascular supply to the deeper layers of the retina. The neurosensory cells connect via specialized neurons (bipolar cells and amacrine cells) to the retinal ganglion cells. The axons of the retinal ganglion cells extend from their cell bodies, located in the most anterior superficial layer of the retina, to the optic nerve. These axons, or nerve fibers, are the primary component of the optic nerve. The superficial retina receives its vascular supply from branches of the central retinal artery, which enters the eye at the optic nerve. The retinal arteries and retinal capillaries are located primarily within the superficial nerve fiber layer. The retinal capillaries are nonfenestrated vessels and comprise the second portion of the blood-retinal barrier. The retinal vasculature is drained entirely via tributaries to a single central retinal vein.

The macula is the central region of the retina. The fovea (the center of the macula) is primarily composed of cones and provides the best central visual acuity (i.e., reading vision) (Fig. A.8). The macula is located temporal to the optic nerve, between the retinal vascular arcades. The macula generally has a slightly more pigmented appearance,

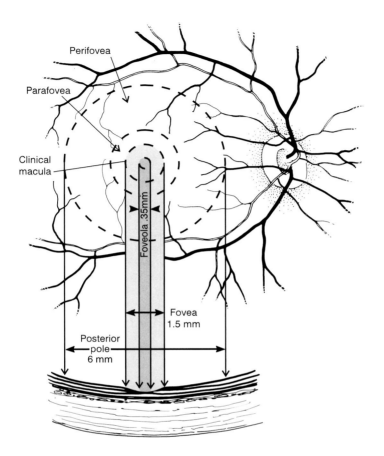

Figure A.8.   Macula and fovea. Note the size and position of the macula and fovea between the superior and inferior temporal arcades of the retinal blood vessels (right eye). (Reprinted with permission from Lemke B. Orbital and ocular anatomy. In: Wright K, ed. Textbook of ophthalmology. Fig. 1.28A. Baltimore: Williams and Wilkins, 1997:38.)

compared to the surrounding retina. If the macular cones are anatomically distorted or dysfunctional, vision may decrease precipitously.

The optic nerve is primarily composed of the axons (the retinal nerve fibers) from the retinal ganglion cells and acts as the neural connection between the neurosensory retina and the brain. The optic nerve "head" is the perpendicular transition of the retinal nerve fibers from the surface of the retina to the optic nerve as they exit the eye. The normal, healthy optic nerve is composed of approximately 1.2–1.5 million neurons or fibers.

General Examination Techniques

G. A. Cioffi

VISUAL ACUITY ASSESSMENT AND PINHOLE TESTING

Analogous to obtaining vital signs in the systemic evaluation, the assessment of visual acuity is perhaps the most critical part of the ophthalmic evaluation. Vision requires not only a healthy functioning eye, but also intact neurologic visual pathways. Accurate visual acuity measurement is dependent on reliable subjective responses from the patient. A variety of eye charts are available for the testing of both distance and near vision. The most common chart used for the assessment of distance vision is the Snellen chart (Fig. B.1). This chart is read at a distance of 20 feet, and the chart should be illuminated at approximately 100 foot candles. Acuity is recorded as a fraction, where the numerator represents the distance to the chart and the denominator represents the distance at which the normal eye can read the specifically sized figures. Each row on the chart has a designated number corresponding to the denominator. Therefore, the letters on the 20/40 row are large enough that a normal eye would see them from 40 feet.

In testing visual acuity, the examiner asks the individual to read progressively smaller lines of letters on the chart. Patients that have difficulty in reading the largest letter on the eye chart (20/400) may be moved closer to the eye chart. A patient who is able to see the 20/400 "E" at 10 feet has a visual acuity of 20/800. For illiterate and non-English speaking patients, the "illiterate E" chart is also available. All the figures on the illiterate E chart are in the shape of the letter E with various orientations (Fig. B.2), and patients are taught to indicate the orientation of the E. Visual acuity should be assessed, whenever possible, with the refractive correction in place (see Chapter 19, "Refractive Errors and Their Correction"). Patients with vision less than 20/400 should be further documented as being able to count fingers at various distances, being able to see only hand motions at various distances, or as having only light perception (able to determine whether a light is on or off).

Documentation of near vision should also be assessed. By convention, near vision is measured at 14 inches and a variety of near vision charts are available. It must be remembered that adults, over the age of 40, have a limited ability to focus on near objects due to presbyopia; these individuals require additional magnification (bifocals or a plus diopter lens) for near vision (see Chapter 19, "Refractive Errors and Their Correction"). Because of presbyopia, visual acuity measurements measured at distance may be more standardized and of more use in the basic ophthalmic examination.

A convenient test which may be used to assess the distance visual acuity in an individual with a refractive error, but without their normal refractive correction, is the pinhole test. The pinhole test eliminates the refractive blur caused by myopia (nearsightedness), hyperopia (farsightedness), and astigmatism (abnormally shaped

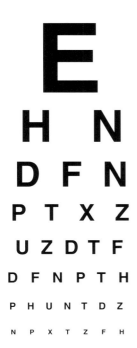

Figure B.1. Snellen visual acuity chart.

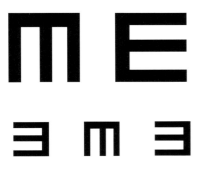

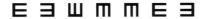

Figure B.2. Illiterate "E" visual acuity chart.

cornea). When the Snellen chart is viewed through an occluder with multiple tiny pinhole openings, only a few centrally aligned rays of light reach the retina. By eliminating the noncentral rays of light, less blur is created on the retina. Centrally aligned light rays are less dependent on focusing by the cornea and lens, therefore refractive errors cause less distortion with use of the pinhole. This allows estimation of the subject's true correctable distance visual acuity.

PUPILLARY RESPONSE TESTING AND AFFERENT PUPILLARY LIGHT DEFECT (MARCUS GUNN PUPIL)

The pupils should be examined under bright and dim light situations for symmetry (equality of size and shape). As well, the reaction of the pupils to a direct light stimulus provides valuable information about both the eye and neural pathways. The pupils should be perfectly round and should react briskly to a direct light stimulus. The afferent pupillary light defect test, or the "swinging flashlight" test, involves assessing the pupillary reaction while alternating direct light stimulation from one eye to the other. In this test, the room lighting is reduced, and the individual is asked to fix on a distant object. Fixation in the distance is important to eliminate the normal pupillary miosis (constriction) associated with close fixation. A bright pen light or transilluminator is shined into the eye from a position slightly below the visual axis, so as not to disrupt the subject's ability to maintain steady fixation in the distance. The speed and extent of the pupillary constriction in each eye is noted. Both the direct response of the pupil in the eye with direct stimulation and the consensual response of the pupil in the contralateral eye should be noted. The pen light is moved quickly across the bridge of the nose to the contralateral eye. A slight enlargement of the pupil may occur as the light is passing over the bridge of the nose. However, once the light is shined in the contralateral eye, both pupils should constrict symmetrically and to the same extent as when the light was shined in the first eye. This test can be repeated by swinging the flashlight back and forth between the two eyes.

In an eye with optic nerve or retinal damage, the direct pupillary response will be lessened, but the consensual pupillary response will remain complete. Therefore, if the swinging flashlight test is performed in an individual with unilateral optic nerve disease, the pupils will dilate when the light is moved to the "bad eye" and constrict when the light is moved to the good eye. This phenomenon is known as a Marcus Gunn or afferent pupillary light defect.

PERIPHERAL VISION ASSESSMENT

Specialized techniques for evaluating the peripheral vision are described elsewhere in this text (see Chapter 34, "Visual Fields"). However, gross assessment of the peripheral vision may be achieved in the office without specialized testing. Even dense visual field abnormalities may be asymptomatic and confrontational testing may be quite informative. More subtle peripheral vision loss may require specialized testing. Patients often will not notice even large visual field abnormalities, because the visual field in the contralateral eye overlaps with the deficient visual field. Therefore, each eye should be tested separately. Confrontation visual field assessment can be performed quickly and easily. For this test, the patient should patch one eye and should be seated facing the examiner at a distance of approximately 3 feet (see Chapter 34, "Visual Fields").

When the patient's left eye is covered, the examiner should close his or her own right eye. The patient is asked to stare directly ahead at the examiner, thus the patient's fixation may be monitored as the examiner and patient are staring "eye to eye." The superior, inferior, temporal, and nasal visual fields can be assessed in this fashion. The examiner presents fingers or hand movements in each of the quadrants asking the patient to subjectively describe either the number of fingers presented or the direction of the hand movement.

EYELID EVERSION

When examining a patient for foreign body sensation, it is important to evert the upper and lower eyelids. Often small particulate matter may be adherent to the posterior surface of the eyelid (the conjunctival surface), and the patient will experience severe foreign body discomfort with each eyelid blink. To identify and remove these foreign bodies, it is necessary to evert the eyelids. The middle layer of each eyelid is composed of a semirigid plate known as the tarsus. The tarsal plate in the upper eyelid extends approximately 8–9 mm from lid margin to the top of the tarsus (see Chapter 10, "Eyelid Malpositions"). The tarsus in the lower eyelid is approximately half this width. To evert the eyelids, topical anesthesia should be instilled in the eye (e.g., tetracaine or proparacaine). For the upper eyelid, the examiner gently grasps the lashes with the thumb and index finger on one hand, and places a cotton-tipped applicator just above the tarsal plate with the other hand (Fig. B.3). The lid is everted by applying downward pressure on the cotton-tipped applicator and lifting the lid margin. The conjunctival surface of the inner lid can then be examined. The lower lid can be everted in a similar fashion, remembering that the tarsus is narrower and the inferior fornix is more accessible. By combining lid eversion with saline irrigation of the superior and inferior conjunctival fornices, most foreign bodies can be removed.

OCULAR MOTILITY ASSESSMENT

Ocular motility should be tested in all patients, especially in settings of ocular, periocular, or facial trauma. When testing ocular motility, the movement of the eyes should be assessed both monocularly and in tandem. The movement of the eyes in all fields of gaze should be assessed. A more detailed description of ocular motility disturbances and assessment of ocular misalignment is found in Chapter 17, "Pediatric and Adult Strabismus," and in Appendix C, "Special Pediatric Examination Techniques." A quick assessment of ocular motility can most easily be performed with a penlight. The reflection of the light on the cornea will help to assess the direction of gaze of the eyes. The light should be held approximately 12 inches from the subject. When the subject is staring straight ahead at the light source, a pinpoint reflection of light should be centered over each pupil if the eyes are aligned properly. The subject is requested to look in each of the six cardinal positions of gaze (left, right, up and right, down and right, up and left, down and left) following the light source. The eyes should move symmetrically and the corneal reflex should remain centered. A discussion of esotropia, exotropia, and other ocular motility disturbances is found in Chapter 17, "Pediatric and Adult Strabismus."

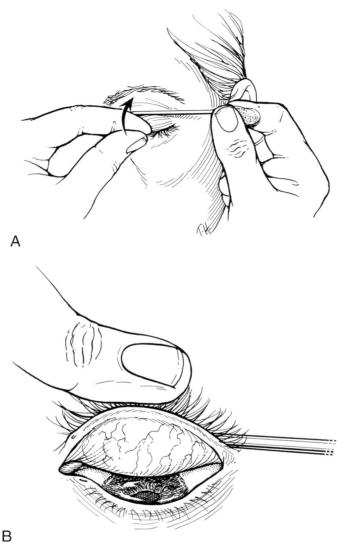

Figure B.3. Upper eyelid eversion. **A.** The lid must be everted above the tarsal plate, approximately 10 mm above the lid margin. **B.** The lid is grasp and everted, exposing the conjunctival surface.

INTRAOCULAR PRESSURE ASSESSMENT

A variety of techniques are available for the assessment of intraocular pressure; however, applanation tonometry remains the gold standard. The applanation tonometer is attached to a slitlamp and measures the force required to flatten the anterior surface of the eye (the cornea) by a standard amount. The greater the force required to flatten

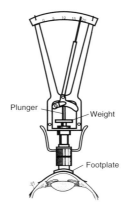

Plunger — Weight

Footplate

Figure B.4. Schiötz tonometer.

the globe, the higher the intraocular pressure. The force is measured in grams which can be converted to intraocular pressure (mm Hg). Although this technique is the gold standard for measuring intraocular pressure, it is not readily available to most nonophthalmologists because of its dependence on a slitlamp biomicroscope.

Schiötz indentation tonometry is more available in most clinic settings. The Schiötz tonometer measures the amount of corneal indentation produced by a predetermined weight which is placed on the eye, while the subject is lying in a supine position (Fig. B.4). With high intraocular pressure, the globe is harder and less corneal indentation occurs. The Schiötz tonometer uses a series of different weights, varying from 5.5 to 15 g, which are attached to a plunger. The plunger rests on the corneal surface and the tonometer measures the amount of indentation on a scale mounted on the top of the tonometer. The scale readings are inversely related to intraocular pressure and are converted to an intraocular pressure reading (mm Hg) by a conversion table provided with the tonometer. Both applanation tonometry and Schiötz tonometry require the use of a topical anesthetic. Because the Schiötz tonometer is portable, it can be used in a variety of clinical settings. However, the accuracy of the Schiötz tonometer is insufficient to monitor the effectiveness of chronic glaucoma therapy. In addition, Schiötz tonometry should be avoided in the setting of ocular trauma if the possibility of globe perforation exists.

Digital palpation of the globe is notoriously inaccurate for assessing the exact intraocular pressure; however, it may be useful in the absence of a formal tonometer. Palpation with comparison between the two eyes can help the examiner determine extreme elevations of intraocular pressure. To perform digital palpation, the patient is asked to gently close both eyes. The examiner then uses the index and middle finger of each hand to palpate the globe through the upper eyelid. The firmness of each eye is compared. With significant elevations of intraocular pressure (40–50 mm Hg), the affected eye will be much harder than the contralateral eye.

HANDHELD LIGHT ANTERIOR SEGMENT EXAMINATION

With a simple transilluminator or handheld penlight, a useful examination of the anterior segment of the eye can be achieved. A penlight can be used to check for pupillary responses as previously described. A penlight is also useful in examining the conjunctiva, eyelid fornices, cornea, anterior chamber, and iris. Swelling, vascular injection, or discoloration of the conjunctiva often require enhanced illumination in order to be detected (see Chapter 15, "Ocular Trauma"). As well, the clarity and integrity of the cornea can be observed. The cornea should have a crystal clear appearance with no opacification (see Chapter 18, "Corneal Abrasions and Corneal Ulcerations"). The anterior chamber is the area between the posterior aspect of the cornea and the anterior surface of the iris. The anterior chamber should be clear and free of debris. The depth of the anterior chamber can be assessed by shining the light from an oblique angle temporal to the eye. In an individual with a very shallow anterior chamber, the temporal iris will project a shadow across the nasal anterior chamber and iris (Fig. B.5). Pharmacological pupillary dilation should be avoided in patients who are suspected of having a narrowed anterior chamber (see Chapter 29, "Glaucoma").

FLUORESCEIN STAINING OF THE CORNEA

Fluorescein is a dye that stains the cornea in any area where the epithelium has been removed, as with a corneal abrasion. Fluorescein also highlights irregularities of the normally smooth anterior surface of the cornea (see Chapter 18, "Corneal Abrasions and Corneal Ulcerations"). Fluorescein is available both as a combination with topical anesthetic drops or on sterile paper strips. The sterile strips must be wet with sterile saline and touched on the interior surface of the lower lid. The yellowish dye will then spread via the tear film over the surface of the eye. Often, corneal staining can be seen with a white light; however, fluorescein dye fluoresces (greenish yellow) under cobalt blue illumination for better visibility. Fluorescein staining may also highlight tiny punctate irregularities of the cornea seen in diseases such as blepharitis and dry eye syndrome.

PHARMACOLOGICAL PUPIL DILATION

Pharmacological dilation of the pupil greatly enhances examination of the posterior segment of the eye. Physicians should not hesitate to dilate the pupil. The diagnostic value of a complete retinal examination through a dilated pupil far outweighs the slight risk of angle closure glaucoma which may be precipitated by dilation. The risk of angle closure is very small in all patients, but especially those under the age of 40. The anterior chamber depth and the associated likelihood of angle closure can be estimated using the oblique illumination techniques previously described. Typically, a sympathomimetic agent (such as phenylephrine 2.5%) and an anticholinergic agent (such as tropicamide 0.5%) can be used to dilate the pupil. A single application of these eyedrops will cause maximal dilation within 20 minutes in most individuals. Repeat dosing may be needed in some subjects, especially those with dark irides. Pupillary dilation will cause blurring of near vision for up to 4–6 hours after instillation of the drops.

FUNDUSCOPIC EXAMINATION: DIRECT OPHTHALMOSCOPY

Direct ophthalmoscopy is an examination technique that should be mastered by every physician. This instrument allows examination with a magnified view of the posterior segment of the eye. Although more sophisticated instrumentation exists, direct ophthal-

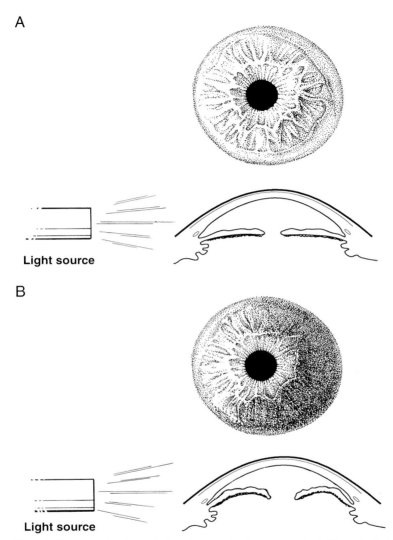

Figure B.5. Oblique illumination anterior chamber depth assessment. **A.** Normal. Note the light transits the entire anterior chamber. **B.** Shallow anterior chamber. Note the shadow on the nasal aspect of the anterior chamber due to the anterior displacement of the iris and lens.

moscopy remains an important part of every ocular examination. With the possible exceptions of small pupils (less than 2 mm) and obstruction of the visual axis which precludes a view of the posterior segment of the eye (such as progressed cataract or vitreous hemorrhage), all eyes can be examined with direct ophthalmoscopy. Examiners should not hesitate to dilate the pupil to gain a better view of the posterior segment of the eye. Diabetic retinopathy and glaucoma are among the most common causes of preventable vision loss, and direct ophthalmoscopy is one of the best techniques to diagnose and monitor these blinding disorders.

The magnification afforded by direct ophthalmoscopy ($15\times$) provides an excellent view of even the finest retinal vessels. Although there are many types of direct ophthalmoscopes, all have multiple apertures for examination through pupils of various sizes, a variable set of objective lenses to focus on the retina, and a source of illumination. Some direct ophthalmoscopes include various color filters for more detailed examination of the posterior segment. An example of this would be the green light (red-free filter) which enhances the contrast of the retinal nerve fiber layer, retinal blood vessels, and retinal hemorrhages.

When the pupil is dilated, a larger aperture and illuminating spot should be used. The ophthalmoscope is held in the examiner's right hand to examine the patient's right eye. The examiner observes the patient's right eye with the examiner's right eye and the patient's left eye with the examiner's left eye.

When examining the posterior segment of the eye with a direct ophthalmoscope, it is preferable to follow a predetermined pattern of examination. The adjustable lens wheel is set between $+7$ to $+10$ diopters initially. A light is then focused through the patient's pupil, and the instrument is moved closer to the eye while observing the red reflex of the fundus. The vessels of the retina are brought into focus by decreasing the dioptric power. Once retinal vessels are identified, the examiner should concentrate on the orientation of the fundus. Following the major vascular arcades to progressively larger vessels will allow localization of the optic nerve head. The optic nerve head should be examined for evidence of abnormalities such as atrophy (pale white discoloration), an enlarged cup/disk ratio, thinning of the neural retinal rim, and neovascularization (delicate new vessel growth on the surface). The edges of the optic nerve should be sharp with a distinct border between nerve and the surrounding retina (see Chapter 28, "Optic Nerve Disorders," and Chapter 29, "Glaucoma"). The vessels exiting the optic nerve should be examined for focal narrowing, emboli, and attenuation (see Chapter 24, "Diabetic Retinopathy," and Chapter 25, "Other Retinal Vascular Diseases"). The examiner can follow each of the four major arcades of vessels into each quadrant. Engorgement of the venous system, narrowing of the arteries, or compression of the arteriovenous conjunctions may all be signs of systemic vascular disease. As well, the examiner can look temporal and slightly inferior to the optic nerve to examine the macular region and fovea. This region is particularly important in diseases such as age-related macular degeneration and diabetes mellitus (see Chapter 24, "Diabetic Retinopathy,"and Chapter 27, "Age-Related Macular Degeneration"). The presence of retinal hemorrhages and exudates are particularly important. The retina in each quadrant can be examined for signs of pathology, such as tears, holes, or pigment clumping. The relative size of retinal changes can be estimated by comparison to the optic nerve, as the normal optic nerve is approximately 1.5 mm in diameter.

Special Pediatric Examination Techniques

A. C. Tongue

INTRODUCTION

Infants and children present special ophthalmic diagnostic challenges. This results from the combination that certain disorders are uncommon and found only in younger individuals and because children may be more difficult to examine. This section presents special examination techniques which should be employed and which will enhance recognition of certain pediatric ocular abnormalities.

EXTERNAL EXAMINATION

Examination of the child's eye and vision system should include inspection of the eyes and periocular area. Asymmetry of external structures such as lid fissures, size and protrusion of the globe or cornea, differences in iris color, and pupil size and configuration should be noted. Children or infants who have any of these conditions should be referred for a complete ophthalmologic evaluation.

Infants with discharge or epiphora (increased tearing) should be evaluated for obstructed tear ducts (Fig. C.1). Neonatal conjunctivitis from other causes needs to be considered and cultures obtained when appropriate (see Chapter 13, "Conjunctivitis"). Purulent conjunctivitis is rarely secondary to nasolacrimal duct obstruction during the first few days of life. A sign of nasolacrimal duct obstruction at birth, or shortly thereafter, is a bluish mass along the superior aspect of the nasal wall due to a distended nasolacrimal sac, referred to as a dacryocele (Fig. C.2). Abnormal tearing may also be associated with glaucoma and corneal disorders (Fig. C.3).

PUPIL EXAMINATION

Examination of the pupil is more difficult in the infant than in the older child or adult. Pupil size should be noted. Unequal pupils should raise the suspicion of Horner's syndrome and particular attention should be paid to the lid on the side of the smaller pupil. In the case of Horner's syndrome, the lid on the affected side will be slightly ptotic. Horner's syndrome may be the result of trauma to the sympathetic plexus, tumor (especially neuroblastoma), or idiopathic.

Direct and indirect pupil reaction should be checked. The observed pupil should constrict when light is directed into it (direct response), or into the opposite pupil (indirect or consensual response).

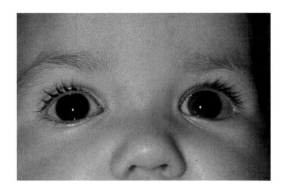

Figure C.1. Nasolacrimal duct obstruction with wet lashes and increased tear lake right eye. (Courtesy of A. Tongue, M.D.)

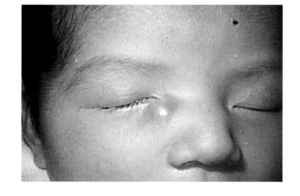

Figure C.2. Congenital dacryocele (nasolacrimal system obstructed at distal and proximal ends with resultant distention of nasolacrimal sac). (See also color section.) (Courtesy of A. Tongue, M.D.)

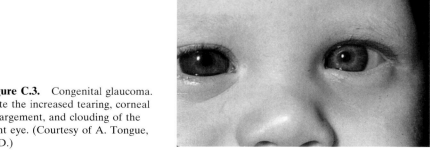

Figure C.3. Congenital glaucoma. Note the increased tearing, corneal enlargement, and clouding of the right eye. (Courtesy of A. Tongue, M.D.)

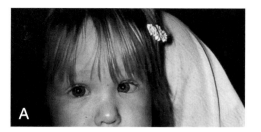
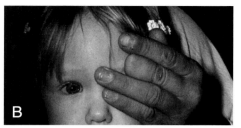

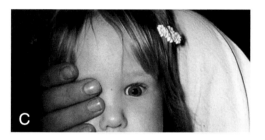

Figure C.4. Afferent pupil defect in patient with optic nerve hypoplasia and esotropia of left eye. Note equal pupils when both eyes are open and exposed to light (**A**). There is no change in pupil size with light exposure of right eye only (**B**). Dilation of pupil with light exposure of left eye only. (**C**). Left pupil constricts more with light stimulation of opposite eye. (Courtesy of A. Tongue, M.D.)

Pupil evaluation for an afferent defect (Marcus Gunn response, described in Appendix B, "General Examination Techniques") is often referred to as the swinging flashlight test. The reaction of the pupil to direct light stimulation is compared to the reaction of the pupil when the light is directed into the opposite, unobserved pupil. In a normal situation, there should be no difference between the pupil constriction from the direct and indirect light stimulation. In cases of afferent pupil defect, the pupil of the affected side constricts more with indirect than direct light stimulation. One of the easier ways of performing this test in children is to shine the ophthalmoscope light simultaneously in both pupils with the room darkened, then to swing the light from one pupil to the other and to watch for dilation or constriction of a pupil. Amblyopia, refractive errors, cataracts, and corneal abnormalities do not cause afferent pupil defects. Optic nerve lesions and retinal lesions can cause an afferent pupil defect. An afferent pupil defect is cause for prompt referral to an ophthalmologist.

In infants, an additional way of looking for an afferent pupil defect is to observe what happens to the pupil of the fixing eye as the other eye is covered (Fig. C.4). If, for example, the pupil of the uncovered eye dilates, an afferent pupil defect may be

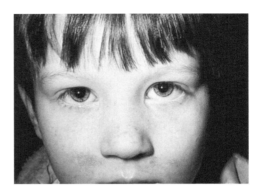

Figure C.5. Hirschberg corneal reflex. Left eye shows the more common slightly nasally displaced reflex. Right corneal reflex is slightly more temporal. Patient has a small angle right esotropia. (Courtesy of A. Tongue, M.D.)

present. The consensual or indirect pupil light stimulation has been removed, and the pupil is dependent on direct light stimulation only. In a normal situation, there should be no pupil dilation when one eye is covered. Individuals with severe amblyopia may also respond with pupil dilation of the amblyopic eye when the nonamblyopic eye is covered, because of lack of accommodation with the amblyopic eye.

Paradoxical pupil reflex is present in some retinal diseases such as Leber's congenital amaurosis. Normally pupils constrict when room lights are turned on and dilate with lights off. The paradoxical pupil dilates with lights on and constricts with lights off.

LIGHT REFLEX TESTS OF HIRSCHBERG AND BRUCKNER

The ophthalmoscope is used to look at the corneal reflex (Hirschberg) and pupillary reflex (Bruckner, red reflex). In neonates and very young infants, the test is mainly performed to detect media opacities or posterior pole (retinal) abnormalities that would change the color of the red reflex. In alert and cooperative infants and children, the test is a valuable tool for detecting refractive errors and small angle strabismus that may lead to amblyopia (see Chapter 17, "Pediatric and Adult Strabismus").

As a screening test for strabismus and refractive errors, the Hirschberg test is valid only if the patient fixes on the light. It is best to perform the test in a semidark room so that the infant or young child is not distracted by other objects and the red reflex is clearly seen. The examiner looks through a direct ophthalmoscope about 1 meter (arms length) away from the patient. The light is focused on the cornea so that a clear corneal reflex is obtained simultaneously in both eyes. The location of the reflex should be symmetrical. In most patients, the reflex is slightly nasal to the center of the pupil, although it may also be slightly temporal to the center of the pupil. If the reflex is not in the same position on the cornea in each eye, and the patient is fixing on the light, the probability of strabismus is very high (Fig. C.5).

In the case of an esotropic eye, the corneal light reflex would be displaced temporally; and in the case of exotropia, the corneal light reflex would be displaced nasally. The degree of strabismus can be estimated by the amount of reflex displacement. If the light reflex is displaced to the pupil margin the deviation is about 15°, or 25–30 diopters. Again, it is important to remember that the patient must fixate on the light source for the test to be valid.

After the corneal reflex is evaluated, attention is directed toward the red reflex

of life, since these are commonly heritable conditions which may be missed unless a cycloplegic refraction is performed. All children with a family history of amblyopia or strabismus should receive careful vision screening at all well-baby and early childhood evaluations.

SUGGESTED READING

Stout, AU, Wright KW. Pediatric eye examination. In: Wright KW, ed. Pediatric ophthalmology and strabismus. St. Louis: C.V. Mosby, 1995:63–73.

Tongue AC, Cibis GW. Bruckner test. Ophthalmology 1981;88:1041–1044.

Wright KW. Introduction to strabismus and the ocular-motor examination. In: Wright KW, ed. Pediatric ophthalmology and strabismus. St. Louis: C.V. Mosby, 1995:1139–1159.

Ophthalmic Diagnostic Codes

DIAGNOSIS	ICD-9 CODES
Acute Angle Closure Glaucoma	365.22
Acute Endophthalmitis	360.01
Acute Follicular Conjunctivitis	372.02
Acute Iridocyclitis	364.00
Amblyopia Unspecified	368.00
Behçet Syndrome	136.1
Blepharitis Unspecified	373.00
Blepharoconjunctivitis Unspecified	372.20
Blurred Vision	368.8
Branch Retinal Artery Occlusion	362.32
Branch Retinal Vein Occlusion	362.36
Burn of Eye and Adnexa Unspecified	940.9
Central Corneal Ulcer	370.03
Central Retinal Artery Occlusion	362.31
Central Retinal Vein Occlusion	362.35
Chalazion	373.2
Chemical Burn to Eye	940.0
Chorioretinitis Due to Toxoplasmosis	130.2
Chorioretinitis Posterior Uveitis	363.20
Chronic Angle Closure Glaucoma	365.23
Chronic Endophthalmitis	360.03
Chronic Follicular Conjunctivitis	372.12
Chronic Iridocyclitis Unspecified	364.10
Congenital Cataract	743.30
Congenital Glaucoma	743.21
Conjunctival Foreign Body	930.1
Conjunctival Hemorrhage	372.72
Contact and Allergic Dermatitis Eyelid	373.32
Contusion of Eye and Adnexa	921.
Contusion of Eyeball	921.3
Contusion of Eyelids and Periocular Area	921.1
Corneal Abrasion	918.1
Corneal Edema Unspecified	371.20
Corneal Foreign Body	930.0
Cortical Senile Cataract	366.15
Cytomegaloviral Retinitis	078.5
Dermatochalasis	374.87
Detachment Retinal Recent or Subtotal	361.05
Detachment Retinal Serous Retinal	361.20
Detachment Retinal Traction Retinal	361.81
Diabetes Mellitus Insulin Dependent	250.51
Diabetes Mellitus Noninsulin Dependent	250.50
Diabetes Mellitus w/o Comp Noninsulin Depen	250.00
Diabetes Mellitus w/o Comp Insulin Depen	250.01

Diabetic Retinopathy Background	362.01
Diabetic Retinopathy Proliferative	362.02
Diplopia	368.2
Disseminated Choroiditis Generalized	363.13
Dry Macular Degeneration	362.51
Endophthalmitis Purulent	360.00
Entropion Unspecified	374.00
Exposure Keratoconjunctivitis	370.34
Disciform Macular Degeneration	362.52
Eyeball Laceration Unspecified	871.4
Filamentary Keratitis	370.23
Giant Cell Arteritis	446.5
Glaucoma Assoc with Pupillary Block	365.61
Glaucoma Assoc with Ocular Trauma	365.65
Glaucoma of Childhood	365.14
Glaucoma Suspect Steroid Responders	365.03
Glaucomatous Atrophy of Optic Disc	377.14
Harada's Disease	363.22
Herpes Simplex	054.
Herpes Simplex Dendritic Keratitis	054.42
Herpes Simplex Dermatitis of Eyelid	054.41
Herpes Simplex Disciform Keratitis	054.43
Herpes Simplex Iridocyclitis	054.44
Herpes Simplex with Ophthalmic Complication	054.4
Herpes Zoster	053.
Herpes Zoster Iridocyclitis	053.22
Herpes Zoster Keratoconjunctivitis	053.21
Herpes Zoster with Ophthalmic Complication	053.20
Homonymous Bilateral Field Defects	368.46
Hordeolum Externum	373.11
Human Immunodeficiency Virus Disease	042.
Hypermetropia	367.0
Hyphema	364.41
Hypopyon	364.05
Ischemic Optic Neuropathy	377.41
Juvenile Rheumatoid Arthritis	714.30
Keratoconjunctivitis Sicca	370.33
Keratoconjunctivitis Unspecified	370.49
Lagophthalmos	374.2
Low Tension Glaucoma	365.12
Macular Degeneration Drusen	362.57
Macular Degeneration Hereditary	362.77
Macular Degeneration Cystoid	362.53
Macular Degeneration Senile	362.50
Marginal Corneal Ulcer	370.01
Migrane Classical	346.00
Myopia	367.1
Narrow Angle Glaucoma	365.02
Neoplasm Choroid Benign	224.6
Neoplasm Choroid Malignant	190.6
Neoplasm Other	238.8
Neoplasm Retina Malignant	190.5
Neurofibromatosis	237.71

Nuclear Sclerosis Cataract	366.16
Ocular Hypertension Borderline Glaucoma	365.04
Ocular Laceration with Prolapse Tissue	871.1
Ocular Pemphigus	694.61
Open Angle Glaucoma Unspecified	365.10
Optic Neuritis Unspecified	377.30
Optic Papillitis	377.31
Orbital Floor Blow out Fracture Closed	802.6
Other Chronic Allergic Conjunctivitis	372.14
Other Mucopurulent Conjunctivitis	372.03
Panuveitis	360.12
Pars Planitis	363.21
Penetrating Wound or Orbit	870.3
Perforated Corneal Ulcer	370.06
Pigmentary Glaucoma	365.13
Posterior Subcapsular Cataract	366.14
Presbyopia	367.4
Primary Iridocyclitis Acute	364.01
Primary Open Angle Glaucoma	365.11
Ptosis of Eyelid	374.3
Recurrent Erosion of Cornea	371.42
Recurrent Iridocyclitis	364.02
Retinal Edema	362.83
Retinal Exudates and Deposits	362.82
Retinal Hemorrhage	362.81
Retinal Ischemia	362.84
Retinal Microaneurysms Nos	362.14
Retinopathy Exudative	362.12
Retinopathy Hypertensive	362.11
Rosacea Acne	695.3
Rosacea Conjunctivitis	372.31
Rubeosis Iridis	364.42
Rupture of Eye Loss of Intraocular Tissue	871.2
Sarcoidosis	135.
Scleritis or Episcleritis Unspecified	379.00
Serous Choroidal Detachment	363.71
Sickle Cell Anemia Unspecified	282.60
Simple Chronic Conjunctivitis	372.11
Steroid Induced Glaucomatous Stage	365.31
Total or Mature Cataract	366.17
Toxocariasis	128.0
Traumatic Cataract Unspecified	366.20
Trichiasis w/o Entropion	374.05
Vascular Sheathing of Retina	362.13
Vernal Conjunctivitis	372.13
Visual Field Defect	368.4
Vitreous Hemorrhage	379.23

INDEX ◉❚